THE WASHINGTON MANUAL®

Pulmonary Medicine
Subspecialty Consult

THIRD EDITION

THE WASHINGTON MANUAL®

Pulmonary Medicine

Subspecialty Consult

THIRD EDITION

Editors

Adam Anderson, MD
Associate Professor of Medicine
Division of Pulmonary and Critical Care Medicine
Washington University School of Medicine
St. Louis, Missouri

Colleen McEvoy, MD
Associate Professor of Medicine
Division of Pulmonary and Critical Care Medicine
Washington University School of Medicine
St. Louis, Missouri

Mary Clare McGregor, MD
Assistant Professor of Medicine
Division of Pulmonary and Critical Care Medicine
Washington University School of Medicine
St. Louis, Missouri

Shail Mehta, MD
Assistant Professor of Medicine
Division of Pulmonary and Critical Care Medicine
Washington University School of Medicine in St. Louis
St. Louis, Missouri

Executive Editor

Thomas M. Ciesielski, MD
Associate Professor of Medicine
Vice Chair of Inpatient Quality and Safety
Department of Medicine
Division of General Medicine and Geriatrics
Washington University School of Medicine
St. Louis, Missouri

Administrative Editor

Rebecca Light, MS
Division of Pulmonary and Critical Care Medicine
Washington University School of Medicine
St. Louis, Missouri

Wolters Kluwer

Philadelphia · Baltimore · New York · London
Buenos Aires · Hong Kong · Sydney · Tokyo

Acquisitions Editor: Joe Cho
Development Editor: Cindy Yoo
Editorial Coordinator: Chester Anthony Gonzalez
Editorial Assistant: Devin Van Gorden
Marketing Manager: Kristen Watrud
Production Project Manager: Jennifer L. Harper
Manager, Graphic Arts & Design: Stephen Druding
Manufacturing Coordinator: Lisa Bowling
Prepress Vendor: Aptara, Inc.

3rd edition

Copyright © 2026 Department of Medicine, Washington University School of Medicine

All rights reserved. This book is protected by copyright. No part of this book may be reproduced or transmitted in any form or by any means, including as photocopies or scanned-in or other electronic copies, or utilized by any information storage and retrieval system without written permission from the copyright owner, except for brief quotations embodied in critical articles and reviews. Materials appearing in this book prepared by individuals as part of their official duties as U.S. government employees are not covered by the above-mentioned copyright. To request permission, please contact Wolters Kluwer at Two Commerce Square, 2001 Market Street, Philadelphia, PA 19103, via email at permissions@lww.com, or via our website at shop.lww.com (products and services).

9 8 7 6 5 4 3 2 1

Printed in Mexico

978-1-9752-3734-9
Library of Congress Cataloging-in-Publication Data available upon request.

This work is provided "as is," and the publisher disclaims any and all warranties, express or implied, including any warranties as to accuracy, comprehensiveness, or currency of the content of this work.

This work is no substitute for individual patient assessment based upon healthcare professionals' examination of each patient and consideration of, among other things, age, weight, gender, current or prior medical conditions, medication history, laboratory data and other factors unique to the patient. The publisher does not provide medical advice or guidance and this work is merely a reference tool. Healthcare professionals, and not the publisher, are solely responsible for the use of this work including all medical judgments and for any resulting diagnosis and treatments.

Given continuous, rapid advances in medical science and health information, independent professional verification of medical diagnoses, indications, appropriate pharmaceutical selections and dosages, and treatment options should be made and healthcare professionals should consult a variety of sources. When prescribing medication, healthcare professionals are advised to consult the product information sheet (the manufacturer's package insert) accompanying each drug to verify, among other things, conditions of use, warnings and side effects and identify any changes in dosage schedule or contraindications, particularly if the medication to be administered is new, infrequently used or has a narrow therapeutic range. To the maximum extent permitted under applicable law, no responsibility is assumed by the publisher for any injury and/or damage to persons or property, as a matter of products liability, negligence law or otherwise, or from any reference to or use by any person of this work.

shop.lww.com

Contributors

Matthew Abbott, MD
Fellow
Division of Pulmonary and Critical Care Medicine
Washington University School of Medicine
St. Louis, Missouri

Adam Anderson, MD
Associate Professor of Medicine
Division of Pulmonary and Critical Care Medicine
Washington University School of Medicine
St. Louis, Missouri

Elissa Arnold, MD
Fellow
Division of Pulmonary and Critical Care Medicine
Washington University School of Medicine
St. Louis, Missouri

Jeffrey J. Atkinson, MD
Professor of Medicine
Division of Pulmonary and Critical Care Medicine
Washington University School of Medicine
St. Louis, Missouri

Michael Beal, MD
Assistant Professor of Radiology
Division of Cardiothoracic Imaging
Washington University School of Medicine
St. Louis, Missouri

Murali M. Chakinala, MD
Professor of Medicine
Division of Pulmonary and Critical Care Medicine
Washington University School of Medicine
St. Louis, Missouri

Alexander C. Chen, MD
Professor of Medicine
Division of Pulmonary and Critical Care Medicine
Washington University School of Medicine
St. Louis, Missouri

Praveen R. Chenna, MD
Associate Professor of Medicine
Division of Pulmonary and Critical Care Medicine
Washington University School of Medicine
St. Louis, Missouri

Stephen Chi, MD
Assistant Professor of Medicine
Division of Pulmonary and Critical Care Medicine
Washington University School of Medicine
St. Louis, Missouri

Vladimir Despotovic, MD
Associate Professor of Medicine
Division of Pulmonary and Critical Care Medicine
Washington University School of Medicine
St. Louis, Missouri

Jonah Graves, MD
Fellow
Division of Pulmonary and Critical Care Medicine
Washington University School of Medicine
St. Louis, Missouri

John Grotberg, MD
Fellow
Division of Pulmonary and Critical Care Medicine
Washington University School of Medicine
St. Louis, Missouri

M. Cristina Vazquez Guillamet, MD
Associate Professor of Medicine
Division of Infectious Diseases
Washington University School of Medicine
St. Louis, Missouri

Rodrigo Vazquez Guillamet, MD
Associate Professor of Medicine
Division of Pulmonary and Critical Care Medicine
Washington University School of Medicine
St. Louis, Missouri

Laura Halverson, MD
Assistant Professor of Medicine
Division of Pulmonary and Critical Care Medicine
Washington University School of Medicine
St. Louis, Missouri

Christian Hendrix, MD
Fellow
Division of Infectious Diseases
Washington University School of Medicine
St. Louis, Missouri

Alison M. Hixon, MD, PhD
Fellow
Division of Infectious Diseases
Washington University School of Medicine
St. Louis, Missouri

Marin H. Kollef, MD
Virginia E. and Sam J. Golman Chair in Respiratory Intensive Care Medicine
Professor of Medicine
Division of Pulmonary and Critical Care Medicine
Washington University School of Medicine
St. Louis, Missouri

Bryan D. Kraft, MD
Associate Professor of Medicine
Director of Medical Critical Care
Washington University School of Medicine
St. Louis, Missouri

James G. Krings, MD
Assistant Professor of Medicine
Division of Pulmonary and Critical Care Medicine
Washington University School of Medicine
St. Louis, Missouri

Kacie Kuykendall, MD
Assistant Professor of Radiology
Mallinckrodt Institute of Radiology
Washington University School of Medicine
St. Louis, Missouri

Zachary Lonjers, MD
Assistant Professor of Medicine
Division of Pulmonary and Critical Care Medicine
Washington University School of Medicine
St. Louis, Missouri

Brandt Lydon, MD
Instructor in Medicine
Division of Pulmonary and Critical Care Medicine
Washington University School of Medicine
St. Louis, Missouri

Patrick B. Mazi, MD
Assistant Professor of Medicine
Division of Infectious Diseases
Washington University School of Medicine
St. Louis, Missouri

Rachel McDonald, MD
Assistant Professor of Medicine
Division of Pulmonary and Critical Care Medicine
Washington University School of Medicine
St. Louis, Missouri

Colleen McEvoy, MD
Associate Professor of Medicine
Division of Pulmonary and Critical Care Medicine
Washington University School of Medicine
St. Louis, Missouri

Mary Clare McGregor, MD
Assistant Professor of Medicine
Division of Pulmonary and Critical Care Medicine
Washington University School of Medicine
St. Louis, Missouri

James McMenimen, MD
Fellow
Division of Pulmonary and Critical Care Medicine
Washington University School of Medicine
St. Louis, Missouri

Shail Mehta, MD
Assistant Professor of Medicine
Division of Pulmonary and Critical Care Medicine
Washington University School of Medicine in St. Louis
St. Louis, Missouri

Nathaniel G. Moulton, MD
Instructor in Medicine
Division of Pulmonary and Critical Care Medicine
Washington University School of Medicine
St. Louis, Missouri

Francisco Novoa, MD
Resident
Division of Medical Education
Washington University School of Medicine
St. Louis, Missouri

Tej M. Patel, MD
Fellow
Division of Pulmonary and Critical Care Medicine
Washington University School of Medicine
St. Louis, Missouri

Andrew Peters, MD
Fellow
Division of Pulmonary and Critical Care Medicine
Washington University School of Medicine
St. Louis, Missouri

Tri Pham, MD
Resident
Division of Infectious Diseases
Washington University School of Medicine
St. Louis, Missouri

Daniel Reynolds, MD
Assistant Professor of Medicine
Division of Pulmonary and Critical Care Medicine
Washington University School of Medicine
St. Louis, Missouri

Tonya D. Russell, MD
Professor of Medicine
Division of Pulmonary and Critical Care Medicine
Washington University School of Medicine
St. Louis, Missouri

Maanasi Samant, MD
Assistant Professor of Medicine
Division of Pulmonary and Critical Care Medicine
Washington University School of Medicine
St. Louis, Missouri

Sahil Sanghani, MD
Chief Resident
Division of Pulmonary and Critical Care Medicine
Washington University School of Medicine
St. Louis, Missouri

Adrian Shifren, MD
Professor of Medicine
Division of Pulmonary and Critical Care Medicine
Washington University School of Medicine
St. Louis, Missouri

Samuel Windham, MD, MS
Research Fellow
Division of Pulmonary and Critical Care Medicine
Washington University School of Medicine
St. Louis, Missouri

Roger D. Yusen, MD, MPH
Associate Professor of Medicine
Division of Pulmonary and Critical Care Medicine
Washington University School of Medicine
St. Louis, Missouri

Department Chair's Note

It is a pleasure to present the third edition of *The Washington Manual Pulmonary Medicine Subspecialty Consult*, which is part of *The Washington Manual® Subspecialty Consult Series*. This pocket-sized book provides a comprehensive approach to the diagnosis and management of a variety of acute and chronic lung diseases. This manual is an excellent medical reference for students, residents, interns, and other practitioners who need access to practical clinical subspecialty information to diagnose and treat patients with asthma, COPD, interstitial lung disease, pulmonary hypertension, cystic fibrosis, pulmonary infections, as well as other common pulmonary conditions. Medical knowledge continues to increase at an astounding rate, which creates a challenge for physicians to keep up with the biomedical discoveries, expansion of genomic and immunologic information, and novel diagnostic and therapeutic strategies that can positively impact patients with lung diseases. *The Washington Manual Pulmonary Medicine Subspecialty Consult, Third Edition* addresses this challenge by concisely and practically providing current scientific information for clinicians to aid them in the diagnosis, investigation, and treatment of common acute and chronic lung diseases.

I would like to personally thank the authors, including house officers, fellows, and attending physicians at Washington University School of Medicine and Barnes-Jewish Hospital. Their commitment to patient care and education is unsurpassed, and their efforts and skill in compiling this subspecialty manual are evident in the quality of the final product. In particular, I would like to acknowledge our editors, Drs. Adam Anderson, Colleen McEvoy, Mary Clare McGregor, and Shail Mehta, who have worked tirelessly to produce another outstanding edition of this manual, as well as our executive editor, Dr. Thomas M. Ciesielski. *The Washington Manual Pulmonary Medicine Subspecialty Consult, Third Edition* will provide practical knowledge that can be directly applied at the bedside and in outpatient settings to improve patient care.

Sincerely,

Victoria J. Fraser, MD
Adolphus Busch Professor
Chair, Department of Medicine
Washington University School of Medicine
St. Louis, Missouri

Preface

This is the third edition of the *Washington Manual® Pulmonary Medicine Subspecialty Consult*, building on prior editions and adding to the long tradition of medical education promoted by *The Washington Manual® of Medical Therapeutics*. The book is intended to provide medical students, residents, fellows, and advanced practice providers a handbook for the evaluation of patients with pulmonary disease and reflect "real-life" clinical experiences. To effectively address our target audience, many of the chapters have been written with the input of medical residents or medical subspecialty fellows and have been coauthored by an attending physician with expertise in the relevant field to ensure that both accurate and relevant information are provided. Given the rapidly changing landscape of medicine, this book should function as a succinct review of pulmonary medicine. Additional reading of primary literature and discussion with seasoned clinicians to provide optimal clinical care are strongly encouraged.

A book such as this is always a collaborative effort. We would like to express our gratitude for the commitment of the key individuals who helped prepare this edition: the residents, fellows, and faculty from across departments and divisions at the Washington University School of Medicine who contributed chapters. We are indebted to Becky Light, whose ability to keep this project on track was nothing short of remarkable. We also thank Katie Sharp for her assistance with publication formalities.

Finally, the editors appreciate the great collaboration that we shared and the love and patience of our families that allowed us to complete this work.

AA
CM
MM
SM

Contents

Contributors v
Department Chair's Note ix
Preface x

1. The Chest Radiograph 1
   Kacie Kuykendall

2. Chest Computed Tomography 10
   Michael Beal

3. Pulmonary Function Testing 20
   Adam Anderson and Jeffrey J. Atkinson

4. Fiberoptic Bronchoscopy 34
   Alexander C. Chen

5. Hypoxemic Respiratory Failure 40
   Tej M. Patel, James McMenimen, and Adrian Shifren

6. Noninvasive Ventilation 50
   Stephen Chi

7. Cough 61
   Daniel Reynolds

8. Asthma 70
   Jonah Graves, Tri Pham, and James G. Krings

9. Chronic Obstructive Pulmonary Disease 83
   Francisco Novoa, Roger D. Yusen, and Rodrigo Vazquez Guillamet

10. Tobacco and Inhalational Abuse 97
    Zachary Lonjers

xii | Contents

11. Community-Acquired Pneumonia **107**
Samuel Windham

12. Nosocomial Pneumonia **115**
M. Cristina Vazquez Guillamet and Marin H. Kollef

13. Mycobacterial Pulmonary Disease **125**
Shail Mehta

14. Fungal Pulmonary Infections **133**
Christian Hendrix and Patrick B. Mazi

15. Viral Respiratory Infections **157**
Alison M. Hixon and M. Cristina Vazquez-Guillamet

16. Cystic Fibrosis **185**
James McMenimen and Jeffrey J. Atkinson

17. Hemoptysis **199**
Rachel McDonald

18. Diffuse Alveolar Hemorrhage **205**
John Grotberg and Bryan D. Kraft

19. Pulmonary Vasculitis **213**
Vladimir Despotovic

20. Pulmonary Embolism and Deep Venous Thrombosis **230**
Elissa Arnold, Sahil Sanghani, and Maanasi Samant

21. Pulmonary Hypertension **244**
Matthew Abbott and Murali M. Chakinala

22. Pleural Diseases **260**
Praveen R. Chenna and Brandt Lydon

23. Sleep-Disordered Breathing **270**
Tonya D. Russell

24. Interstitial Lung Disease **277**
Andrew Peters and Mary Clare McGregor

25. Occupational Lung Disease 293
    Adam Anderson

26. Antineoplastic Therapy–Induced Pulmonary Disease 308
    Colleen McEvoy

27. Solitary Pulmonary Nodule 314
    Nathaniel G. Moulton and Michael Beal

28. Lung Transplantation 324
    Laura Halverson and James McMenimen

Index 345

The Chest Radiograph

Kacie Kuykendall

GENERAL PRINCIPLES

- The CXR is ubiquitous in medicine and remains among the hardest of diagnostic studies to master. The key to proficiency lies in reviewing all CXRs ordered. Close interaction with radiology staff is invaluable in building ones' skills and homing in on a specific diagnosis.
- Using a consistent search pattern will allow for systematic and comprehensive analyses.
- At the Mallinckrodt Institute of Radiology (MIR), we try to initially read all CXRs without any clinical history. The clinical information is reviewed after the initial perusal so as to avoid bias and ensure subtle, clinically relevant findings are not overlooked.
- The importance of prior CXRs for comparison cannot be stressed enough. Understanding a finding often relies on knowing whether it is acute, subacute, or chronic. An area of consolidation, for example, could represent a community-acquired pneumonia on a CXR. If the area is stable from 1 year ago, low-grade adenocarcinoma or radiation changes (if applicable) become more likely.

INITIAL ASSESSMENT

Patient Position and Study Quality
- Initial evaluation begins with assessment of patient position and quality of the study.
- This evaluation includes assessing the film for:
  - Rotation
  - Degree of inspiration
  - Patient position
  - Radiation dose

Patient Rotation
- A common method of assessing for the presence of rotation is to evaluate the relationship of the medial heads of the clavicles to the spinous processes of the vertebral bodies. When truly straight, each clavicular head will be equidistant to the adjacent spinous process.
- If the patient is rotated, the mediastinal borders will be altered. Rotation can be confused for mediastinal widening. Lack of appreciation for patient rotation can result in needless workup of perceived mediastinal changes.

Degree of Inspiration
- The degree of inspiration will affect the density of the lungs.
- As a general rule, the diaphragm should be crisp, and the peak should be rounded.

- For those who prefer counting ribs, 10 posterior ribs and 6 anterior ribs should be seen on an inspiratory study.

Patient Position
- Erect versus supine positioning is pertinent, as it will alter the interpretation of air–fluid interfaces, blood flow distribution, and caliber of the pulmonary vessels. Cephalization, for example, can be appreciated only on an upright film.
- The air–fluid level in the gastric fundus often allows one to understand whether the CXR is upright, supine, or decubitus.

Radiation Dose
- Radiation dose of a CXR has become more challenging in the digital era.
- As a general rule, the optimally exposed CXR allows visualization of the vertebral bodies and disk spaces through the mediastinal structures and also allows visualization of the pulmonary vessels through the heart and diaphragm.
- With new digital techniques, postprocessing allows the technologist to manipulate the image to achieve this same effect. The reader, therefore, must be careful that he/she can see through both the heart and mediastinum but that the image does not look too pixilated. Should pixilation occur, the reader must be aware that an insufficient radiation dose was used.

CXR Views
- There are a number of different variations of a CXR that may be obtained to evaluate thoracic pathology. These include the posteroanterior (PA) view, the lateral (LAT) view, the anteroposterior (AP) view, and the lateral decubitus (LD) view.
- All of these views share the concept of a point source which results in a fan x-ray beam. The result is magnification of structures which are farther from the detector. A good analogy is the shadow created by your hand on a classroom desk from an overhead light bulb. If you lift your hand off the desk, the shadow becomes bigger and fuzzier.

Posteroanterior View
The **PA view** is acquired with the patient in a standing position during full inspiration. The patient faces the detector, which is in contact with the anterior chest wall. The x-ray beam is directed toward the cassette from a distance of 6 ft, which results in minimal magnification of the heart.

Lateral View
- The **LAT view** is also taken with the patient standing during full inspiration at a distance of 6 ft. The arms are lifted. By convention, the patient's left side is placed in contact with the detector, and the beam is directed from right to left to reduce magnification of the heart.
- LAT views are useful for evaluating lesions behind the heart, diaphragm, or mediastinum that may be hidden on PA views.
- The left diaphragm can be differentiated from the right diaphragm on this view by locating the loss of the left diaphragmatic border when in contact with the cardiac silhouette or by locating the right posterior ribs (which will appear magnified and larger since they are farther from the cassette).

- It is important to note that magnification is about the same between the PA and LAT views. If a lesion is found on one view, the relationship with a landmark (e.g., aortic arch) can be used to localize it on the other.

Anteroposterior Views
- **The AP views** are usually taken with portable machines and are most often used to image the chest in patients who cannot have formal PA and LAT views, such as intensive care unit or intraoperative patients.
- These studies are conducted with the cassette behind the patient, in contact with his/her back. The x-rays are directed from front to back, often at a distance of <6 ft. The patient is often in a sitting or supine position and unable to perform a full inspiration.
- AP views often result in increased lung attenuation (from lack of complete inspiration) and increased magnification of mediastinal and cardiac structures (from increased distance between these structures and the cassette).
- It is important to understand that magnification of anterior structures occurs in the AP view to prevent inappropriate interpretation of an enlarged mediastinum or cardiac silhouette.

Lateral Decubitus Views
- **LD views** are taken with the patient lying on the ipsilateral side. For example, a left LD is taken with the left side down.
- There are four clinical situations in which a decubitus view might be helpful.
  - When evaluating whether the ipsilateral effusion is mobile
  - When evaluating whether a contralateral pneumothorax is present
  - When the contralateral lung has a concomitant pneumonia with an effusion
  - When the ipsilateral lung collapses normally. If it does not, one might suspect a radiolucent obstructing foreign body within the airway

GENERAL APPROACH TO CXR INTERPRETATION

- A systematic approach to the CXR reduces the risk of missed pathology.
- Although there are many systems for evaluating CXRs, the schema used here is arranged so that often-neglected areas are addressed first, and more common areas that may divert attention are addressed last.
- The PA CXR is addressed in detail, but any view can be read in a similar or slightly modified fashion.

Osseous Structures

The first structures surveyed are the **osseous structures** of the thorax, including the ribs (anterior and posterior aspects), the sternum (including signs of previous sternal splitting surgeries), the shoulder girdle (including the clavicles and scapulae), and the spine (both the vertebrae and disk spaces). The skeletal survey should look for clues to understanding the other findings, including fractures, metastases, or previous surgery.

Upper Abdomen

Next, the **upper abdomen** is inspected. On an upright film any gas collections are evaluated, including the stomach bubble and the colon. Displacement of these structures may be indicative of organomegaly. An abnormal shape of the gas may be indicative of free intraperitoneal gas. The upright PA film is the study of choice for evaluating the presence of free air in the abdomen which is seen as a thin crescent under the diaphragm.

The Diaphragm

The **diaphragm** is evaluated next. The hemidiaphragms are smooth hemispherical structures, with the right diaphragm being 2–3 cm higher than the left owing to the presence of the liver below. The hemidiaphragms should be evaluated for shape (flattened in hyperinflation), sharpness (obscured with pleural effusions), and general symmetry (eventration, paralysis, or hernia through the hemidiaphragm leads to asymmetry).

The Mediastinum

Evaluation of the **mediastinum** usually follows and is one of the more complex parts of the CXR evaluation because it includes so many thoracic structures.

Mediastinal Lines

The nine key lines of the mediastinum should be assessed for any focal distortion or displacement.

- The interfaces of the lungs, the anterior and posterior junction lines
- The right paratracheal stripe
- The left subclavian artery reflection
- The concave aorticopulmonary window
- The descending aorta
- The left and right paravertebral lines
- The azygoesophageal recess

Mediastinal Borders

- The nine lines are followed by the right and left mediastinal borders.
- The right border is formed (from bottom to top) by the right atrium, the ascending aorta, and superior vena cava.
- The left border is formed (from bottom to top) by the left ventricle, left atrial appendage, main pulmonary artery, and aortic knob.
- Both global cardiac and chamber enlargement should be noted. Global cardiac enlargement can be determined by calculating the cardiothoracic ratio—the width of the cardiac shadow on a PA view should be less than half the internal width of the bony thorax at its widest point. Any ratio >50% usually signifies cardiac enlargement.
- Although chamber enlargement is often the cause of an enlarged cardiac shadow, a pericardial effusion gives a similar appearance and should always be considered, especially when there is an acute change in apparent cardiac size.
- The LAT film can be especially helpful in differentiating chamber enlargement versus pericardial effusion. On an LAT film, the pericardium is usually seen as a 2-mm stripe between two lucent arcs. In the presence of an effusion, this stripe is thickened. This finding is fairly specific and is often referred to as the sandwich or Oreo cookie sign.

Mediastinal Masses
- Mediastinal masses are often noted on this portion of the evaluation. The mediastinum is broken up into three different compartments, anterior, middle, and posterior for convenience of differential diagnosis. While various methods for dividing the mediastinum exist, a commonly used method is to define the compartments as follows:
    - **Anterior mediastinum** as the compartment between the sternum and an imaginary line drawn directly anterior to the trachea and posterior to the inferior vena cava. The differential for anterior mediastinal masses is usually headed by thymic lesions (thymoma and germ cell tumors) and lymphoma.
    - **Middle mediastinum** as the compartment from the trachea to a vertical line drawn 1 cm behind the anterior edge of the vertebral bodies. The differential for middle mediastinal masses most commonly includes foregut duplication cysts (esophageal or bronchogenic) or lymphadenopathy, but a hiatal hernia should be considered if an air–fluid level is present.
    - **Posterior mediastinum** as the remaining space. Most posterior mediastinal masses are neurogenic in nature such as a schwannoma or neurofibroma.

The Aorta
The **aorta** should also be evaluated on the CXR. All of its portions (ascending, arch, and descending) evaluated for enlargement (possible aneurysm), calcification (atherosclerotic disease), and tortuosity (hypertensive disease).

The Hila
The **hila** are then reviewed. Their shape, size, and density are important and may indicate the presence of disease. The left hilum should be higher than the right owing to the fact that the left pulmonary artery courses above the left mainstem bronchus and the right pulmonary artery arises below the right mainstem bronchus.

The Pleural and Extrapleural Spaces
- The **pleural space** (between the parietal and visceral pleurae) and **extrapleural spaces** (between the parietal pleura and chest wall) are also carefully inspected.
- First, the pleura along the diaphragm is inspected from the cardiophrenic to the costophrenic angles. Next, the pleura lining the LAT margin of the lung is followed upward to the apex, and then over and down the mediastinal contour to the cardiophrenic angle where the inspection began.
- By following the pleural markings, the fissures of the lungs (including fluid collecting or tracking into them) and even accessory fissures can be evaluated.
- Careful examination of these spaces allows for the detection of small pleural effusions, pneumothoraces, pleural thickening or calcification, and masses.
- LAT films are more sensitive than PA films for the detection of small pleural effusions. Whereas ~175 mL of fluid is needed to produce blunting of the costophrenic angles on PA views, as little as 75 mL can be detected in the costophrenic angle on an LAT view.

Extrapulmonary Masses
- Extrapulmonary masses (pleural and extrapleural) can be difficult to distinguish from pulmonary masses on PA films.
- A number of features may assist in differentiating between the two types of masses.
  - First, a second view can be obtained (a mass overlying the lungs on a PA view may be noted to be extrapulmonary on an LAT view).
  - Second, the interface between the lesion and the lung is sharp with an extrapulmonary mass because they are superimposed structures.
  - Third, the angle between the chest wall and an extrapulmonary lesion is obtuse (>90 degrees).
- The incomplete border sign can be useful as well. In this sign, only 270 degrees of a round mass are seen. This comes from the fact that the last 90 degrees is the portion that is arising from the pleura or chest wall. As a general rule this sign denotes an extrapulmonary mass.

Medical Devices
Medical devices should be carefully evaluated. Commonly encountered medical devices include endotracheal tubes (ETs), nasogastric tubes, central venous catheters (including dialysis catheters), Swan–Ganz catheters, pacing and defibrillating devices, coronary artery stents, chest tubes, various peritoneal shunts, and surgical staple lines or wires.

Endotracheal Tubes
ET tips should be assessed for proper location, ideally 4 cm from the carina in the midtrachea with a minimal safe distance of 2 cm from the carina. Malpositioned ET tubes may ventilate only one lung if advanced too far, leading to contralateral lung collapse, or may enter the pharynx or dislodge into the esophagus if placed too superiorly. ET tubes move with changes in chin position. When the patient flexes, the tip advances. In other words, the "hose follows the nose."

Nasogastric Tubes
Nasogastric tubes should be evaluated for proper positioning.

Central Access Devices
- Central venous catheters need to be evaluated for proper course and tip placement in the superior vena cava, with special attention for pneumothorax after placement.
- Swan–Ganz catheter tips should be assessed for proper location in the pulmonary artery and should not be advanced any more distally than the proximal interlobar pulmonary arteries (tip should remain within mediastinal shadow). Improper placement can lead to complications such as pulmonary infarction, pulmonary artery perforation, or pneumothorax.

Lungs
The **lungs** are the last to be evaluated. A focused, consistent approach is best. Working from bottom to top, the lungs are compared to each other. With the exception of the slightly elevated right hemidiaphragm and the asymmetric cardiac shadow, the lungs should be similar in appearance at each level of inspection. Any differences in the density of the film or the vascular markings are an indication of possible pulmonary pathology.

Final Steps
Again, it must be emphasized that once the evaluation is complete, it is essential to **evaluate old films and compare them with the current study**. This comparison allows for a more detailed understanding of the pathology being evaluated and may affect management in a significant fashion (e.g., a rapidly growing mass will be managed differently than a mass that has been stable for a number of years). Before concluding the CXR assessment, the study should be reviewed with a radiologist, or the final report should be reviewed. This way any subtle findings can be addressed and reviewed.

COMMONLY USED FINDINGS FOR EVALUATING LUNG DISEASE

Radiographic Densities
- The key to understanding findings on a CXR relies on understanding the five main densities detected by radiography: Air, Fat, Fluid, Calcium, Metal. The densities are listed from darkest (air) on a radiograph to the whitest (metal). Metal attenuates the x-ray beam the most while air attenuates it the least.
- Only by juxtaposing two different densities, (e.g., heart and lung) can one see borders. Knowledge of normal borders allows for distinction from pathology. When a normal border is lost or a new border is present, pathology is suspected.

Radiographic Signs
Another basic tenet is the understanding that certain findings are frequently associated with a specific disease process. This association is often referred to as a sign.

The Silhouette Sign
- One common reason for ordering CXRs is to exclude pneumonia. The silhouette sign can be useful for this indication.
- Normally, the lungs attenuate the x-ray beam less than the heart and mediastinum. As a result, the lungs appear black and provide nice contrast with the white central structures. When the lung becomes filled with fluid (as in pneumonia), the border with the heart is effaced. This loss of the normal border is known as the silhouette sign.
- This silhouette will vary on the location of lung pathology; see Table 1-1 for anatomic locations of silhouette signs.

TABLE 1-1 ANATOMIC LOCATIONS OF SILHOUETTE SIGNS

Lung Pathology	Silhouette Sign (Loss of Border)
Right upper lobe	Ascending aorta and right tracheal lung interface
Right middle lobe	Right heart border
Right lower lobe	Right diaphragm
Left upper lobe	Aortic knob
Lingula	Left heart border
Left lower lobe	Left diaphragm and descending aorta

Luftsichel Sign

A hyperlucent crescent adjacent to the aorta, often indicative of a hyperexpanded left lower lobe associated with left upper lobe collapse. This finding has been labeled the **luftsichel** sign (meaning air crescent in German). Often, the luftsichel sign is easier to appreciate on a CXR than the actual lobar collapse itself.

Air Bronchogram Sign

- Often times the bronchi are visualized within a consolidation. This finding is known as the air bronchogram sign. Consolidation refers to filling of the alveoli by fluid. The air bronchogram sign can be explained by the contrast of the air-filled bronchi (dark) against the consolidation (white). Inflammation adjacent to the airway may result in dilatation of the airway (akin to an ileus). This feature may accentuate the air bronchogram.
- When acute, this may be indicative of pulmonary edema, pneumonia, or pulmonary hemorrhage.
- When more chronic, one needs to think about low-grade adenocarcinoma or an inflammatory air–space process such as organizing pneumonia, radiation pneumonitis, or eosinophilic pneumonia.

Lobar Collapse

- Helpful findings in identifying lobar collapse (lobar atelectasis) include movement of lung fissures and crowding of pulmonary vessels or bronchi. Less specific signs include airway deviation, mediastinal shift, changes in adjacent lung density, and narrowing of the rib spaces. These findings occur because lobar collapse is associated with volume loss.
- Although pneumonia, lobar collapse, and pleural effusion may all appear white on a CXR, only lobar collapse will have volume loss.
- Volume loss is important to differentiate from volume gain because it is indicative of a different differential diagnosis.
- There are helpful findings indicating volume gain:
  - Mediastinal shift **away** from the lesion
  - Airway deviation **away** from the lesion

Pneumothorax

- Another common indication for CXR is the evaluation of pneumothorax. Certain radiologic findings can help with identification.
- There are two essential signs of a pneumothorax:
  - Presence of a white visceral pleural line
  - Absence of lung markings peripheral to this pleural line
- There are other radiologic findings that may be helpful:
  - Total or subtotal lung collapse
  - The deep sulcus sign (larger costophrenic recess on the side of the pneumothorax potentially with an inverted diaphragm)
  - Displacement of mediastinal structures
- Pneumothorax will move with changes in patient position. As a result, the pneumothorax is better seen apically on an upright view and better seen over the diaphragm and costophrenic angle on a supine view.

- In fact, this mobility can be useful in distinguishing a medial pneumothorax from a pneumomediastinum. The medial pneumothorax should move with a change in position.
- In larger patients, skin folds are often confused with a pleural line. These are differentiated by the fact that skin folds form a dark line due to intervening gas in the fold.

Diffuse Lung Disease
- Evaluation of diffuse lung disease is also a common clinical question, and its proper understanding relies on the interpretation of the predominant pattern on CXR.
- Diffuse disease can present as a generalized linear (reticular) pattern, a nodular pattern, a reticulonodular pattern, or a consolidative pattern.
- Although much has been written about trying to distinguish interstitial from alveolar disease, this can be very tricky on CXR alone. As a general rule, reticular processes tend to be interstitial.
- Knowing the chronicity of the process is extremely helpful, as acute diffuse reticular disease is usually secondary to pulmonary edema or viral pneumonia. More chronic reticular disease suggests a more chronic disease, such as fibrosis.
- When the pattern assumes a more nodular form, pneumonia and malignancy are more likely.

Chest Computed Tomography

Michael Beal

GENERAL PRINCIPLES

- Common indications for a CT scan of the chest are broken into two main categories: those patients with abnormal CXR findings requiring further evaluation, and those patients with a normal CXR but with suspicion for occult disease.
  - Common abnormal radiographic findings prompting a follow-up CT include staging of bronchogenic carcinoma; evaluation of a nodule, mass, or opacity; and characterization of infiltrative lung disease, mediastinal, pleural, or chest wall abnormalities.
  - Common radiographically occult diseases include the evaluation of potential metastases, suspected aortic dissection, hemoptysis, bronchiectasis, infiltrative lung disease, endocrine abnormalities, or source of infection.
- Similar to the interpretation of CXR, it is important not to bias your interpretation of the CT scan based solely on the patient's known clinical history. While an understanding of the clinical scenario is important to focus on specific areas of the study, careful attention must be paid to the entirety of the examination to avoid missing pertinent findings.
- Comparison to prior CT studies is also essential to both characterize the time progression of lesions, and to determine whether subtle findings truly represent pathology.

INITIAL ASSESSMENT

Ordering a CT

- Not all chest CT examinations are performed in the same way. Many CT departments use a variety of protocols to scan the thorax. These protocols are created to convey to the technologists information on radiation technique, reconstruction techniques, and methods of contrast use and enhancement. The protocols are usually based on clinical scenarios, such as aortic dissection, pulmonary embolism, or interstitial lung disease, and providing a meaningful indication for the examination will help ensure that the proper protocol is used.
- There are several important aspects to be considered when preparing the patient for a CT scan, including the area to be scanned, the use of contrast, and the patient's ability to tolerate the contrast.

Body Region
- The region of the body to be scanned should be documented and will typically consist of a combination of the chest, abdomen, and pelvis. This decision

will be made by the referring physician based on clinical context and may be adjusted by the radiologist as needed.
- Increasingly, insurance restrictions do not allow for the changing of the region to be scanned by anyone but the referring clinician.
- A chest CT tends to scan from the thoracic inlet through the adrenal gland.
- An abdomen CT tends to cover the dome of the diaphragm through the iliac crests.
- A pelvic CT scans from the iliac crest through the pubic symphysis.

Contrast
- It is necessary to understand when the use of contrast is appropriate. A scan can be ordered with contrast, without contrast, or with and without contrast depending on the indication for the study.
- Contrast can be administered intravenously (most common) or orally (rare for thoracic conditions). As a general rule, IV contrast is indicated for patients with suspected hilar, mediastinal, or pleural abnormalities and in patients with potential vascular abnormalities such as a pulmonary embolus. It can help distinguish lymph nodes from hilar vessels, underscore the vascular component of arteriovenous malformations, and identify the enhancing rim characteristic of empyemas.
- A noncontrast scan is generally indicated for assessing lung disease, ruling out pulmonary metastases, and for assessing nodules.
- A chest CT scan with and without contrast is typically only indicated for evaluation and differentiation of an aortic dissection or intramural hematoma, initial evaluation of pulmonary arteriovenous malformations, or characterization of a known mediastinal mass.
- There are four important considerations to understand if a patient can receive contrast: renal function, allergy, vascular access, and volume status.
- Contrast agents are excreted by the kidneys; one must assess renal function prior to ordering a contrast-enhanced study.
  - Many centers use a serum creatinine level because of its ease in acquisition and it can be converted via a simple equation to creatinine clearance, which is an estimation of the glomerular filtration rate (GFR). Generally, IV contrast should be avoided in patients with a clearance of <30 mL/min.
  - Of note, patients on dialysis can receive contrast media since the contrast will be filtered in their next dialysis session.
- It is also important to assess for a history of a reaction to contrast when preparing a patient for CT. Patients should be specifically asked about iodinated contrast material, as many do not consider contrast a type of medication.
  - Shellfish allergy alone is not a contraindication to the use of IV contrast.
  - The severity of any reaction to contrast agents should also be characterized.
  - Generally, a patient with a history of itching or hives following prior contrast administration can receive premedication, whereas a patient with a history of prior serious contrast reactions such as laryngeal edema or anaphylaxis should not receive contrast despite premedication. The reactions can be somewhat idiosyncratic and tend to get more severe over time.
  - Premedication typically consists of a combination of corticosteroid and antihistamine.

- When ordering a study with contrast, the vascular access of the patient is an important and potentially limiting consideration. Although convention may vary by institution, typically central access or peripheral antecubital access with a 20-gauge line or larger is required. Specific questions about access requirements are best addressed through consultation with the radiology department.
- It is also important to remember that contrast is a bolus of fluid volume. Because of the osmolality, the contrast dose is equivalent to over 1 L of normal saline and may cause problems for patients with pulmonary edema or cardiac issues. **As a general guideline, if the patient could not tolerate a 1-L bolus of saline, they should not receive IV contrast.**

CT Scans and Protocols
High-Resolution CT
- High-resolution CT (HRCT) is a scanning protocol often used to diagnose diffuse lung diseases, bronchiectasis, emphysema, and focal lung lesions.
- HRCT does not require contrast and obtains detailed images that are comparable to gross tissue inspection.
- HRCT uses thin slices to improve resolution and view the fine details of the pulmonary parenchyma.
- In many centers, HRCT is performed in both inspiration and expiration.

Low-Dose CT
- Low-dose CT reduces the total radiation dose but still results in readable images in the majority of patients.
- This type of scan is typically indicated for lung cancer screening, children, or if multiple follow-up examinations are required.
- Low-dose CT may be limited by patient size, as reduced radiation dose, and larger patient size both result in increased image noise and poorer resolution.

Other Protocols
Various protocols also exist for the evaluation of pulmonary embolus, aortic dissection, and thoracic aorta pathology. The appropriate use of these protocols is best clarified through consultation with a radiologist.

Preparing the Patient
- Patients can be hesitant about CT scans, which usually stem from concern regarding the radiation dose and specifics of the procedure. It is helpful to relate the radiation exposure to that of natural background radiation, where one conventional chest CT is approximately equal in exposure to 2 years of natural background radiation.
- It is also helpful to explain to patients that the scan can be interrupted or terminated at any time if problems arise and that they will be able to communicate with the radiographer in the control room through an intercom.
- Claustrophobic patients may find it beneficial to close their eyes during the examination.
- Patients should also be aware of the need for controlled breathing throughout the study, as this reduces image noise due to diaphragmatic movement.
- All clothing with zippers and all metallic objects should be removed to prevent confusion when interpreting the image.

- Patients should be made NPO 4 hours prior to their scheduled scan as IV contrast material can occasionally be pro-emetic. Four hours allow the stomach to be cleared of contents so the risk of aspiration can be reduced.

GENERAL APPROACH TO CT INTERPRETATION

- When starting the CT analysis, prior imaging studies and the clinical history should be examined to focus the interpretation and the differential diagnosis.
- The use of prior imaging to aid in the interpretation of the current chest CT cannot be stressed enough, as it is extremely useful in determining the time course of certain lesions and bringing subtle abnormalities to light.
- The characterization of lesions into acute or chronic is also essential to narrow the differential diagnosis and assess for change over time.

Window Levels and Window Width

- CT has much better contrast discrimination than a standard CXR. Levels of CT attenuation that are often able to be differentiated include (from dark to light): air, fat, fluid, muscle, enhancing organ, bone, and metal. The density levels of these items are assigned values known as a Hounsfield unit (HU). The density of water is arbitrarily set to a value of 0 HU and the scale increases/decreases with corresponding radiodensity.
- Chest CT scans will often load with multiple series to view. These series are typically broken up by windowing technique or the use of contrast.
  - Since the human eye is unable to differentiate between the 2000 shades of gray that can be seen on a CT scan, windowing is used in areas of the body with similar density.
  - Windowing narrows the HU pixel range that will be displayed (decreases the potential number of shades of gray) so that each shade can be differentiated easier by the human eye. With fewer shades of gray to be displayed, contrast between the fine tissue details is maximized.
- Routine window settings for chest CT include one for the lung parenchyma, bone, and the mediastinum.

Basic Anatomy

- Identification of the correct anatomical structures must first start with an understanding of patient positioning.
- When viewing a CT scan, imagine that you are standing at the patient's feet looking toward the head as he or she lies supine on a table. This way the patient's left side is on image right, and right side is on image left.
- The patient is supine, so the vertebral column is at the bottom of the image and the chest wall is at the top.
- There may be circumstances where an image is taken in the prone position, where image right is the patient's right and image left is the patient's left. The top of the image is the vertebral column, and the bottom is the chest wall.
- Knowledge of the positioning is not only important for identifying anatomy, but also aids in distinguishing gravity-related changes (i.e., dependent atelectasis) from pathologic findings such as inflammation or fibrosis.

- Images are also reconstructed in the coronal and sagittal planes. The coronal plane is as if you are looking at the patient from the front, and the sagittal plane is as if you were looking at the patient from the left side.
- Differentiating an expiratory CT from an inspiratory CT may also be required and is best done through inspection of the shape of the trachea on corresponding levels. In the expiratory CT, the membranous portion of the trachea will flatten so that the trachea does not resemble an "O," as it does during inspiration.
- The identification of normal structures on the chest CT is required to be able to identify any abnormal structures or pathology. This is best carried out by grouping structures into the mediastinum, hila and lungs, pleura, chest wall, and diaphragm.

Mediastinal Anatomy

- The mediastinum is the tissue compartment situated between the lungs, bounded anteriorly by the sternum and posteriorly by the spine.
- Superiorly, structures are identified with reference to the trachea. The esophagus lies posterior to the trachea at this level, and the great arterial branches of the aorta lie anterior and lateral to the walls of the trachea. At this level, the great arterial branches will be seen from anatomic right to left as the innominate artery (brachiocephalic artery), left carotid artery, and left subclavian artery.
- Anterior to these great arterial vessels will be the great veins, with the left brachiocephalic vein coursing across the mediastinum as the most anterior great vessel.
- The thyroid gland can also be identified caudally near the level of the thoracic inlet. Because of its iodine content, the thyroid is usually very bright.
- The aorta, superior vena cava, pulmonary arteries, and lymph node groups are important to identify. Usually, the aortic arch is easily identified crossing from the anterior to posterior mediastinum lateral to the trachea. The superior vena cava is seen anterior and to the anatomic right of the trachea.
- The thymus may also be seen anterior to the aortic arch and posterior to the sternum. Other notable structures at this level are the main pulmonary arteries and the azygos vein, which can be seen passing over the right main bronchus and emptying into the superior vena cava.
- Important lymph node groups to identify and assess for enlargement or pathology include the paratracheal chain, subcarinal nodes, and aortopulmonary window nodes. Lymph nodes with a short axis >1 cm are considered enlarged, with an exception in subcarinal nodes where >1.5 cm is considered enlargement.
- The paracardiac mediastinum includes the chambers of the heart and origins of the great vessels. The main pulmonary artery can be seen arising most anterior and rising from the right ventricle. It can be followed to its split into left and right pulmonary branches.
- The superior vena cava can also be visualized as it enters the right atrium. Identification of the aortic root as it projects out of the left ventricle can be helpful since coronary arteries may be seen as they originate near the aortic valve cusps and can be assessed for calcification. The aortic root originates between the main pulmonary artery and right atrium.
- The most posterior portion of the heart is the left atrium, and most anterior is the right ventricle. The remaining heart chambers can be identified with relation to these structures and their outflow tracts. The inferior vena cava may also be identified caudally near the diaphragm as it courses into the right atrium.

- Assessment of the retrosternal space for the internal mammary arteries and veins, and lymph nodes may also be useful in certain scenarios.
- Enlarged vessels may indicate superior vena cava obstruction, and enlarged lymph nodes always indicate pathology (most commonly breast cancer or lymphoma).

Hila and Lung Anatomy
- The anatomy of the pulmonary hila is visualized well on contrast-enhanced CT, which aids in the diagnosis of endobronchial lesions, surrounding masses, and vascular lesions.
- Vascular anatomy often follows airway anatomy, so evaluation of these structures can take place concomitantly. The anatomy of the right and left hila with a focus on airway anatomy will be reviewed here separately.
- The right hilum can be tracked as the right mainstem bronchus branches from the trachea at the level of the carina.
- The right pulmonary artery passes anterior and inferior to the bronchus at this level.
- The right upper lobe bronchus will first be seen branching off about 1 cm distal to the carina with the right superior pulmonary vein directly anterior to this structure. This upper lobe bronchus will further branch into anterior, posterior, and superior segmental branches.
- After the upper lobe bronchus branches, the right airway will continue as bronchus intermedius. At the lower level of bronchus intermedius, the right middle lobe bronchus arises anteriorly just caudal to the right pulmonary artery and can be followed branching into medial and lateral segments.
- Distal to the branching of the middle lobe bronchus, bronchus intermedius becomes the right lower lobe bronchus, and gives rise to the superior segment and the basal segmental bronchi (anterior, medial, lateral, and posterior). These segments vary in their appearance and are not always visible on CT.
- The left hilum can also be tracked as the left main bronchus courses from the trachea at the level of the carina. The left pulmonary artery passes superior to the left main bronchus at this level and will then descend posteriorly.
- The left main bronchus takes a longer course than the right before branching, and first branches off as the left upper lobe bronchus, which courses anterolaterally from its origin.
- The left superior pulmonary veins are anteromedial to the bronchus at this level. The upper lobe bronchus further branches into a lingular bronchus (which gives rise to superior and inferior segments) and anterior and apicoposterior segments.
- The left lower lobe bronchus is relatively symmetrical with the right lower lobe bronchus, and branches into a superior segment and three basal segments (anteromedial, lateral, and posterior).

Pleural, Diaphragm, and Chest Wall Anatomy
- The pleura, diaphragm, and chest wall are visualized well on contrast enhanced chest CT imaging and are most efficiently evaluated with soft tissue (mediastinal) windows.
- When assessing the pleura and diaphragm, it is important to remember that the diaphragmatic space extends well below the lung bases and scans must continue all the way down to this angle to be completely assessed.

- The visceral and parietal layers of the pleura are not normally visible on CT. The parietal (superficial) and visceral (deep) layers lie internal to the ribs and the innermost intercostal muscles and are separated from these structures by a layer of extrapleural fat.
- Identification of the diaphragmatic crura is also important to avoid mistaking them with enlarged lymph nodes or masses, as they can take on a rounded appearance. The crura are tendinous structures that extend inferiorly from the diaphragm to attach to the vertebral column.
- There are several physiologic openings in the diaphragm that should also be identified. These include the aortic hiatus, esophageal hiatus, and foramen of the inferior vena cava.
  - The aortic hiatus is most posterior and is bounded anteriorly by the crura and posteriorly by the spine. It is usually found at vertebral level T12. The azygos and hemiazygos veins, thoracic duct, intercostal arteries, and splanchnic nerves also pass through the aortic hiatus.
  - The esophageal hiatus is more anterior in the diaphragm and is located in the muscular part of the diaphragm. It arises around the level of the T10 vertebrae and also contains both vagal nerve trunk branches.
  - The foramen of the inferior vena cava arises around the level of the T8 vertebrae and is anterior and to the right of the esophageal hiatus.
- Gross inspection of the chest wall is important to identify any abnormalities that may also be clues to the diagnosis. Knowledge of the anatomy of the axillary space is particularly helpful in identifying abnormal lymph nodes and other pathology.
- When patients are scanned with both arms by their side, the axilla is bordered by the fascial coverings of pectoralis major and minor anteriorly; the chest wall and serratus anterior medially; the latissimus dorsi, teres major, and subscapularis posteriorly; and the biceps brachii and coracobrachialis laterally.
  - The axillary space also contains physiologic lymph nodes, axillary vessels, and nerves such as the brachial plexus and intercostals.
  - Normal lymph nodes in this region can be as large as 1.5 cm in the short axis, but with the appropriate clinical context lymph nodes >1 cm may be cause for concern.
  - Pathologic lymph nodes are best identified by direct comparison for symmetry in the axillae.
- Inspection of the supraclavicular area, breasts, and superior sulci should also take place with a concern for enlarged lymph nodes and masses.

APPROACH FOR READING CHEST CT

- With knowledge of the key anatomy, an organized approach for evaluating the chest CT is required to identify all findings. It is important to adhere to a consistent search pattern every time a chest CT is evaluated, as obvious findings may take attention away from less obvious findings that are equally important.
- Inspection should begin with the transaxial images in the soft tissue window.
- Because the beginner often neglects the soft tissues of the thoracic wall, these tissues should be evaluated first, followed by the mediastinum.

- Images should then be switched to the transaxial lung window with evaluation of the lung parenchyma, pleura, and bones.

Soft Tissue Window
- Inspection of the thoracic wall will occur first in the soft tissue window. Close attention should be paid to the axilla and breasts for enlarged lymph nodes and masses.
- The mediastinum should then be evaluated for pathologic masses or anatomical abnormalities. It may be easiest to orient yourself relative to the aortic arch or trachea.
- Cranially from the aortic arch (supra-aortic mediastinum), careful attention should be paid to the presence of enlarged lymph nodes, thyroid lesions or enlargement, and vessel abnormalities. When evaluating the space caudally from the aortic arch to the superior aspect of the heart (subaortic mediastinum), focus should be paid to the aortopulmonary window, subcarinal space, and anterior aortic space for the presence of enlarged lymph nodes.
- As you extend caudally into the paracardiac mediastinum, the hilar region should be assessed for configuration and vessel caliber, lobulation, and enlargement.
- The heart should also be assessed for signs of coronary atherosclerosis or chamber dilations, and the descending aortic space evaluated for pathologic lymph node enlargement.
- When analyzing lymphadenopathy or a mass on CT, pay attention to the location and the attenuation of the abnormality. Both will be helpful in generating differential diagnoses and will be useful in communicating with other specialists. A fatty mass in the anterior mediastinum, for example, is less likely to be malignant than one in the middle mediastinum.

Lung Window
- The lung window is very wide and allows for assessment of the parenchyma, pleura, and bones.
- The lung parenchyma should be assessed first with evaluation for the normal branching pattern and caliber of vessels along with the interlobar fissures and presence of bullae.
- Careful attention should be paid for any nodules (<3 cm), masses (>3 cm), consolidation, or infiltrate.
- The pleura should then be assessed for the presence of abnormalities such as thickening, enhancement, calcification, plaques, pleural fluid, or pneumothorax.
- Finally, the bones (ribs, scapula, and vertebrae) should be evaluated for normal marrow structure, spinal stenosis, or signs of osteoarthritis such as osteophyte formation. Focal lytic or sclerotic processes and fractures should also be identified.

Basic Lung Parenchymal Patterns
- Narrowing the differential diagnosis of lung disease on CT also requires an organized schema and is best delineated by characterizing the dominant pattern, distribution within the secondary lobule, and distribution within the lung.
- The dominant pattern is assessed first with other findings serving to narrow the differential diagnosis. This dominant finding should be grouped into reticular, nodular, high-attenuation, or low-attenuation patterns.

Reticular Pattern

The reticular pattern displays too many lines and is usually from thickened interlobular septae.

- Smooth septal line thickening is most often due to interstitial pulmonary edema (Kerley B lines) or lymphangitic carcinomatosis. Occasionally, it may be seen with viral pneumonias.
- Nodular septal line thickening is most often due to sarcoidosis, silicosis, or lymphangitic carcinomatosis.
- Irregular septal line thickening is a finding most often seen with fibrosis (usually nonspecific interstitial pneumonia).

Nodular Pattern

With a nodular pattern, the distribution of the nodules is key to narrowing the differential diagnosis, and identifying pleural nodules can help with this process.

- Centrilobular nodules are nodules in the center of the secondary pulmonary lobule, which do not touch the pleura. The most likely differential diagnosis consisting of hypersensitivity pneumonitis, infection, or respiratory bronchiolitis.
- The presence of a tree-in-bud pattern, of irregular and often nodular branching structures most identifiable in the lung periphery, can narrow this differential diagnosis to endobronchial spread of infection (usually mycobacterial or bacterial), aspiration, or airway disease associated with infection (such as bronchiectasis, cystic fibrosis, or allergic bronchopulmonary aspergillosis [ABPA]).
- Perilymphatic nodules are distributed along the bronchovascular bundles and the pleura. These nodules are characteristic of sarcoidosis, silicosis, and lymphangitic carcinomatosis.
- If nodules are present with a random distribution, the likely differential diagnosis is miliary TB, fungal infection, sarcoidosis, or the hematogenous spread of metastases.

High-Attenuation Pattern

- A high-attenuation pattern can be characterized as ground glass opacity (GGO) or consolidation with a large degree of overlap between the two.
- GGO occurs when there is a hazy increase in lung opacity without obscuring the underlying vessels and is broken down into acute versus chronic.
  - Acute GGO occurs in cases such as pulmonary edema, pneumonia, or pulmonary hemorrhage.
  - Chronic GGO may be due to organizing pneumonia, hypersensitivity pneumonitis, chronic eosinophilic pneumonia, alveolar proteinosis, lung fibrosis, and pulmonary adenocarcinoma.
  - The location of GGO in the lung is helpful in distinguishing these etiologies.
- **Crazy paving** is another term used to describe the distribution of GGO and occurs when it is combined with smooth septal thickening, resembling a pattern of paving stones or irregular shapes and lines. The differential diagnosis is similar to GGO. Of note, however, is the classic association of this pattern with alveolar proteinosis.

- Consolidation refers to filling in of the alveolar air spaces with loss of visualization of the pulmonary vessels.
  - As with GGO, the differential is very much based on the chronicity of the finding.
  - When chronic, one must consider atypical infection, pulmonary adenocarcinoma, inflammatory pneumonia (organizing pneumonia or eosinophilic pneumonia), or congenital lesions (such as sequestration).

Low-Attenuation Pattern
- A low-attenuation pattern occurs due to emphysema, cystic lung disease, honeycombing, or bronchiectasis.
- Cystic lung disease is defined as radiolucent areas with a wall thickness <4 mm and is most often due to pneumatoceles, honeycombing, Langerhans cell histiocytosis (LCH), lymphocytic interstitial pneumonia, or lymphangioleiomyomatosis.
- Honeycombing occurs with usual interstitial pneumonia (UIP), interstitial fibrosis, or end-stage sarcoidosis.
- Bronchiectasis can occur with cystic fibrosis, ABPA, immune deficiency, mycobacterial disease, or a prior infection causing focal bronchiectasis. With bronchiectasis, care should be taken to exclude a central obstructing mass.
- Mosaic attenuation refers to scattered dark (low-attenuation) areas within normal lung akin to a tile mosaic. Visualization of attenuated vasculature in the darker areas helps to prevent confusion with GGO.
- In mosaic attenuation, the darker areas are abnormal secondary to:
  - Small airway disease (most notably bronchiolitis obliterans).
  - Small vessel disease (most notably chronic pulmonary embolism).

Pulmonary Function Testing

Adam Anderson and Jeffrey J. Atkinson

GENERAL PRINCIPLES
- Pulmonary function tests (PFTs) are an integral part of a pulmonary evaluation and management.
- PFTs can be divided into spirometry (measurement of air movement in and out of the lungs), plethysmography (measurement of lung volumes), and diffusing capacity (measurement of gas exchange within the lungs).
- The availability of user-friendly pulmonary function testing devices has resulted in widespread use of on-site PFTs and home testing resulting in an increased need for formal training in collecting and interpreting valid pulmonary function measurements.
- PFTs are best interpreted in relation to an individual's clinical presentation and not in isolation. All parts of the PFTs should be used when evaluating a patient.
- It is important to remember that PFTs **do not** make pathologic diagnoses such as emphysema or pulmonary fibrosis. They provide physiologic measurements identifying ventilatory defects and, in doing so, support the existence of the relevant disease process and aid in the evaluation of its treatment.
- This text assists with evaluation of basic spirometry, diffusing capacity, and lung volumes and will allow the reader to identify common ventilatory defects using the data provided by PFTs.

NORMAL VALUES AND REFERENCE RANGES
- The results of PFTs are interpreted by comparing them to reference values representing normal healthy subjects.
- These normal or **predicted values** take into account many variables, most importantly age, height, gender, and self-described race/ethnicity.
- However, they neglect other influencing variables that may have effects, including air pollution, socioeconomic status, and others.
- The most utilized reference equations are from the global lung initiative (GLI), and a 2022 equation that is weighted to allow removal of self-described race from interpretation will likely replace previous versions.

Percent Predicted Method
- Traditionally, but without scientific basis, pulmonary function laboratories have arbitrarily set normal ranges for each predicted value.
- The lower and upper limits of normal for each predicted value are set as 80% and 120% of the predicted value, respectively.

- The measured values for each pulmonary function variable are compared with the predicted values of each variable and expressed as "percent of predicted."
- **Measured values that fall within the 80–120% range of predicted values are considered normal.**
- This method permits easy instruction and is still in widespread use but is no longer recommended because it results in misdiagnosis in younger and older individuals.

The Lower Limit of Normal Method

- The currently preferred method for defining normal range of each predicted (normal) value uses a percentile-based approach.
- **Using this method, measured values less than the Lower Limit of Normal (LLN) (5th percentile of the healthy population defined as 1.64 standard deviations below the mean) are considered abnormal.**
- Severity is then determined by the number of standard deviations the result is from the mean (z-score) because these values have a normal distribution.
- **A z-score of −1.64 to −2.5 is mild, −2.5 to −4 is moderate, and < −4 is severe.**
- The LLN method can lead to more precise diagnoses of chronic obstructive pulmonary disease (COPD), especially in the elderly.[1] The percent predicted method may overdiagnose COPD in elderly patients while underdiagnosing young patients.[2]
- The LLN method standardizes severity assessments, which have historically been determined by individual pulmonary function laboratories and often differ for spirometry, lung volume, and DLCO testing within the same lab.[3]
- If the PFT testing software does not produce a z-score, the percent predicted method can be utilized.

STANDARDIZATION OF PULMONARY FUNCTION TESTS

- To obtain useful information from PFTs, the adequacy of both the testing equipment and the test results should be scrutinized.
- The American Thoracic Society (ATS) publishes guidelines for the standardization of spirometry, including recommendations on equipment calibration, validation of results, measurement of parameters, and acceptability and reproducibility criteria for the data obtained.[4]
- Because most PFTs are obtained from dedicated PFT labs, this text describes the standardized criteria for interpretation of PFT data and excludes details on equipment setup and testing techniques.
- Only when all the acceptability and reproducibility criteria are met can PFTs be interpreted with confidence.
- If acceptability and reproducibility criteria are not met, interpretation should note lack of confidence and alternative testing should be considered to confirm abnormalities.
- Up to eight patient efforts may be performed; after this, patient fatigue affects the data obtained.
- The results with the maximum pulmonary function are always used for interpretation.

Acceptability Criteria

PFTs should initially be assessed for acceptability that is best determined by studying the flow–volume loops.

Acceptability criteria for PFTs include the following:

- Freedom from artifacts particularly in the first second (coughing, glottic closure, early termination, leak, variable effort)
- Good starts (i.e., the initial portion of the curve that is most dependent on patient effort is free from artifact)
- Satisfactory end expiratory flow (at least a 1-second plateau in the volume–time curve)

Reproducibility Criteria

Once the minimum of three acceptable flow–volume loops has been obtained, the reproducibility of the PFTs should be assessed.

Reproducibility criteria for PFTs include the following:

- The two largest forced vital capacity (FVC) measurements should be within 0.15 L of each other.
- The two largest forced expiratory volumes in 1 second (FEV$_1$) measurements should be within 0.15 L of each other.

NORMAL PULMONARY FUNCTION TESTS

Flow–Volume Loops

- Normal PFTs are defined by a normal-shaped flow–volume loop; please see Figure 3-1.[5]

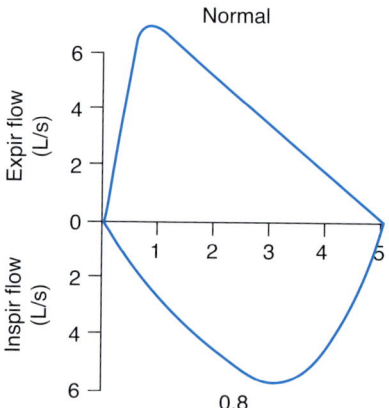

Figure 3-1 Normal flow–volume loop. (Reproduced with permission from Scanlon PD. *Hyatt's Interpretation of Pulmonary Function Tests*. 5th ed. Philadelphia, PA: Lippincott Williams & Wilkins; 2019. Figure 2.7.)

- The flow–volume loop is the plot of the FVC maneuver.
- The FVC maneuver involves the patient taking a maximum inspiration followed by a maximum and forceful expiration.
- The flow–volume loop portion of pulmonary function testing is also known as spirometry.
- The expiratory limb of a normal flow–volume loop has a rapid peak and a gradual decline in flow back to zero.
- The inspiratory limb should have a rounded shape.

FEV_1 and FVC

- Normal pulmonary function is also defined by the measured values for the FVC and the FEV_1.
- **FVC** is defined as the maximum volume of air that is **forcefully** exhaled after a maximum inspiration.
- **FEV_1** is defined as the maximum volume of air exhaled during the **first second** of the FVC.
- The measured values for FEV_1 and FVC are compared to the predicted values for FEV_1 and FVC. **Values above the LLN (or 80–120% of predicted) are considered normal.**

Lung Volumes

- Lung volumes are measured separately from the flow–volume loop.
- Lung volume measurement requires two separate maneuvers; a test to measure functional residual capacity and a test to measure vital capacity without a forced exhalation.
- Like the FEV_1 and FVC, measured lung volumes are compared to the predicted values.
- **Lung volumes above the LLN (or between 80% and 120% predicted) are considered normal.**
- The most important lung volumes for this discussion are total lung capacity (**TLC**), and residual volume (**RV**).
  - **TLC** is defined as the volume of air in the lung after complete maximal inspiration.
  - **RV** is defined as the volume of air left in the lungs after complete maximal expiration.

EVALUATING PULMONARY FUNCTION TEST PATTERNS

There are normal, obstructive, and restrictive patterns observed on PFTs, which will be discussed in detail. The following algorithm will allow for characterization of the disease pattern, see Figure 3-2.[6,7]

OBSTRUCTIVE VENTILATORY DEFECTS

- An obstructive ventilatory defect (OVD) exists when there is a disproportionate decrease in the FEV_1 when compared to the FVC.
- **An FEV_1:FVC ratio <LLN (or <0.7) defines an OVD.**

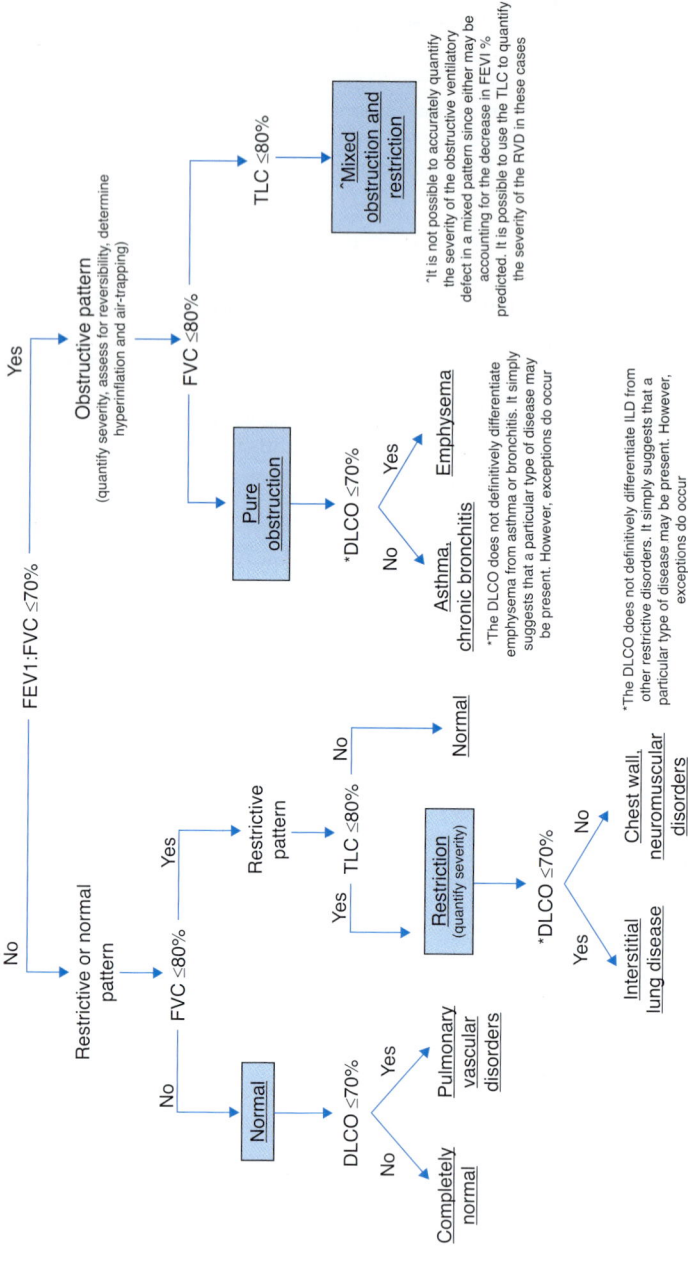

Figure 3-2 Evaluation of pulmonary function tests. DLCO, diffusing capacity for carbon monoxide; FVC, forced vital capacity; TLC, total lung capacity. (Data from Pellegrino R, Viegi G, Brusasco V, et al. Interpretive strategies for lung function tests. *Eur Respir J.* 2005;26:948–968.)

TABLE 3-1 QUANTIFYING THE SEVERITY BY PERCENTILE FOR AN OBSTRUCTIVE VENTILATOR DEFECT

Severity	FEV_1 z-Score
Mild	<–1.64 but >–2.5
Moderate	<–2.5 but >–4
Severe	<–4

- The FVC may be reduced in an OVD, but the FEV_1 is always reduced to a greater degree.
- The ATS cautions against diagnosing an OVD in individuals who have a decreased FEV_1:FVC ratio but normal measured FEV_1 and FVC, because this pattern can on occasion be seen in healthy subjects.
- OVDs indicate airflow limitation and imply airway narrowing.
- In emphysema, for example, the narrowing is believed to be the result of decreased elastic support of smaller airways from alveolar septal destruction, whereas in chronic bronchitis and asthma, mucosal inflammation and excess luminal mucus are common etiologies.
- Once the diagnosis of an OVD has been made, the defect needs to be fully characterized by performing the following:
  - Quantifying the severity of the OVD
  - Assessing the reversibility of the obstruction
  - Determining whether there is hyperinflation
  - Determining whether there is air trapping

Quantifying an Obstructive Ventilatory Defect

Quantifying the severity of the OVD is done by utilizing the z-score for the FEV_1 (Table 3-1).

Assessing for Bronchodilator Reversibility

- Assessing for reversibility of an obstruction requires spirometry be performed both before and after bronchodilator administration.
- **Positive reversibility of the airway obstruction is indicated by a change in pre- versus postbronchodilator FEV_1 or FVC of more than 10% of the predicted value** ([post-BD value – pre-BD value] × 100/predicted value).
- Previous methods utilized an absolute increase in the postbronchodilator FEV_1 by both ≥12% and ≥200 mL to indicate a positive response.
- These criteria are best applied when active therapy is not present (e.g., no albuterol for 4 hours but are also likely altered by long-acting bronchodilators as well).
- The lack of reversibility during a PFT does not indicate there will be no significant clinical response to bronchodilator therapy, but rather that baseline reversibility is not elevated.
- Although asthma is typically a reversible OVD, bronchodilator responsiveness during a PFT is not pathognomonic for asthma, nor does the absence exclude asthma.

Determining if Hyperinflation Is Present
- **Hyperinflation** denotes that at maximum inspiration or expiration the lungs are at a greater volume than is expected for an individual. In physiologic terms, the individual's TLC *or* RV is increased.
- The presence of **hyperinflation** is determined by comparing the measured TLC *or* RV to the predicted TLC *or* RV: **TLC z-score >1.64 (or >120% of predicted).**

Determining if Air Trapping Is Present
- **Air trapping** denotes that during expiration, there is dynamic collapse of airways resulting in incomplete exhalation of air.
- **RV z-score >1.64 or (120% of predicted).**

The Flow–Volume Loop in Obstructive Ventilatory Defects
- OVDs change the shape of the flow–volume curve. The expiratory curve still has a rapid initial peak, but the terminal portions of the expiratory flow drop progressively with worsening obstruction.
- As a result, the expiratory limb of the curve takes on a progressively increasing concavity. Eventually, there is also a decrease in the peak expiratory flow at the initial portion of the curve.
- In severe disease, there is an initial rapid but reduced peak followed by a precipitous drop in flow and a very gradual taper of the flow to zero, see Figure 3-3.[5]
- When lung volumes are measured the curve on PFT reports will reflect measured values and may shift leftward, if hyperinflation and/or air trapping is present.

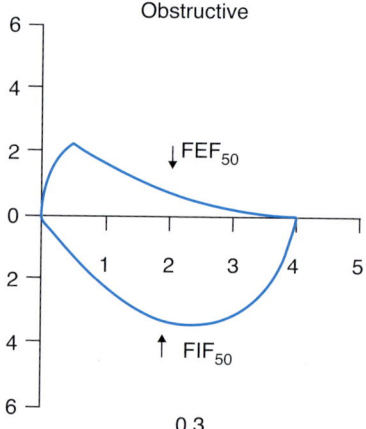

Figure 3-3 Obstructive lung disease flow–volume loop. (Reproduced with permission from Scanlon PD. *Hyatt's Interpretation of Pulmonary Function Tests*. 5th ed. Lippincott Williams & Wilkins; 2019. Figure 2.7.)

UPPER AIRWAY OBSTRUCTION

- The OVDs discussed so far all represent obstruction at the level of smaller, more distal airways. Obstruction of the larger, more central airways (trachea and major bronchi) presents differently and is most easily identified on inspection of the inspiratory and expiratory limbs of the flow–volume loop.
- Three forms of upper airway obstruction can be discerned:
  - Fixed obstruction
  - Variable intrathoracic obstruction
  - Variable extrathoracic obstruction

Fixed Upper Airway Obstruction

- When a central airway contains a fixed obstruction, the cross-sectional area of the obstructed airway does not change throughout the respiratory cycle (hence its characterization is *fixed*).
- The obstruction is present during both inspiration and expiration, and both limbs of the flow–volume loop are almost equally affected.
- There is characteristic truncation of both the inspiratory and expiratory flow limbs with the resulting "box" shape on the flow–volume loop, see Figure 3-4.[5]

Variable Upper Airway Obstruction

- When an airway contains a variable obstruction, manifestation of the obstruction is dependent on both the location of the obstruction (within or external to the thorax) and the phase of the respiratory cycle (inspiration or expiration). Extrathoracic is anatomically defined as above the sternal notch.

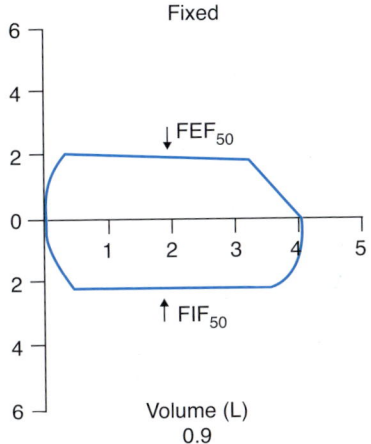

Figure 3-4 Fixed upper airway obstruction flow–volume loop. (Reproduced with permission from Scanlon PD. *Hyatt's Interpretation of Pulmonary Function Tests.* 5th ed. Lippincott Williams & Wilkins; 2019. Figure 2.7.)

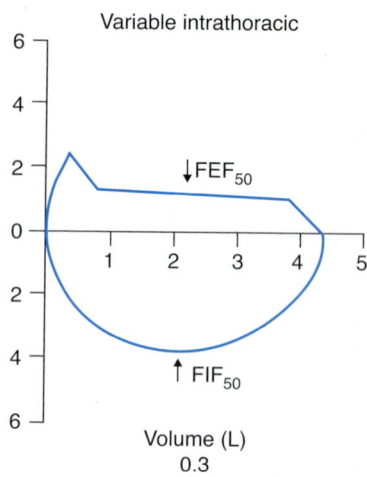

Figure 3-5 Variable intrathoracic obstruction flow–volume loop. (Reproduced with permission from Scanlon PD. *Hyatt's Interpretation of Pulmonary Function Tests*. 5th ed. Lippincott Williams & Wilkins; 2019. Figure 2.7.)

- Changes in the cross-sectional area of the obstructed airway vary with both inspiration and expiration and intra- or extrathoracic location of the obstructing lesion.
  - In variable **intrathoracic** obstruction, the expiratory limb is primarily affected.
  - During forced expiration, pleural pressure exceeds the intrathoracic airway pressure. As a result, the airway narrows, and the obstruction worsens. During forced inspiration, the pleural pressure is negative, the airway widens, and the obstruction is relieved. Thus, only the expiratory limb is truncated, see Figure 3-5.[5]
  - In variable **extrathoracic** obstruction, the inspiratory limb is primarily affected.
  - During forced inspiration, atmospheric pressure exceeds the extrathoracic airway pressure. As a result, the airway collapses, and the obstruction worsens. During forced expiration, the airway pressure increases, and the obstruction is relieved. Thus, only the inspiratory limb is truncated, see Figure 3-6.[5]

RESTRICTIVE VENTILATORY DEFECTS

- A restrictive ventilatory defect (RVD) exists when there is a reduction of maximum lung inflation, manifested by a reduction in TLC. Therefore, **a TLC < LLN (or <80% of predicted) defines an RVD**.
- The presence of an RVD may be suspected using spirometry when the FVC is reduced but remains in proportion to the reduction in FEV_1. In these cases, the FEV_1:FVC ratio will be normal or increased.

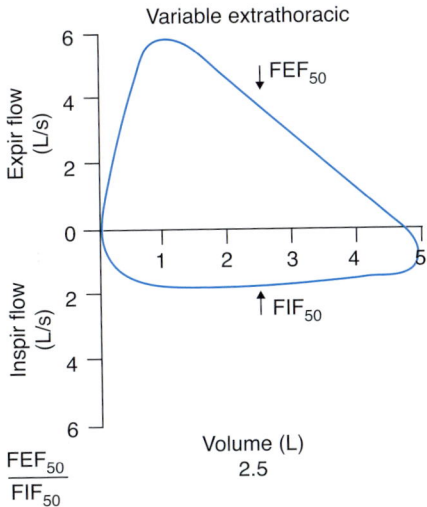

Figure 3-6 Variable extrathoracic obstruction flow–volume loop. (Reproduced with permission from Scanlon PD. *Hyatt's Interpretation of Pulmonary Function Tests.* 5th ed. Lippincott Williams & Wilkins; 2019. Figure 2.7.)

- To diagnose an RVD definitively, however, lung volumes should be obtained to quantify the TLC.
- An RVD is not specific for any individual disease and can result from many disorders classified into three categories (intrinsic, extrinsic, neuromuscular):
  - Intrinsic lung disease which affects the lung parenchyma
  - Extrinsic lung disease, such as disorders of chest wall or pleura that limit expansion of the lungs or cause compression
  - Neuromuscular disease that impairs the respiratory muscles
- For example, in pulmonary fibrosis, the restriction is the result of the fibrosis of the alveolar walls and "stiffening" of the lung parenchyma. In muscular dystrophy, weakened diaphragmatic and thoracic muscles are the etiologies. An RVD can also be caused by removal of lung tissue (lobectomy, pneumonectomy) as this results in a decrease in the TLC compared to predicted normal.
- Once the diagnosis of an RVD has been made, the defect needs to be quantified, which is done using the FVC or the TLC by the z-score or percent predicted, see Table 3-2.

The Flow–Volume Loop in Restrictive Ventilatory Defects

- The proportions of the flow–volume loop are essentially unchanged in RVDs.
- The curve is often narrowed and shifted to the right, reflecting the smaller lung volumes associated with RVDs, see Figure 3-7.[5]
- Although peak expiratory flow is decreased, note that at each measured lung volume, flow is often greater than in normal lungs.

TABLE 3-2 QUANTIFYING THE SEVERITY BY PERCENTILE FOR A RESTRICTIVE VENTILATORY DEFECT

Severity	FVC z-Score	TLC z-Score
Mild	<−1.64 but >−2.5	<−1.64 but >−2.5
Moderate	<−2.5 but >−4	<−2.5 but >−4
Severe	<−4	<−4

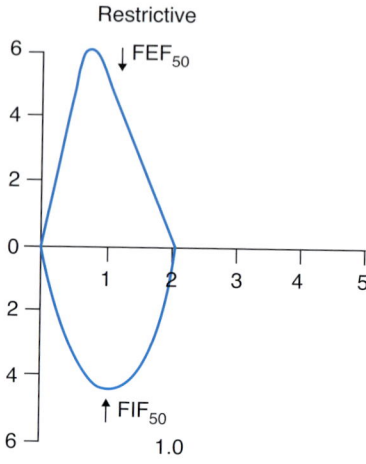

Figure 3-7 Restrictive lung disease flow–volume loop. (Reproduced with permission from Scanlon PD. *Hyatt's Interpretation of Pulmonary Function Tests.* 5th ed. Lippincott Williams & Wilkins; 2019. Figure 2.7.)

DIFFUSING CAPACITY

- Diffusing capacity is often measured as part of a PFT. It is performed separately from spirometry and lung volume measurement.
- It is a measure of the integrity of the alveolar–capillary membrane across which gas exchange takes place.
- The diffusing capacity is a nonspecific measurement and provides only a physiologic assessment of the **efficiency of gas exchange**.
- Any disease affecting the lung ventilation, pulmonary interstitium, circulation or available hemoglobin can alter the diffusing capacity.
- The gas used to measure diffusing capacity is carbon monoxide, so the diffusing capacity is expressed as **diffusing capacity of the lung for carbon monoxide (DLCO)**.
- The measured value is often adjusted to eliminate the effects of the hemoglobin concentration and/or baseline carboxyhemoglobin if these are known.[8] The adjusted value is expressed as the **adjusted DLCO ($DLCO_{ADJ}$)**.

- Calculation of the $DLCO_{ADJ}$ is not mandatory but desirable.
- Measured values of DLCO and $DLCO_{ADJ}$ are compared to the LLN or predicted values.
- **Percent predicted values for DLCO or $DLCO_{ADJ}$ between 70% and 120% are considered normal.**
- The reason for the wide range in normal DLCO and $DLCO_{ADJ}$ is the large amount of variability between different measurements in the same individual at any given time. This is the only PFT test where a mean of two separate efforts is utilized.
- Of note, the finding of normal PFTs with an isolated decrease in $DLCO_{ADJ}$ should raise a high index of suspicion for disease in the pulmonary vascular system.
- Similar to lung volumes a surgical resection of part of the lung will reduce DLCO values as the capillary bed for gas exchange is smaller than predicted.

OTHER PULMONARY FUNCTION TESTS

Maximal Voluntary Ventilation

- Maximal voluntary ventilation (MVV), reported in liters per minute, is defined as the maximum amount of air that can be breathed in and out in 1 minute.
- For patient comfort, it is usually measured over 12 seconds and the value extrapolated to 1 minute.
- MVV is a very nonspecific measurement and can be reduced in either restrictive or obstructive disorders.
- MVV is often used to assess patient's respiratory musculature prior to surgery to help predict postoperative pulmonary complications.
- MVV is very effort dependent and requires good patient instruction.
- It is also a reflection of lung volume changes, lung–thorax compliance, and airway resistance. Therefore, MVV may be a less-than-accurate predictor of respiratory strength and endurance.
- Average values for males and females are 140–180 L/min and 80–120 L/min, respectively.
- However, interpretation is more complicated because MVV is proportional to FEV_1 and will decrease when FEV_1 is reduced.
- In the setting of a reduced FEV_1 a reduced MVV is expected to be proportional, so the following equation is utilized. **Predicted MVV = FEV_1 × 40 (note some sources use FEV_1 × 35).**

Methacholine Challenge Testing

- Asthma is defined as a reversible obstructive airway disease. Therefore, in individuals suspected of having asthma, PFTs may appear normal, without evidence of obstruction.
- In individuals where PFTs are normal but asthma is strongly suspected clinically, bronchial provocation testing is indicated to induce airway constriction and allow for the diagnosis (and further management) of asthma.
- Other individuals who should be considered for bronchial provocation testing include those with[9]:
  - Chronic cough
  - Wheezing

- Intermittent dyspnea
- Workplace-related cough/wheezing/dyspnea
- Exercise-associated cough/wheezing
• The methacholine challenge test is a direct, chemical test of airway responsiveness. It allows for a semiquantitative assessment of airway reactivity but gives no insight into the stimulus responsible for the reactivity in an individual.
• The advantage of the test is that it has good reproducibility.
• The disadvantage is that multiple factors can affect the test, including the following:
  - Medications (bronchodilators, steroids, antihistamines, β-agonists, cholinesterase inhibitors)
  - Respiratory infection
  - Exposure to sensitizers (allergens or chemicals)
• The test begins with the administration of a sterile saline aerosol followed by the measurement of the FEV_1 twice (as a baseline).
• Increasing concentrations of methacholine diluted in sterile saline are then administered to the patient at 5-minute intervals, and the FEV_1 is measured twice after each increase in concentration. The greater of the two FEV_1 measurements is utilized.
• The concentrations range from 0.003 to 16 mg/mL of methacholine in sterile saline and are roughly doubled each time until either a positive response is obtained or a maximum concentration is achieved (Table 3-3).
• **A positive methacholine challenge is defined as a decrease in FEV_1 from baseline of >20% at a methacholine concentration of <8 mg/mL.**
• The methacholine concentration resulting in a positive challenge is reported as the PC20 (provocative concentration causing a 20% fall in FEV_1), for example, a decrease in FEV_1 from baseline occurring at a methacholine concentration of 0.5 mg/mL is reported as a PC20 = 0.5 mg/mL.
• **A negative methacholine challenge occurs if there is no change from baseline, or any decrease in FEV_1 from baseline is <20% and a concentration of >8 mg/mL has been reached.**

TABLE 3-3 METHACHOLINE DILUTION SCHEDULE

Dose Number	Methacholine Concentration (mg/mL)
0	0 (baseline)
1	0.031
2	0.0625
3	0.125
4	0.025
5	0.5
6	1
7	2
8	4
9	8
10	16 (maximum)

- When patients undergoing bronchial provocation testing are on inhaled corticosteroids, a decrease in FEV_1 from baseline of >20% at a methacholine concentration of 16 mg/mL may be considered a positive methacholine challenge test.[10]

REFERENCES

1. Roberts SD, Farber MO, Knox KS, et al. FEV1/FVC ratio of 70% misclassifies patients with obstruction at the extremes of age. *Chest.* 2006;130(1):200–206.
2. Hardie JA, Buist AS, Vollmer WM, Ellingsen I, Bakke PS, Mørkve O. Risk of over-diagnosis of COPD in asymptomatic elderly never-smokers. *Eur Respir J.* 2002;20(5):1117–1122.
3. Stanojevic S, Kaminsky DA, Miller MR, et al. ERS/ATS technical standard on interpretive strategies for routine lung function tests. *Eur Respir J.* 2022;60(1):2101499.
4. Graham BL, Steenbruggen I, Miller MR, et al. Standardization of Spirometry, 2019 Update. An Official American Thoracic Society and European Respiratory Society Technical Statement. *Am J Respir Crit Care Med.* 2019;200(8):e70–e88.
5. Hyatt RE, Scanlon PD, Nakamura M. *Interpretation of Pulmonary Function Tests.* 4th ed. Lippincott, Williams & Wilkins; 2014:4–21.
6. Al-Ashkar F, Mehra R, Mazzone PJ. Interpreting pulmonary function tests: recognize the pattern, and the diagnosis will follow. *Cleve Clin J Med.* 2003;70(10):866, 868, 871–873.
7. Pellegrino R, Viegi G, Brusasco V, et al. Interpretative strategies for lung function tests. *Eur Resp J.* 2017;49:948–968.
8. Graham BL, Brusasco V, Burgos F, et al. 2017 ERS/ATS standards for single-breath carbon monoxide uptake in the lung. *Eur Respir J.* 2005;26:720–735.
9. Crapo RO, Casaburi R, Coates AL, et al. Guidelines for methacholine and exercise challenge testing—1999. This official statement of the American Thoracic Society was adopted by the ATS board of directors, July 1999. *Am J Respir Crit Care Med.* 2000;161:309–329.
10. Sumino K, Sugar EA, Irvin CG, et al; American Lung Association Asthma Clinical Research Centers. Methacholine challenge test: diagnostic characteristics in asthmatic patients receiving controller medications. *J Allergy Clin Immunol.* 2012;130(1):69–75.

Fiberoptic Bronchoscopy

Alexander C. Chen

GENERAL PRINCIPLES

- Fiberoptic bronchoscopy (FOB) was developed by Shigeto Ikeda in the 1960s.
- FOB has become a vital procedure for pulmonologists, with nearly 500,000 procedures performed in the United States every year.[1]
- The rise of the field of interventional pulmonology has increased the diagnostic and therapeutic range of the bronchoscope.
- As technology has improved, indications for FOB have increased (Table 4-1).
- Most contraindications are relative, and potential reward must merit the possible risk (Table 4-2). The major absolute contraindication is a significant increase in intracranial pressure (ICP), as coughing during the procedure can further increase ICP leading to brain herniation.

TABLE 4-1 INDICATIONS FOR FIBEROPTIC BRONCHOSCOPY

Inspection of	Evaluation, Diagnosis, or Management of		Other
• Upper aerodigestive tract, larynx, vocal cords, and related structures	• Chronic cough • Wheezing • Pneumonia	• Tracheoesophageal fistula • Tumor • Tracheobronchial stenosis	• Assisting in intubation and extubation • Assisting percutaneous tracheostomy • Brachytherapy
• The major conductive airways	• Persistent pulmonary infiltrates • Disrupted bronchial tree secondary to trauma • Thermal or chemical inhalational injury • Anastomotic sites after lung transplantation • Position/patency of an endotracheal/tracheostomy tube	• Foreign body • Persistent atelectasis • Lymphadenopathy • Pulmonary nodule	• Intralesional injection of drugs • Brachytherapy • Stent placement • Surveillance for rejection after lung transplantation

TABLE 4-2	RELATIVE CONTRAINDICATIONS TO BRONCHOSCOPY

Relative Contraindication

Life-threatening arrhythmias
Severe hypoxemia
Recent myocardial infarction
Unstable angina
Uncorrected bleeding diathesis
Severe pulmonary hypertension
Thrombocytopenia
Superior vena cava syndrome
Unstable cervical spine

Pre-bronchoscopy Evaluation

- In an American College of Chest Physicians (ACCP) survey, a majority of operators obtain a preprocedure chest radiograph, coagulation studies, and complete blood count. Less than one-half obtain an EKG, arterial blood gas, electrolytes, or pulmonary function tests.[2] Routine preprocedure labs are not absolutely indicated unless specific concerns exist.
- Cardiac evaluation in patients with known coronary disease undergoing elective bronchoscopy can be considered, and guidelines have been published by the American College of Cardiology/American Heart Association.[3]

Procedural Medications

- Medications are commonly used before and during bronchoscopy to facilitate a safe, comfortable, and successful procedure. There are no convincing data that antisialogogues (such as atropine) are efficacious, and because of the side effects, they are not recommended on a routine basis.[4]
- Bronchoscopy procedures may be performed under General Anesthesia or moderate sedation.
- The type of sedation administered may depend on institutional preferences, complexity of the procedure, and physician preferences. For moderate sedation:
  - Benzodiazepines play a central role in providing amnesia and anxiolysis. Midazolam given parenterally is often used for its fast onset of action and short half-life.[4] Lorazepam has been used as a preprocedure medication with improved patient satisfaction at 24 hours versus placebo.
  - Opiates decrease the laryngeal reflexes and cough response and provide some anxiolysis.
    - Fentanyl given parenterally is commonly used, again due to short onset of action.[4]
    - Meperidine has been used pre- and intraprocedurally, but its use is increasingly discouraged because of its active metabolites, long half-life, and increased risk of seizures.
    - New hypnotic agents and benzodiazepines with ultra-short durations of action are being explored for use in moderate sedation cases.[5]

- Propofol is a sedative-hypnotic drug with rapid onset and very short duration of action.[6] Recovery time after an infusion is only minutes.
  - Titration of propofol takes experience to avoid the most common side effect of hypotension.
  - Many institutions require anesthesia support for administration during procedures, and therefore it is often not used during routine bronchoscopies performed without Anesthesia support.

Monitoring
- The operator is ultimately responsible for the care and safety of the patient during the bronchoscopy.
- Additional assistance is required, including at least one respiratory therapist or nurse. A second assistant can be either a second respiratory therapist or a procedural nurse.
  - Assistants monitor the patient, record vital signs, administer, and record medications, handle specimens, and assist with the bronchoscope and other equipment.
  - Special assistance is also needed when the patient is on a mechanical ventilator as insertion of a bronchoscope creates increased airway resistance.
- Equipment for monitoring and supporting the patient should include continuous pulse oximetry and EKG, vascular access, supplemental oxygen, suction, and an automated blood pressure cuff.
- Additional equipment that should be immediately available includes supplies needed for endotracheal intubation, cardiopulmonary resuscitation, vascular access, and needle decompression of pneumothorax.

Technique
- The most common patient position is supine, in bed, with the operator standing at the patient's head.
- A transoral approach is often used, sometimes with insertion of a laryngeal mask airway or endotracheal tube, and sometimes with no artificial airway. A transnasal or transtracheostomy approach may also be utilized.
- During insertion of the bronchoscope, the operator should note abnormalities of the upper airway, false and true vocal cords, and glottic area. After passage through the cords, the trachea and tracheobronchial tree are examined to at least the first subsegmental level. Topical anesthesia to the upper aerodigestive tract, glottic area, and bronchial tree can be accomplished by the application of lidocaine, benzocaine, tetracaine, or historically, cocaine.
  - Lidocaine is the most commonly used topical anesthetic for FOB because of its fast onset of action and wide therapeutic window. It is applied in the glottic area, as well as directly on the tracheobronchial tree.[6]
  - Safety for lidocaine is well established at doses <7 mg/kg.[6]
  - Operators must be aware of the risk of methemoglobinemia when using topical anesthetics, even in small amounts. When it occurs, it can be reversed by administration of methylene blue.
- The bronchoscope is most commonly held using the nondominant hand with additional guidance at the mouth or nose (depending on bronchoscope insertion site) using the dominant hand. Rotation of the scope is controlled by

rotation of the bronchoscopist's hand and flexion, and extension of the scope is determined by managing the thumb lever on the bronchoscope.
- Attention should be made to maintain the bronchoscope position within the central lumen of the tracheobronchial tree and off of the wall to optimize the view when performing airway inspection.
- Maintaining a relatively straight bronchoscope will improve maneuverability and translation of rotational forces from the handle to the tip of the bronchoscope.
- After examination of the airways, diagnostic or therapeutic procedures may be attempted.

Postprocedure
- After the procedure, the patient requires monitoring in a postprocedure area until they have recovered from sedation.
- A patient cannot drive home from the procedure and should not operate machinery or perform other potentially dangerous activity after the procedure.
- A postprocedure chest radiograph is generally obtained at the discretion of the bronchoscopist, often depending on the type of procedure that was performed.

DIAGNOSIS
- A list of diagnostic uses of bronchoscopy can be seen in Table 4-1.
- Airway inspection is the mainstay of FOB and is generally performed with each procedure.
- Tumors, cysts, source of hemoptysis, signs of infection, foreign bodies, and altered airway anatomy are some of the more common abnormalities encountered during inspection.
- Bronchoalveolar lavage (BAL) consists of wedging the end of the FOB in a distal airway, followed by instillation of sterile saline through the bronchoscope with subsequent aspiration back through the bronchoscope, in 50-mL aliquots.
  - BAL is most useful for obtaining microbiologic cultures in diagnosing typical and atypical infections.
  - Cytology can be sent to aid in diagnosis of infection, malignancy, and occasionally diffuse lung disease.
  - Cell count can show a preponderance of macrophages (normal), neutrophils, lymphocytes, eosinophils, or a fairly even mix of cell types, which are indicative of different disease states.
  - Successively bloodier BAL return aliquot may be suggestive of diffuse alveolar hemorrhage.
- Transbronchial lung biopsy is performed by passing biopsy forceps through the bronchoscope and into the lung, with the goal of sampling the distal airways parenchyma.
  - Biopsies are examined by experienced pathologists and can diagnose a wide range of pulmonary pathology.
  - Transbronchial biopsies are generally performed using fluoroscopic guidance as the area being sampled is too distal for direct visualization, though this is not absolutely necessary.
- Endobronchial biopsy is performed by passing biopsy forceps through the bronchoscope and sampling airways lesions in the larger airways under direct visualization.

- Transbronchial needle aspirations (TBNA) are used to take cytologic samples from enlarged mediastinal lymph nodes, mediastinal masses, or peripheral lung lesions.
- Endobronchial ultrasound has led to a marked increase in the range of diagnostic uses of FOB.
  - Endobronchial ultrasound using a linear array ultrasound is becoming the standard of care for diagnosis of mediastinal lymphadenopathy and masses, replacing traditional TBNA, and can also be used for sampling masses within 3–4 cm of the large airways in experienced hands. It is also superior to other modalities for imaging the structure of the trachea and mainstem bronchi.
  - Radial endobronchial ultrasound consists of a small, high-frequency ultrasound probe that can be guided through the bronchoscope into the distal airways, and advanced under fluoroscopic guidance with the goal of obtaining a real-time ultrasound image of a distal pulmonary nodule, allowing for biopsy and needle aspiration.
- Along with radial endobronchial ultrasound, 3D navigational systems, thin and ultrathin bronchoscopes, and robotic bronchoscopy systems have been developed that are being increasingly used to sample pulmonary nodules.[7,8]

TREATMENT

- A list of therapeutic uses of bronchoscopy is seen in Table 4-1.
- Advances in the field of interventional pulmonology have led to a large increase in the therapeutic uses of FOB, several of which are listed below. Some of these procedures are performed solely by these bronchoscopic specialists, while some are also performed by general pulmonologists.
  - Tracheobronchial narrowing from malignancy, strictures, or other pathology can be alleviated by stent placement or balloon dilatation, though the latter's effects are much less permanent.
  - Cryotherapy can remove malignancies or other airway obstructions. During cryotherapy, a probe is placed on the obstruction at extremely low temperatures, in essence freezing the obstruction to the probe and allowing for extrication.[9]
  - Argon plasma coagulation can be used to stop focal bleeding or obliterate obstructive airway lesions, neodymium:yttrium aluminum garnet (Nd:YAG) lasers may also do the latter.
  - Foreign body removals are usually performed using biopsy forceps or other tools and sometimes occur under fluoroscopic guidance depending on the density of the foreign body.
  - Therapeutic aspiration of secretions is sometimes performed in the presence of atelectasis with respiratory failure.[9]
  - Management of anastomotic stricture or dehiscence after lung transplantation can generally be managed by debridement or stenting.
  - Placement of one-way endobronchial valves may be an option for patients with persistent air leaks.
  - Placement of one-way endobronchial valves are also being used in carefully selected patients for bronchoscopic lung volume reduction in patients with emphysema.

COMPLICATIONS

- FOB is overall very safe, with a reported mortality of 0–0.013%.[10,11]
- Major complications (pneumothorax, pulmonary hemorrhage, or respiratory failure) occur in <1% of procedures.[10]
- After bronchoscopy, the patient may experience low-grade fever, cough, hypoxemia, sore throat, hoarseness, or low-grade hemoptysis.
- Pneumothorax occurs in ~4% of patients after transbronchial lung biopsy,[11] and is usually detected by postprocedure chest radiograph.

REFERENCES

1. Ernst A, Silvestri GA, Johnstone D; American College of Chest Physicians. Interventional pulmonary procedures: guidelines from the American College of Chest Physicians. *Chest.* 2003;123(5):1693–1717.
2. Prakash UB, Offord KP, Stubbs SE. Bronchoscopy in North America: the ACCP survey. *Chest.* 1991;100(6):1668–1675.
3. Eagle KA, Brundage BH, Chaitman BR, et al. Guidelines for perioperative cardiovascular evaluation for noncardiac surgery. Report of the American College of Cardiology/American Heart Association Task Force on Practice Guidelines. Committee on Perioperative Cardiovascular Evaluation for Noncardiac Surgery. *Circulation.* 1996;93(6):1278–1317.
4. Wahidi MM, Jain P, Jantz M, et al. American College of Chest Physicians consensus statement on the use of topical anesthesia, analgesia, and sedation during flexible bronchoscopy in adult patients. *Chest.* 2011;140(5):1342–1350.
5. Pastis NJ, Yarmus LB, Schippers F, et al. Safety and efficacy of remimazolam compared with placebo and midazolam for moderate sedation during bronchoscopy. *Chest.* 2019;155(1):137–146.
6. Matot I, Kramer MR. Sedation in outpatient bronchoscopy. *Respir Med.* 2000;94(12):1145–1153.
7. Chen AC, Chenna P, Loiselle A, Massoni J, Mayse M, Misselhorn D. Radial probe endobronchial ultrasound for peripheral pulmonary lesions. A five year institutional experience. *Ann Am Thorac Soc.* 2014;11:578–582.
8. Chen AC, Pastis NJ Jr, Mahajan AK, et al. Robotic bronchoscopy for peripheral pulmonary lesions: a multicenter pilot and feasibility study (BENEFIT). *Chest.* 2021;159(2):845–852.
9. Mehishi S, Raoof S, Mehta AC. Therapeutic flexible bronchoscopy. *Chest Surg Clin N Am.* 2001;11(4):657–690.
10. Jin F, Mu D, Chu D, Fu E, Xie Y, Liu T. Severe complications of bronchoscopy. *Respiration.* 2008;76(4):429–433.
11. Pue CA, Pacht ER. Complications of fiberoptic bronchoscopy at a university hospital. *Chest.* 1995;107(2):430–432.

Hypoxemic Respiratory Failure

Tej M. Patel, James McMenimen, and Adrian Shifren

GENERAL PRINCIPLES

Definition
Respiratory failure refers to an inability of the respiratory system to meet the oxygenation, ventilation, or metabolic requirements of a patient.

Classification
- **Hypoxemic respiratory failure (type 1 respiratory failure)** is characterized by a partial pressure of oxygen (P_aO_2) less than 60 mm Hg with normal or decreased partial pressure of carbon dioxide (P_aCO_2). This will be the focus of this chapter.
- **Hypercapnic respiratory failure (type 2 respiratory failure)** is characterized by a P_aCO_2 greater than 50 mm Hg and arterial pH less than 7.30.
- It is important to understand the nuanced difference between **hypoxia** and **hypoxemia**.
  - **Hypoxia** refers to impaired oxygen delivery or utilization at the cellular level resulting in anaerobic metabolism.
  - **Hypoxemia** refers to a decrease in oxygen content in the arterial blood, which includes both oxygen bound to hemoglobin and/or dissolved the blood.
- There are four basic classes of hypoxia:
  - **Hypoxemic hypoxia:** low P_aO_2 and arterial oxygen saturation (S_aO_2) leads to decreased oxygen delivery to tissues.
  - **Anemic hypoxia:** decreased oxygen carrying capacity due to decreased hemoglobin leads to decreased oxygen delivery to tissues.
  - **Circulatory hypoxia:** decreased cardiac output impairs oxygen delivery to tissues.
  - **Cytotoxic hypoxia:** impaired utilization of oxygen at the cellular level within tissues. Note that cytotoxic hypoxia can occur without the presence of hypoxemia.
- In clinical practice, hypoxia cannot readily be measured and thus hypoxemia is often used as a surrogate for hypoxia.

Pathophysiology
- It is good practice to determine the alveolar (A)–arterial (a) pressure gradient of oxygen, referred to as the A-a gradient, when evaluating hypoxemic respiratory failure.

- To determine the A-a gradient, you first need to calculate the alveolar P_AO_2, using the alveolar gas exchange equation:
  - $P_AO_2 = (P_B - P_{H2O}) \times FiO_2 - P_aCO_2 \div RQ$
    - P_{atm}: barometric pressure (P_B), varies with altitude, at sea level generally 760 mm Hg
    - P_{H2O}: partial pressure of humidified water, generally 47 mm Hg
    - FiO_2: fraction of inspired oxygen, generally 0.21 breathing room air
    - RQ: ratio of carbon dioxide production to carbon dioxide consumption, generally averaged to 0.8
  - The A-a gradient is determined by subtracting the measured arterial P_aO_2 from the calculated P_AO_2.
  - A normal A-a gradient varies based on the patient age and supplemental oxygen, as both age and supplemental oxygen can alter the A-a gradient.

Etiology

- Hypoxemic respiratory failure results from one of five basic pathophysiologic mechanisms.
- These can be differentiated in part using the A-a gradient.
  - Decreased inspired oxygen:
    - Decreased P_B (normal A-a gradient)
    - Low FiO_2 (normal A-a gradient)
  - Alveolar hypoventilation (normal A-a gradient)
  - Diffusion limitation (increased A-a gradient)
  - Ventilation/perfusion (V/Q) mismatch (increased A-a gradient):
    - True pulmonary shunts (V/Q = 0)
    - Shunt-like states (0.8 > V/Q > 0)
  - Anatomic right-left shunt (increased A-a gradient)
- Multiple pathophysiologic mechanisms may be at play in a single hypoxemic patient at any given time.
- The most common cause of hypoxemic respiratory failure is V/Q mismatch.
- The causes of hypoxemic respiratory failure are shown Figure 5-1.[1]

Decreased Barometric Pressure or Fraction of Inspired Oxygen

- The partial pressure of inspired oxygen (P_iO_2) can be determined by: $P_iO_2 = FiO_2 (P_B - P_{H2O})$.
- In conditions such as high altitude, a low P_B decreases the P_iO_2. A reduced P_iO_2 decreases the driving pressure for oxygen diffusion across the alveolar–capillary membrane resulting in hypoxemia without increasing the A-a gradient.
- Decreased FiO_2, such as during a house fire, decreases the FiO_2 lower than that of room air (21%) resulting in hypoxemia without increasing the A-a gradient.

Alveolar Hypoventilation

- Reduction in alveolar ventilation will increase the partial pressure of alveolar carbon dioxide (P_ACO_2).
- The alveolar gas equation demonstrates that increase in P_ACO_2 results in decreases in P_AO_2 resulting in hypoxemia without increasing the A-a gradient.
- Hypoxemia related to hypoventilation can be reversed by an increase in FiO_2 using supplementary oxygen, or by an increase in alveolar ventilation.

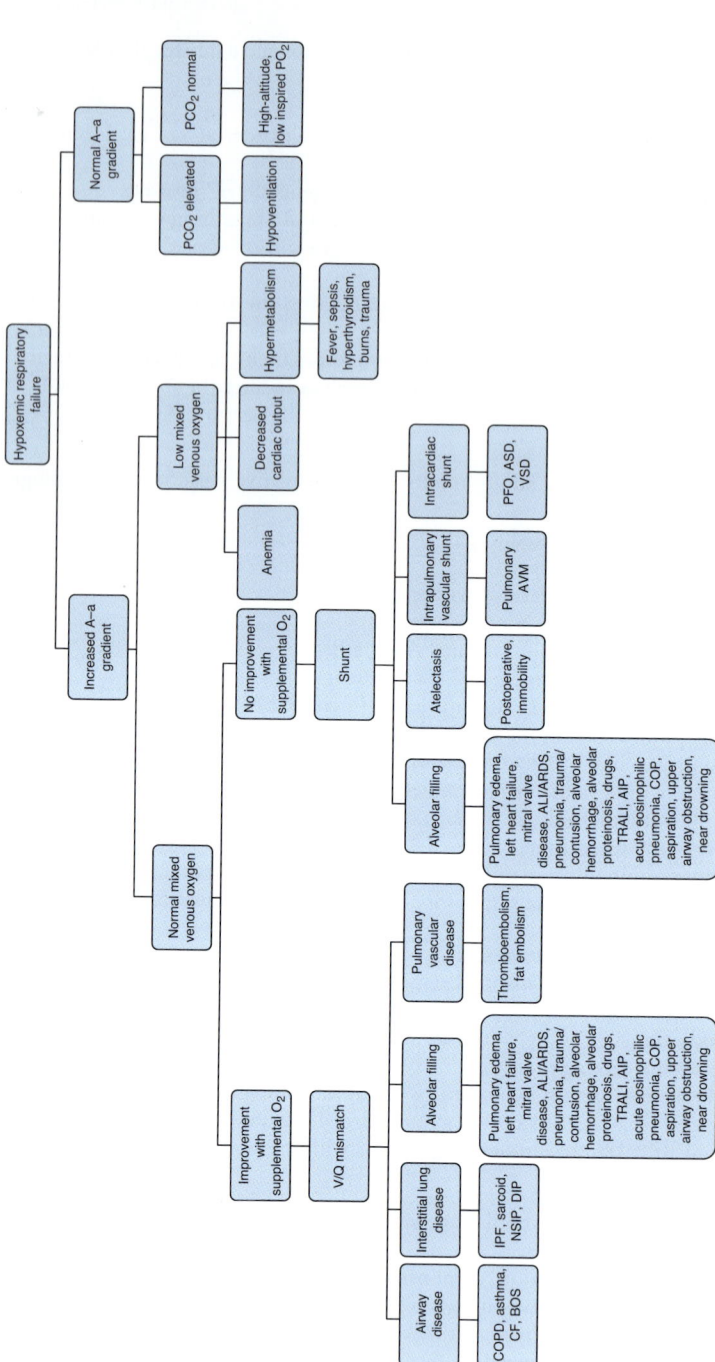

Figure 5-1 Etiology and approach to hypoxemic respiratory failure. (From Kollef M, Isakow W. *The Washington Manual of Critical Care.* 2nd ed. Lippincott Williams & Wilkins; 2012:42.)

General Principles | 43

Diffusion Limitation
- Diffusion of gas across a membrane is governed by Fick's Law: $V_{gas} + (A \times D \times [P1 - P2]) \div T$
  - V_{gas} = volume of diffusing gas
  - A = surface area available for diffusion
  - D = diffusion coefficient of the gas
  - P1 – P2 = difference in partial pressures of the gas across the membrane
  - T = thickness of the membrane
- In healthy subjects at rest, a single red blood cell (RBC) will spend approximately 0.75 seconds moving through a pulmonary capillary in contact with an alveolus.
- Oxygen is a perfusion-limited gas. Therefore, the P_aO_2 in the alveolus equilibrates quickly with that in the capillary. This takes approximately 0.25 seconds.
- Thus, there is considerable diffusion reserve if other variables in Fick Law are compromised.
- Diffusion of oxygen across the alveolar–capillary membrane is rarely the sole reason for hypoxemia.
- However, in conditions where cardiac output is increased (i.e., exercise) the RBC spends significantly less time in contact with the alveolus. In these instances (e.g., interstitial lung disease), impaired diffusion may contribute to the development of hypoxemia with an increased A-a gradient.
- Diffusion limitation will correct with increased FiO_2 using supplementary oxygen.

Ventilation/Perfusion Mismatch
- **V/Q mismatch** is the most common cause of hypoxemic respiratory failure.
- Ventilation, perfusion, and V/Q ratio are nonuniform in human lungs.
- There is regional heterogeneity of V/Q ratio within the lung, with both ventilation and perfusion being higher at the lung base, and lower at the lung apex.
- V/Q ratios are higher at the lung apex and lower at the lung base.
- In general, homeostasis results in an overall lung V/Q ratio of close to 1, with normal (matched) lung V/Q being around 0.8.
- **Pulmonary shunt** (V/Q = 0) and **dead space ventilation** (V/Q → ∞) represent the extremes of no ventilation or no perfusion to an alveolus respectively.
- Low V/Q ratios produce hypoxemia by decreasing P_AO_2 and subsequently P_aO_2, and refer to clinical circumstances in which alveoli receive either no perfusion (true shunt, V/Q = 0) or reduced perfusion relative to ventilation (shunt-like state 0.8 > V/Q > 0).
- Low V/Q mismatch is a form of right-left shunt (discussed below) and is characterized by a widened A-a gradient.
- High V/Q mismatch leads to **dead space** in which inhaled air does not participate in gas exchange reducing the amount of carbon dioxide that can be exhaled, resulting in hypercapnia.

Right-left Shunts
- Right-to-left shunting occurs when deoxygenated mixed venous blood does not participate in gas exchange within alveoli, resulting in return of deoxygenated blood to the systemic circulation and subsequent arterial hypoxemia.

- Shunts may be of two general types (see Figure 5-1):
  - Anatomic, where blood physically bypasses the alveoli/lungs.
  - Physiologic, where blood flows through the alveoli but gas exchange is impaired.
- Anatomic right-left shunts include openings between the atria, ventricles, and/or great vessels that allow blood to flow directly from the venous to the arterial circulation, bypassing the lungs.
- They also include pulmonary arteriovenous malformations (AVMs), direct communications between a pulmonary artery and pulmonary vein, bypassing the pulmonary capillary bed and hence the alveoli.
- Physiologic shunts include true shunts (V/Q = 0) or shunt-like states (0.8 > V/Q > 0) discussed above.
- Right-left shunting is characterized by a widened A-a gradient and **inability to completely correct with supplemental oxygen,** especially when the shunt fraction is greater than 30%.

Low Mixed Venous Oxygen Content
- Typically, the mixed venous oxygen content of blood returning to the right side of the heart does not affect the P_aO_2 significantly.
- However, **in the setting of shunt or shunt-like states,** subjects may become hypoxemic secondary to low mixed venous oxygen.
- Disease states that lower mixed venous oxygen are shown in Figure 5-1.

DIAGNOSIS

Clinical Presentation
History
Although hypoxemia can be asymptomatic, profound hypoxemia may present with different clinical signs and symptoms of variable severity. The presenting clinical symptoms can provide some insight into the etiology of hypoxemic respiratory failure, as well as guide the diagnostic evaluation.

- Copious airway secretions and abundant expectoration (among other clinical signs) can occur in **pulmonary edema.**
- Cough and purulent sputum (among other clinical signs) can occur in **pneumonia.**

Physical Examination
Manifestations of hypoxemia include, but are not limited to, cyanosis, restlessness, confusion, anxiety, delirium, tachypnea, tachycardia, hypertension, cardiac arrhythmias, and/or tremor. All of these clinical signs are both insensitive and nonspecific.

Diagnostic Criteria
Hypoxemic respiratory failure is defined as P_aO_2 less than 60 mm Hg and/or S_aO_2 less than 89%.

Diagnostic Testing
- Initial diagnostic testing will likely include pulse oximetry, CXR, and arterial blood gas (ABG).
- Further diagnostic testing will depend on the patient's comorbidities, clinical presentation, and the physical exam findings.

Laboratory Evaluation
- A standard complete blood count (CBC) should be obtained as changes in hemoglobin can alter oxygen delivery.
- A drug screen (serum or urine) can assist in some cases of hypoventilation.
- If that patient is believed to have acute respiratory distress syndrome (ARDS), it is prudent to obtain more specific labs to diagnose the cause.
- Infectious evaluation (blood, sputum, and urine) should always be performed if the possibility of infection is entertained.
- If diffuse alveolar hemorrhage is suspected, a vasculitis work-up would consist of antineutrophil cytoplasmic antibody (ANCA), antinuclear antibody (ANA), anti-glomerular basement membrane (anti-GBM), rheumatoid factor (RF), complement levels, cryoglobulins, and other pertinent testing.

Imaging
- **CXR:** a standard two-view posterior–anterior (PA) and lateral CXR is always preferred to a portable CXR and is more sensitive for detecting and characterizing underlying lung pathology. However, the clinical situation must be taken into account.
- **CT chest:** depending on the clinical situation, a CT of the chest can help narrow the differential diagnosis for hypoxemic respiratory failure. A noncontrast CT scan almost always suffices, with the exception of suspicion for pulmonary embolus in which case a CT pulmonary angiogram is indicated.

Diagnostic Procedures
Transthoracic Echocardiogram with bubble study: a cardiac ultrasound may assist in evaluation of some causes of hypoxemia, such as congestive heart failure, cardiac or pulmonary anatomic right to left shunts, valvular heart disease, or pericardial disease. Note that in patients with unexplained hypoxemic respiratory failure, it is important to obtain a bubble study to rule out right to left shunts.

TREATMENT

- Treatment of hypoxemic respiratory failure involves treatment of the underlying cause, as well as general and respiratory supportive care.
- The therapeutic goal is to ensure adequate oxygenation of vital organs.
- For conscious, spontaneously breathing patients, supplemental oxygen is one of the most important initial treatments for hypoxemic respiratory failure.
- The inspired oxygen concentration should be the lowest amount of supplemental oxygen that results in a **P_aO_2 of ≥60 mm Hg** or an **S_aO_2 ≥90%**. Higher arterial oxygen tensions are of no proven benefit.
- Appropriate oxygen delivery generally involves slowly increasing the FiO_2 with monitoring of both P_aO_2 and P_aCO_2.
- The FiO_2 should be increased to a goal P_aO_2 of 60–70 mm Hg or an S_aO_2 of ≥90%.
- Although there is concern for CO_2 retention (and resultant worsening respiratory acidosis) in chronic obstructive pulmonary disease (COPD) patients with CO_2 retention when oxygen is administered, these patients are at greater risk from acute hypoxemia than hypercapnia. Therefore, the goals of oxygen therapy

in COPD patients are the same as for other subjects, although some sources advocate for using an S_aO_2 of >88% in these cases.

Oxygen Delivery Devices
- The selection of the appropriate noninvasive delivery system depends on the stability of the patient, availability of devices, and level of respiratory support required.
- For the critically ill or unstable patient, a planned, controlled intubation is always more desirable than emergent intubation.
- Predefined criteria for intubation and mechanical ventilation are broad and nonspecific. Mechanical ventilation is not covered in this chapter.
- Oxygen delivery devices for hypoxemic respiratory failure can broadly be divided into two classes.
  - **Low-flow devices:** nasal cannulas and face masks
  - **High-flow devices:** Venturi masks and high-flow nasal cannulas

Low-Flow Oxygen Delivery Devices
Low-flow oxygen delivery devices provide a variable FiO_2 based on the size of the oxygen reservoir, the rate at which the reservoir is filled, and the ventilatory pattern of the patient.

Nasal Cannulas
- These low-flow systems provide insufficient gas to replace an entire inspired tidal volume (V_t). As a result, **a large part of each inhaled breath is composed of ambient (room air) gas.**
- **Nasal cannulas are appropriate in patients with minimal or no respiratory distress, or those who are unable to tolerate a facemask.**
- The benefits include allowing the patient to eat, drink, and speak.
- Their main disadvantage is that the exact FiO_2 is unknown. This is because the oxygen flow rate, the patient's inspiratory flow rate, and the inhaled V_t all influence the final FiO_2.
- Nasal cannulas deliver flow rates of 1–6 L/min.
- As a general rule, for every liter per minute delivered, the oxygen concentration increases by approximately 3% above that of room air (21%). Therefore, with a normal V_t, the commonly utilized **nasal cannula flow rates of 1–6 liters per minute (L/min) provide an FiO_2 of 24–40%.**
- At flow rates greater than 6 L/min, flows become increasingly turbulent and oxygen delivery is no more effective than when delivered at 6 L/min. In addition, patients in respiratory distress may have higher peak inspiratory flow rates than 6 L/min. When the patient inspiratory flow rate exceeds that delivered by the nasal cannula, room air is entrained into the lungs, resulting in a reduction in oxygen delivery.

Reservoir Nasal Cannulas
- Reservoir nasal cannulas are low-flow systems that can either increase the percentage of oxygen delivered compared to nasal cannulas or act as oxygen-conserving devices.
- The reservoirs facilitate conservation of oxygen by storing oxygen from exhalation for delivery during subsequent inhalation.

Treatment

- The reservoirs trap the initial portion of expired gas from the large conducting airways that contain a high percentage of oxygen (anatomic dead-space gas that did not participate in gas exchange in the alveoli).
- The reservoirs also receive a continuous flow of oxygen from the oxygen source.
- The combination of oxygen from the source and the reservoir results in a higher FiO_2 during the subsequent inspiration and allows for total flow rates to be reduced.

Simple Facemasks
- These low-flow systems also provide a means of delivering a higher FiO_2 than can be achieved via nasal cannula.
- Two types of facemask exist: those with and those without an oxygen reservoir.
- To avoid accumulation of expired air within the mask, and subsequent retention of CO_2, the oxygen flow rates should be greater than 5–6 L/min.
- **Simple facemasks generally provide an FiO_2 of 35–60%.**

High-Flow Oxygen Delivery Devices
High-Flow Nasal Cannulas
- High-flow nasal cannula systems (e.g., Optiflow, Airvo) allow oxygen to be delivered at rates that exceed a patient's inspiratory flow rate.
- Using an air/oxygen blender, active humidifier, single heated tube, and nasal cannula, warm humidified **oxygen flows of up to 60 L/min can be delivered nasally.**
- High oxygen flow rates allow for the elimination of room air during inspiration enabling patients to breathe high fractions of oxygen without dilution by ambient air. An **FiO_2 of up to 100% can be effectively delivered.**
- High-flow nasal cannula systems provide physiologic benefits including:
  - positive airway pressures between 3 and 7 cm H_2O that assist in preventing atelectasis.
  - dead space washout of waste gasses such as CO_2.
  - increased V_t.

Venturi Masks
- These high-flow systems deliver precise oxygen concentrations.
- They utilize the **Venturi effect,** the reduction in pressure resulting from air flowing through a constricted section of a conduit. Oxygen passes through a narrow orifice under pressure into a larger tube, creating a subatmospheric pressure. This drop in pressure results in a shearing force that draws room air into the delivery system through several openings (entrainment ports) in the tubing.
- Oxygen concentration is adjusted by changing both the size of the entrainment ports and the oxygen flow.
- The **maximum FiO_2 achievable is 50%.**
- This type of mask provides a constant FiO_2 independent of changes in inspiratory flow rate.
- It allows for easy stepwise increases or decreases in FiO_2 as oxygen delivery is titrated to P_aO_2 or S_aO_2.
- The main disadvantage is that the FiO_2 provided by these masks is limited and may be insufficient to maintain appropriate oxygen saturations in sicker patients.

Nonrebreather Facemasks
- These high-flow systems consist of a facemask that provides a constant flow of oxygen into an attached reservoir bag, resulting in an FiO_2 of greater than 60% at 6 L/min oxygen flow.
- **Each liter per minute of flow over 6 L/min increases the inspired oxygen concentration by around 10%.**
- **Placed correctly, the oxygen concentration can reach almost 100%.**
- This type of mask is most appropriate for spontaneously breathing patients who require the highest possible oxygen concentration.
- The disadvantages of nonrebreather facemasks include oxygen toxicity, inability to feed patients owing to the tight seal required, limitation of speech, patient discomfort, and inability to provide aerosolized treatments.

Other Therapies
- **Incentive spirometry** assists patients with deep breathing. The deep inspiration is believed to help prevent the development of significant atelectasis. In the setting of elective surgery, it should be started prior to the operative procedure and continued postoperatively. Ideally, patients would use incentive spirometer 10 or more times per hour.
- **Pulmonary flutter valves** (i.e., Aerobika, Acapella) assist patients with clearance of secretions and mucus in an effort to improve pulmonary ventilation and oxygenation.
- **Mobilization** and **ambulation,** through both maintenance of an upright position and exercise, may help prevent atelectasis.

MONITORING, PATIENT EDUCATION, AND FOLLOW-UP

- Oxygen should continually be weaned to a goal P_aO_2 of 60–70 mm Hg or a goal S_aO_2 of ≥90% while the patient is hospitalized and treated for their underlying ailment.
- Patients should be educated on their specific disease and what to expect in relation to long-term oxygen therapy if needed.
- Long-term oxygen therapy is indicated in patients with a P_aO_2 ≤55 mm Hg or S_aO_2 ≤88% at rest or that develops with exertion. However, this recommendation is based on patients with COPD and may not apply to all patients with hypoxemic respiratory failure.
- Prior to discharge, a patient should be assessed for a requirement for long-term oxygen therapy both at rest and with exertion since these requirements often differ.
- A 6-minute walk can provide this information by allowing for titration of oxygen at rest and with exercise. Oxygen can then be prescribed as needed.
- If chronic oxygen therapy needs to be administered as an outpatient, patients should be educated on the use of long-term oxygen, and the dangers associated with oxygen administration (specifically the harms of smoking or cooking with open flames when oxygen is present).
- Concentrated sources of oxygen promote rapid combustion, and when exposed to open flames, highly concentrated oxygen can result in explosions.
- The amount of oxygen required to maintain oxygen saturations ≥88% can vary over time.

- Patients discharged on oxygen should be followed in the outpatient setting within 2–6 weeks depending on the etiology of their hypoxemic respiratory failure and their oxygen requirements on discharge.
- In patients requiring ongoing oxygen therapy, a 6-minute walk should be performed at least yearly to ensure an adequate oxygen prescription.
- In certain cases, an ABG may be clinically indicated at follow-up.

REFERENCE

1. Kollef M, Isakow W. *The Washington Manual of Critical Care*. 2nd ed. Lippincott Williams & Wilkins; 2012.

Noninvasive Ventilation

Stephen Chi

GENERAL PRINCIPLES

Definition

- **Noninvasive ventilation** (NIV) refers to the delivery of ventilatory support without invasive airway devices.
- This definition excludes any modality that invasively bypasses the upper airway, such as laryngeal masks, endotracheal tubes, and tracheostomies.
- While often used interchangeably with **noninvasive positive pressure ventilation** (NIPPV), historically NIV also referred to negative pressure ventilation devices such as the "iron lung" and cuirass ventilators which apply negative pressure to an external shell around the patient.
- For the purposes of this chapter, NIV denotes positive pressure ventilatory support administered through a face mask, nasal mask, or similar device.

Clinical Application

- NIV requires the patient to wear a tight-fitting mask that forms a seal around the patient's mouth and/or nose.
- Masks are typically equipped with one-way valves to prevent backflow of air and humidity to the ventilator, as well as antiasphyxiation valves that open to allow ambient air into the mask if circuit airflow stops.
- Long-term outpatient use of NIV is increasingly common in the management of obstructive sleep apnea (OSA), obesity hypoventilation syndrome (OHS), chronic obstructive pulmonary disease (COPD), and neuromuscular disorders.
- In the acute inpatient setting, NIV is often utilized to avoid risks associated with endotracheal intubation and invasive mechanical ventilation (IMV). NIV does not replace the need for IMV in many clinical scenarios, however, and **should not delay intubation if emergently indicated**.
- While IMV and NIV share similar physiologic principles, several key differences should be noted:
  - NIV can be rapidly initiated and discontinued at the bedside, making short-term trials of NIV a reasonable option in patients without clear contraindications (Table 6-1).[1,2]
  - While still associated with discomfort and claustrophobia, NIV is generally much less uncomfortable than IMV delivered via endotracheal devices. Continuous sedation is therefore not mandatory while on NIV unlike most instances of IMV.
  - Ensuring lung-protective or low tidal volume ventilation is not feasible in the absence of sedation or a true volume-controlled mode.
  - Secretion management is impaired by the presence of a tight-fitting mask, whereas patients on IMV can undergo tracheal suctioning.

TABLE 6-1	CONTRAINDICATIONS TO NONINVASIVE VENTILATION

Absolute Contraindications
Cardiac or respiratory arrest
Need for urgent/emergent intubation
Inability to fit NIV mask

Relative Contraindications
Active vomiting/hematemesis
Hemodynamic instability
Severe encephalopathy (Glasgow Coma Scale <10)
Inability to protect airway/clear secretions
High risk for aspiration
Facial surgery or trauma/burns
Fixed upper airway obstruction
Undrained pneumothorax

Adapted from Kollef M, Isakow W. *The Washington Manual of Critical Care*. 3rd ed. Wolters Kluwer/Lippincott Williams & Wilkins; 2017 and Mehta S, Hill NS. Noninvasive ventilation. *Am J Respir Crit Care Med*. 2001;163:540–577.

- ○ **Mask leak is a major limitation of NIV.** Leak tends to worsen in the setting of facial hair, high set pressures, or patient–ventilator asynchrony as patients may close their glottis or mouth in response to unwanted breaths. Care should be taken to ensure an adequate mask seal and promote patient initiation of breaths.

CLASSIFICATION

- IMV and NIV devices have analogous modes (i.e., how the ventilator triggers, delivers, and cycles each breath) and terminology, however, there is no standardization between manufacturers regarding specific nomenclature.
- Modes commonly seen in clinical practice include **continuous positive airway pressure** (CPAP), **bilevel positive airway pressure** (BiPAP), and **average volume-assured pressure support** (AVAPS).
- Modes are primarily distinguished by the types of pressures delivered during the respiratory cycle, with additional settings such as flow rate, fraction of inspired oxygen (FiO_2), and cycling criteria dependent on the mode and machine.
- **Expiratory positive airway pressure** (EPAP) is the pressure against which the patient exhales at the end of inhalation and is functionally identical to **positive end-expiratory pressure** (PEEP).
- **Inspiratory positive airway pressure** (IPAP) is the ventilatory pressure support the patient receives when a breath is initiated, lasting until the breath is cycled. Note that the IPAP refers to the **total pressure administered during inhalation,** in contrast to IMV in which the inspiratory pressure setting classically describes **pressure administered above PEEP.** Bilevel NIV settings of 10 cm H_2O (IPAP) and 5 cm H_2O (EPAP) are therefore equivalent to IMV pressure

support ventilation settings of 5 cm H_2O (pressure support) over 5 cm H_2O (PEEP).
- NIV modes should be tailored to each patient's situation, and pressures titrated according to clinical response, in order to maximize chances of NIV success.

Continuous Positive Airway Pressure
- CPAP maintains a set positive pressure throughout the entire respiratory cycle (i.e., inhalation and exhalation) and is not ventilatory support in a strict physiologic sense as ventilation remains fully dependent on patient effort.
- CPAP "stents open" the upper airway by providing continuous pressure within the airway, leading to its widespread outpatient usage in treatment of OSA.
- Newer home CPAP machines offer "auto-CPAP" modes which adjust the level of positive pressure over time to minimize apneic events as patients progress through sleep stages.
- Despite not providing ventilatory support, CPAP has therapeutic benefits in both hypoxemic and hypercapnic respiratory failure.
  - Hypoxemic respiratory failure:
    - PEEP **recruits underventilated or collapsed lung,** thereby preventing atelectasis and hypoxemia.
    - Continuous airway pressure **increases partial pressure of oxygen in the alveoli (PAO_2)**. In the alveolar gas equation, $PAO_2 = FiO_2 * (P_B - P_{H2O}) - (PaCO_2/R)$, P_B denotes barometric pressure which is augmented by pressure delivered from the ventilator through the mask. At a given FiO_2, increasing this mean airway pressure will increase the partial pressure of inspiratory oxygen and therefore oxygen tension in the alveoli (PAO_2).
    - Patients can receive up to 100% FiO_2 via CPAP machines through oxygen bleed-in or connection to high-flow oxygen sources.
    - PEEP **decreases left ventricular afterload and preload** alleviating hypoxemia driven by cardiogenic pulmonary edema (CPE).
  - Hypercapnic respiratory failure:
    - CPAP therapy decreases hypoventilation seen in OSA/OHS by **preventing airway collapse**.
    - Patients with severe obstructive lung disease may develop dynamic hyperinflation driven by prolonged exhalation and inability to fully exhale, particularly in the context of respiratory distress. The positive elastic recoil pressure resulting from hyperinflation is termed intrinsic PEEP and contributes to increased work of breathing, respiratory acidosis, and hypercapnia. **Delivery of extrinsic PEEP overcomes intrinsic PEEP,** lessening work of breathing and hypercapnia.[3]
- From a practical standpoint, **CPAP is commonly used for treatment of uncomplicated hypoxemic respiratory failure and OSA/OHS,** whereas alternative NIV modes are preferred for the management of other forms of respiratory failure and respiratory fatigue.

Bilevel Positive Airway Pressure
- **BiPAP** is CPAP with a second level of pressure support during inspiration, akin to pressure support ventilation for mechanically ventilated patients.

- BiPAP at minimum requires operators to set IPAP and EPAP levels, measured in cm H_2O.
  - By convention BiPAP settings are referred to as the IPAP followed by the EPAP, for example, 12 cm H_2O and 5 cm H_2O.
  - The greater the difference between the IPAP and the EPAP, the greater the theoretical ventilatory support the patient receives.
  - Progressively higher levels of IPAP and EPAP are less likely to be tolerated by the patient, and more likely to cause excessive mask leak.
- Additional settings on BiPAP include FiO_2, cycling criteria, backup respiratory rate, and rise time.
  - FiO_2 up to 100% can be delivered through connection to high-flow oxygen sources.
  - Cycling criteria determine how the ventilator ends the inspiratory phase and transitions from IPAP to EPAP. Many hospital-administered machines cycle based on a fixed inspiratory time, whereas home units often cycle by measuring when the inspiratory flow falls to a set percentage of the peak inspiratory flow. Earlier cycling (shorter inspiratory time) will lower tidal volumes and allow for longer expiratory phases, whereas later cycling will provide more ventilatory support with respect to higher tidal volumes and mean airway pressures.
  - BiPAP machines with spontaneous/timed (S/T) modes have the option to set a backup respiratory rate. Exceeding the patient's spontaneous respiratory rate may increase minute ventilation but carries substantial risk of patient–ventilator asynchrony and discomfort.
  - Rise time controls how quickly the ventilator transitions from EPAP to IPAP during the inspiratory phase. This setting is primarily adjusted for patient comfort.
- In addition to the therapeutic benefits of CPAP, BiPAP treats respiratory failure through ventilatory support:
  - Pressure support directly **alleviates work of breathing and augments tidal volume and minute ventilation,** which can be further enforced via the backup rate if available.
  - Bilevel positive pressure ventilation further recruits atelectatic lung and increases mean airway pressure compared to CPAP alone.
- BiPAP therefore has utility for the **management of hypoxemic respiratory failure, hypercapnic respiratory failure, and increased work of breathing,** and is preferred in most acute clinical scenarios over CPAP alone.

Average Volume-Assured Pressure Support

- **AVAPS** is a newer mode of NIV that leverages variable pressure settings to target a goal tidal volume, analogous to pressure-regulated volume control modes on IMV.
- In addition to the settings described for BiPAP, AVAPS operators must also set a target tidal volume (Vt) and an IPAP range, that is, a minimum IPAP and maximum IPAP.
  - AVAPS will automatically titrate IPAP within the specified range until Vt is achieved. The algorithm by which AVAPS and similar modes perform this titration is proprietary to each manufacturer.
  - Certain ventilators also have the option of setting an EPAP range which will be simultaneously adjusted to maintain upper airway patency.

- Auto-titrating modes such as AVAPS have the benefits of improved patient comfort and variable levels of support as the patient's respiratory effort changes, such as providing higher pressure support during deep sleep or decreasing pressure support as the patient's clinical condition improves.
- Although the combination of Vt and a backup rate may appear to guarantee a minimum minute ventilation, this should not be relied upon in clinical practice. Gradual titration of pressure support, patient–ventilator asynchrony, and mask leak may prevent consistent Vt delivery, and close monitoring of patient tolerance and actual minute ventilation is still required.
- AVAPS may be suboptimal in patients with high intrinsic respiratory drive, such as asthmatic patients, patients with primary metabolic acidosis, and patients with central neurologic injury. If patients can achieve tidal volumes above Vt without assistance, AVAPS will serially decrease pressure support until reaching the minimum IPAP, which risks allowing the patient to fatigue despite receiving NIV.
- AVAPS otherwise has similar utility to BiPAP in the **management of hypoxemic and hypercapnic respiratory failure,** although this mode may not be readily available.

SPECIFIC DISEASE INDICATIONS FOR NONINVASIVE VENTILATION

- NIV's efficacy has been best studied and demonstrated in CPE and hypercapnic respiratory failure from COPD.
- NIV may also improve outcomes in other conditions by **avoiding risks associated with intubation and IMV,** such as hemodynamic compromise peri-intubation, infectious complications including ventilator-associated pneumonia, and adverse effects of sedation.
- In general, a trial of NIV is reasonable for most situations unless a frank contraindication is identified, or immediate intubation is warranted.

Cardiogenic Pulmonary Edema
- CPE is characterized by left ventricular failure leading to excess extravascular fluid in the pulmonary interstitium and alveoli, resulting in atelectasis and decreased lung compliance.
- NIV effectively treats CPE by recruiting atelectatic lung, unloading respiratory muscles, and reducing left ventricular preload and afterload to facilitate forward cardiac flow.
- Two large meta-analyses of randomized controlled trials in CPE found that NIV therapy with CPAP or BiPAP compared to standard medical care was associated with significantly lower hospital mortality and endotracheal intubation rates.[4,5] These studies notably did not find evidence for increased risk of cardiac ischemia or hypotension among patients treated with NIV, which had been historically reported as potential contraindications.
- **CPAP is recommended for patients presenting with CPE and hypoxemic respiratory failure** unresponsive to initial medical therapies.
- Initial therapy with BiPAP should be considered in patients presenting with concurrent hypercapnic respiratory failure or markedly increased work of breathing.

Chronic Obstructive Pulmonary Disease
- NIV has increasingly become standard of care in the initial management of acute exacerbations of chronic obstructive pulmonary disease (AECOPD) leading to hypercapnic respiratory failure.
- Multiple randomized controlled trials and meta-analyses have consistently shown significant decreases in mortality, endotracheal intubation rate, hospital-associated complications, and inpatient length of stay when AECOPD is treated with NIV in addition to standard therapies.[6–8]
- In AECOPD requiring ventilatory support, first-line treatment with NIV compared to IMV is similarly associated with lower mortality, hospital-acquired infections, cost, and inpatient length of stay.[9]
- **BiPAP is the preferred NIV modality** with the most published data supporting its use in AECOPD, although CPAP and AVAPS modes have also shown positive results.
- NIV should be initiated in patients with AECOPD in whom respiratory acidosis persists (pH <7.35) despite other first-line medical therapies.
- NIV can also facilitate extubation and weaning of COPD patients from IMV. Randomized controlled trials in this population have demonstrated lower rates of mortality, weaning failure, and nosocomial pneumonia, as well as decreased ICU and hospital length of stay.[10,11]

Postextubation Respiratory Failure
- Postextubation respiratory failure occurs in 10–20% of mechanically ventilated patients and carries a poor prognosis.
- Among patients at high risk of postextubation respiratory failure, **prophylactic** NIV applied immediately after extubation decreases rates of reintubation and mortality compared to standard oxygen therapy alone.[12–14]
  - High-risk criteria vary by study and commonly include **advanced age >65, chronic cardiopulmonary disease, and prolonged mechanical ventilation**.
  - Prophylactic high-flow oxygen therapy is another respiratory support modality that has been studied extensively in postextubation respiratory failure, and its efficacy compared to NIV remains the subject of active research. The choice of whether to use high-flow oxygen, NIV, or a combination of these therapies to prevent postextubation respiratory failure must be guided by clinician discretion of whether patients are likely to tolerate NIV or require positive pressure ventilatory support.[15]
- NIV has not shown consistent clinical benefit as a rescue therapy for patients who have already developed postextubation respiratory failure and may instead cause harm by inappropriately delaying reintubation. If NIV is attempted in patients with established postextubation respiratory failure, trials should be short and a low threshold for reintubation must be maintained.[16,17]
- **Prophylactic NIV should be strongly considered in patients at high risk for postextubation respiratory failure.**

Chest Wall Deformity and Neuromuscular Disease
- Patients with neuromuscular disease or thoracic deformities may present with hypoxemia related to poor secretion clearance or hypercapnia from respiratory muscle weakness or sleep-disordered breathing.

- NIV can be an appropriate first-line therapy for patients presenting with both acute and chronic respiratory failure resulting from these disorders.[18]
- **AVAPS and other auto-titrating modes may be ideal** in this patient population.
  - NIV treatment in neuromuscular disorders tends to be chronic once initiated, making patient comfort a high priority.
  - Pressure support requirements are expected to change with disease progression as well as physiologic respiratory variation, which are exaggerated in the setting of neuromuscular weakness. Auto-titrating modes provide more flexibility to both patients and providers with less need for frequent adjustment of IPAP and EPAP settings.
- NIV can be considered in patients with chest wall trauma who remain hypoxemic despite regional anesthesia.
- Several small randomized controlled trials support using NIV for patients with isolated chest trauma, rib fractures, and hypoxemia with a trend towards lower mortality and endotracheal intubation rates.[19–21]
- Additional research is required on the optimal NIV mode and patients with higher trauma severity scores or polytrauma, who were typically excluded from these studies.

Acute Hypoxemic Respiratory Failure Trauma

- The use of NIV in acute hypoxemic respiratory failure unrelated to the above conditions is not clearly beneficial, with studies showing conflicting results. Treatment failure is more common in the setting of higher illness severity, pneumonia, and acute respiratory distress syndrome (ARDS).[22–24]
- Immunocompromised patients may be an exception, as meta-analyses have suggested decreases in mortality, nosocomial pneumonia, and endotracheal intubation rates among immunocompromised patients receiving early NIV for hypoxemic respiratory failure. These findings were not replicated in more recent randomized controlled trials, however.[25,26]
- Current societal recommendations are that NIV can be an alternative to endotracheal intubation in carefully selected patients with acute hypoxemic respiratory failure, particularly immunocompromised patients. Clinical discretion and close monitoring are required, and IMV should be pursued if the patient does not improve clinically within 1–2 hours of NIV initiation.

Asthma

- Data is lacking on the use of NIV for the treatment of acute asthma exacerbations.[12]
- **Routine use of NIV is not recommended for asthmatic patients,** and trials of NIV must be undertaken judiciously and with frequent reassessment.
- Severe respiratory acidosis in the setting of an acute asthma exacerbation should be treated with intubation and IMV.

Palliative Noninvasive Ventilation

- NIV may alleviate dyspnea in end-of-life circumstances.[27,28]
  - Relief of dyspnea with NIV must be weighed against potential discomfort and claustrophobia from face-mask ventilation.
  - NIV may limit disposition options at end of life.

- Effective communication and clarification of the patient's goals of care are necessary to determine whether to initiate palliative NIV and set appropriate expectations.

INITIATION OF NONINVASIVE VENTILATION

- NIV should only be initiated in locations with experienced staff, including readily available respiratory therapists to titrate settings, assess tolerance, and monitor for decompensation requiring more invasive mechanical support. In practice, this tends to restrict NIV usage to intensive care units or designated respiratory wards.
- Absolute and relative contraindications to NIV should be reviewed before any trial of NIV (Table 6-1).
- Table 6-2 lists common starting settings for NIV. These settings should be further individualized for each patient and clinical scenario.
- Once patient tolerance has been established, NIV settings should be titrated in a stepwise manner with attention to patient comfort and clinical response.
- Suggested titration increments:
  - CPAP: Increase by 1–2 cm H_2O up to maximum of 20 cm H_2O.
  - IPAP: Increase by 2–3 cm H_2O up to maximum of 20–25 cm H_2O.

TABLE 6-2 INITIAL SETTINGS FOR COMMON NONINVASIVE VENTILATION MODES			
	CPAP	**BiPAP**	**AVAPS**
Expiratory positive airway pressure	5 cm H_2O	4–5 cm H_2O	4–5 cm H_2O
Inspiratory positive airway pressure	N/A	10–12 cm H_2O	Minimum EPAP + 4 cm H_2O Maximum 20 cm H_2O
Tidal volume	N/A	N/A	6–10 mL/kg ideal body weight
Inspiratory time	N/A	0.8–1 seconds	0.8–1 seconds
FiO_2	0.21–1	0.21–1	0.21–1
Backup rate	N/A	10–12 breaths/min	10–12 breaths/min

AVAPS, average volume-assured pressure support; BiPAP, bilevel positive airway pressure; CPAP, continuous positive airway pressure; EPAP, expiratory positive airway pressure N/A, not applicable.

Adapted from British Thoracic Society Standards of Care Committee. Non-invasive ventilation in acute respiratory failure. *Thorax*. 2002;57:192–211; Kollef M, Isakow W. *The Washington Manual of Critical Care*. 3rd ed. Wolters Kluwer/Lippincott Williams & Wilkins; 2017.

- (IPAP – EPAP): Increase by 2–3 cm H_2O up to maximum of 15 cm H_2O. Changes to EPAP and IPAP should be coordinated to avoid unintended changes in ventilatory support.
- Inspiratory time: Adjust by 0.1–0.2 seconds to alter inspiratory to expiratory ratio as clinically indicated.

SPECIAL CONSIDERATIONS AND MONITORING

- Ensuring appropriate mask fit is crucial to minimizing air leak and optimizing patient–ventilator synchrony.
- Patient discomfort and claustrophobia are major limitations to the use of NIV. Tolerance of NIV can be improved by adjusting flow rates, titrating to the minimum pressure needed for clinical response, trialing different mask types, and allowing brief breaks from NIV if clinically feasible. Sedation is generally not administered given the risk of respiratory suppression, although dexmedetomidine is a notable exception that may be utilized with appropriate monitoring.
- In addition to standard vital sign monitoring, observed tidal volume and minute ventilation on the NIV device should be regularly assessed to guide titration of IPAP, EPAP, and inspiratory time.
- Check an arterial blood gas within the first hour after initiation. Venous blood gas may be a reasonable alternative in isolated hypercapnic respiratory failure. Blood gas values usually improve within the first 1–2 hours if NIV is likely to succeed.
- Clinical stabilization and improvement should occur within the first 4–6 hours of NIV.
- Patients treated with prolonged NIV should be examined for pressure injuries or skin necrosis resulting from mask usage.
- Ventilator-induced lung injury is not exclusive to IMV and can occur with any form of positive pressure ventilation, including NIV. Excessively high tidal volumes on NIV should prompt immediate reassessment of pressure settings or alternative respiratory support.
- Do not hesitate to intubate the patient if NIV is failing. Inappropriate delay in intubation predisposes to rapid clinical deterioration and significant morbidity and mortality.

REFERENCES

1. Kollef M, Isakow W. *The Washington Manual of Critical Care*. 3rd ed. Wolters Kluwer/Lippincott Williams & Wilkins; 2017.
2. Mehta S, Hill NS. Noninvasive ventilation. *Am J Respir Crit Care Med*. 2001; 163(2):540–577.
3. O'Donoghue FJ, Catcheside PG, Jordan AS, Bersten AD, McEvoy RD. Effect of CPAP on intrinsic PEEP, inspiratory effort, and lung volume in severe stable COPD. *Thorax*. 2002;57(6):533–539.
4. Berbenetz N, Wang Y, Brown J, et al. Non-invasive positive pressure ventilation (CPAP or bilevel NPPV) for cardiogenic pulmonary oedema. *Cochrane Database Syst Rev*. 2019; 4(4):CD005351.
5. Mariani J, Macchia A, Belziti C, et al. Noninvasive ventilation in acute cardiogenic pulmonary edema: a meta-analysis of randomized controlled trials. *J Card Fail*. 2011; 17(10):850–859.

6. Osadnik CR, Tee VS, Carson-Chahhoud KV, Picot J, Wedzicha JA, Smith BJ. Noninvasive ventilation for the management of acute hypercapnic respiratory failure due to exacerbations of chronic obstructive pulmonary disease. *Cochrane Database Syst Rev.* 2017;7(7):CD004104.
7. Chandra D, Stamm JA, Taylor B, et al. Outcomes of noninvasive ventilation for acute exacerbations of chronic obstructive pulmonary disease in the United States, 1998–2008. *Am J Respir Crit Care Med.* 2012;185(2):152–159.
8. Brochard L, Mancebo J, Wysocki M, et al. Noninvasive ventilation for acute exacerbations of chronic obstructive pulmonary disease. *N Engl J Med.* 1995;333(13):817–822.
9. Lindenauer PK, Stefan MS, Shieh MS, Pekow PS, Rothberg MB, Hill NS. Outcomes associated with invasive and noninvasive ventilation among patients hospitalized with exacerbations of chronic obstructive pulmonary disease. *JAMA Intern Med.* 2014;174(12):1982–1993.
10. Nava S, Ambrosino N, Clini E, et al. Noninvasive mechanical ventilation in the weaning of patients with respiratory failure due to chronic obstructive pulmonary disease: a randomized controlled trial. *Ann Intern Med.* 1998;128(9):721–728.
11. Burns KEA, Stevenson J, Laird M, et al. Non-invasive ventilation versus invasive weaning in critically ill adults: a systematic review and meta-analysis. *Thorax.* 2022;77(8):752–761.
12. Rochwerg B, Brochard L, Elliott MW, et al. Official ERS/ATS clinical practice guidelines: noninvasive ventilation for acute respiratory failure. *Eur Respir J.* 2017;50(2):1602426.
13. Lin C, Yu H, Fan H, Li Z. The efficacy of noninvasive ventilation in managing postextubation respiratory failure: a meta-analysis. *Heart Lung.* 2014;43(2):99–104.
14. Nava S, Gregoretti C, Fanfulla F, et al. Noninvasive ventilation to prevent respiratory failure after extubation in high-risk patients. *Crit Care Med.* 2005;33(11):2465–2470.
15. Thille AW, Muller G, Gacouin A, et al. Effect of postextubation high-flow nasal oxygen with noninvasive ventilation vs high-flow nasal oxygen alone on reintubation among patients at high risk of extubation failure: a randomized clinical trial [published correction appears in *JAMA* 2020 Feb 25;323:793]. *JAMA.* 2019;322(15):1465–1475.
16. Esteban A, Frutos-Vivar F, Ferguson ND, et al. Noninvasive positive-pressure ventilation for respiratory failure after extubation. *N Engl J Med.* 2004;350(24):2452–2460.
17. Keenan SP, Powers C, McCormack DG, Block G. Noninvasive positive-pressure ventilation for postextubation respiratory distress: a randomized controlled trial. *JAMA.* 2002;287(24):3238–3244.
18. Benditt JO. Respiratory care of patients with neuromuscular disease. *Respiratory Care.* 2019;64(6):679–688.
19. Bollinger CT, Van Eeden SF. Treatment of multiple rib fractures. Randomized controlled trial comparing ventilatory with nonventilatory management. *Chest.* 1990;97(4):943–948.
20. Hernandez G, Fernandez R, Lopez-Reina P, et al. Noninvasive ventilation reduces intubation in chest trauma-related hypoxemia: a randomized clinical trial. *Chest.* 2010;137(1):74–80.
21. Karcz MK, Papadakos PJ. Noninvasive ventilation in trauma. *World J Crit Care Med.* 2015;4(1):47–54.
22. Ferreyro BL, Angriman F, Munshi L, et al. Association of noninvasive oxygenation strategies with all-cause mortality in adults with acute hypoxemic respiratory failure: a systematic review and meta-analysis. *JAMA.* 2020;324(1):57–67.
23. Antonelli M, Conti G, Moro ML, et al. Predictors of failure of noninvasive positive pressure ventilation in patients with acute hypoxemic respiratory failure: a multi-center study. *Intensive Care Med.* 2001;27(11):1718–1728.
24. Frat JP, Thille AW, Mercat A, et al. High-flow oxygen through nasal cannula in acute hypoxemic respiratory failure. *N Engl J Med.* 2015;372(23):2185–2196.
25. Gristina GR, Antonelli M, Conti G, et al. Noninvasive versus invasive ventilation for acute respiratory failure in patients with hematologic malignancies: a 5-year multicenter observational survey. *Crit Care Med.* 2011;39(10):2232–2239.

26. Lemiale V, Mokart D, Resche-Rigon M, et al. Effect of noninvasive ventilation vs oxygen therapy on mortality among immunocompromised patients with acute respiratory failure: a randomized clinical trial. *JAMA*. 2015;314(16):1711–1719.
27. Azoulay E, Demoule A, Jaber S, et al. Palliative noninvasive ventilation in patients with acute respiratory failure. *Intensive Care Med*. 2011;37(8):1250–1257.
28. Nava S, Ferrer M, Esquinas A, et al. Palliative use of non-invasive ventilation in end-of-life patients with solid tumours: a randomised feasibility trial. *Lancet Oncol*. 2013;14(3):219–227.

Cough

Daniel Reynolds

GENERAL PRINCIPLES

- Cough is a protective mechanism to prevent aspiration.
- Cough is a common symptom that is a substantial driver of outpatient care visits.
- Chronic cough has been estimated to be the presenting symptom in over 30% of all respiratory patient visits in the United States.
- There is a strong female predominance in chronic cough, accounting for up to two-thirds of patients.
- Chronic cough is associated with poor quality of life and high health care costs.
- A diagnostic framework to approach cough is essential in management.

Classification

Cough is classified based on the duration of symptoms, which can help provide a framework for diagnosis.

- *Acute* cough is defined as less than 3 weeks.
- *Subacute* cough is defined as greater than 3 weeks, and less than 8 weeks.
- *Chronic* cough is defined as greater than 8 weeks.

Acute Cough

Acute cough can be divided into three main categories: infectious, exacerbation of underlying disease, and exposure related.

Infectious

- *Viral infections* of the upper respiratory tract are the most common cause of acute cough. Rapid diagnostic testing with a respiratory viral panel via polymerase chain reaction (PCR) can rapidly lead to a diagnosis.
  - Common respiratory viruses include rhinovirus/enterovirus, respiratory syncytial virus, and a variety of others including influenza, adenovirus and parainfluenza.
  - SARS-CoV-2, the virus responsible for COVID-19 is also a commonly encountered cause of an infectious viral cough.
  - Viral infections typically present as part of the common cold with symptoms including rhinorrhea, sneezing, irritation of the throat, lacrimation, and nasal congestion. Fever may or may not be a presenting symptom. Cough may be productive of mucus or nonproductive.
    - Coughing usually presents on day 4 or 5 after infection.
    - Further imaging with these acute symptoms is often unnecessary; however, imaging should be pursued in high-risk patients including those that are immunocompromised and those with underlying structural lung disease.

- *Bacterial pneumonia* is also a common cause of acute infectious cough, and it typically presents with cough, fevers, and shortness of breath. Imaging is typically necessary and reveals pulmonary infiltrates.
- *Viral or bacterial rhinosinusitis* can also result in postnasal drainage leading to acute cough.
  - Viral rhinosinusitis can be difficult to distinguish from bacterial sinusitis.
  - Viral rhinosinusitis can be symptomatically managed with antihistamines and nasal decongestants, while bacterial sinusitis typically requires antibiotics.

Exacerbation of Underlying Disease Process

- *Allergic rhinitis* is an IgE-mediated syndrome characterized by paroxysms of sneezing, nasal congestion, and irritation of the eyes and nose.
  - Symptoms are often improved by using nonsedating antihistamines and avoiding offending allergens.
  - Glucocorticoid nasal sprays, such as inhaled fluticasone, are an effective treatment for allergic rhinitis.
- Chronic obstructive pulmonary disease (COPD) *exacerbation* may result from smoking, air pollutants, allergens, and infections.
  - *Streptococcus Pneumoniae, Heamophilus influenza,* and *Moraxella catarrhalis* are among the most common bacterial pathogens isolated in COPD exacerbations.
  - Viral infections are also a common etiology leading to an exacerbation of COPD.
  - Antibiotics may be prescribed if the acute cough is accompanied by worsening shortness of breath, increased oxygen requirements, increased sputum production, or change in the character of sputum.

Exposure

- *Occupation* or *environmental* exposures may also be contributors to cough.
- A thorough history, such as workplace exposures, household exposures such as pets or new carpeting, change in medications, will help pinpoint this diagnosis.

Chronic Cough

Chronic cough is a condition of neural dysregulation. While the differential diagnosis of chronic cough is broad, the most common etiology in nonsmokers is typically due to upper airway cough syndrome (postnasal drip), asthma, and gastroesophageal reflux. Table 7-1 outlines etiologies of chronic cough. Chronic cough can cause impaired quality of life and is a significant economic burden on the patient and health care systems. Refractory chronic cough is intractable to standard of care treatment and typically requires a multidisciplinary team including pulmonologists, ENT, and allergists.

Upper Airway Cough Syndrome (Postnasal Drip)

- Symptoms may include nasal discharge, frequent throat clearing, and a sensation of nasal discharge dripping into the back of the throat.
- Physical exam may show secretions in the nasopharynx, and presence of cobblestoning.
- However, postnasal drip may be silent, leaving a practitioner with nonspecific symptoms to help guide treatment.

TABLE 7-1 ETIOLOGIES OF CHRONIC COUGH

Most Common
- Upper airway cough syndrome
- Asthma
- Gastroesophageal reflux
- COPD with chronic bronchitis
- Angiotensin-converting enzyme inhibitor use
- Environmental triggers—Cough hypersensitivity syndrome
- Tobacco use
- Nonasthmatic eosinophilic bronchitis
- Bronchiectasis

Less Common
- Postinfectious bronchospasm
- Pertussis
- Interstitial lung disease
- Malignancy
- Arteriovenous malformation
- Chronic aspiration

Rare
- Sarcoidosis
- Tuberculosis
- Irritation of external auditory canal
- Tracheal diverticula
- Cystic fibrosis
- Hyperthyroidism
- Carcinoid syndrome
- Psychogenic cough

- Therefore, when there is a lack of alternative cause of a patient's cough, empiric therapy for upper airway cough syndrome should be attempted before extensive workup of alternate cough etiologies.

Asthma
- The clinical spectrum of symptoms includes recurrent episodic wheezing, chest tightness, breathlessness, and cough, particularly at nighttime and/or in the early morning.
- Persistent cough, particularly nighttime cough, may be a sign of poorly controlled asthma.
- *Cough variant asthma* will often present with cough and may progress to encompass other common asthma symptoms.

Gastroesophageal Reflux Disease
- Symptoms include heartburn or a sour taste in the mouth, but some patients may also lack these symptoms. Empiric therapy is often reasonable when cough is of unclear etiology.
- Prolonged esophageal pH monitoring is generally considered the gold standard for confirmation of GERD.

COPD with Chronic Bronchitis
- The most common cause of chronic cough in smokers.
- Defined as cough productive of sputum ≥3 months' duration in at least 2 consecutive years in the absence of any other lung disease.
- Usually found with extensive smoking history, often greater than 1 pack per day for more than 20 years.
- Spirometry is necessary to establish the diagnosis of COPD.

ACE Inhibitors
- ACE inhibitors are a well-known cause of a chronic nonproductive cough.
- Usually begins within 1 week of starting treatment but can be seen up to 6 months later.
- Mechanism is not entirely clear, but it is believed that accumulation of bradykinin may stimulate afferent nerve fibers in the airway.
- Cessation of the medication is both diagnostic and therapeutic.
- Angiotensin II receptor blockers (ARBs) are not typically associated with cough and can be substituted for an ACE-inhibitor.

Bronchiectasis
- Bronchiectasis occurs less frequently than the other above-listed causes.
- Bronchiectasis is the result of repeated damage from chronic infections and airway inflammation in the bronchial tree that leads to irreversible dilatation of the affected airways.
- This anatomical alteration can lead to easily collapsible airways, poor mucus excretion, and chronic infection.
- Most patients will produce chronic mucopurulent sputum at baseline that becomes more purulent during acute infectious processes.

Nonasthmatic Eosinophilic Bronchitis
- Increasingly recognized as a cause of chronic cough.
- Patients often have atopic sensitivities, elevated sputum eosinophils, and airway inflammation.
- Although similar characteristics can be seen in patients with cough-variant asthma, patients with eosinophilic bronchitis do not demonstrate airway hyperresponsiveness.
- Inhaled glucocorticoids are mainstay of treatment.

Cough Hypersensitivity Syndrome
- Characterized by dysregulation of neural pathways and receptors in central nervous system, vagal afferent sensory nerves and ganglia.
- Cough may be triggered by low levels of thermal, mechanical, or chemical exposure.

Less Common Causes of Cough
- Postinfectious chronic cough
  - Following a viral respiratory infection can occur, and last more than 8 weeks.
  - COVID-19 can lead to a variety of prolonged symptoms, so-called "long COVID," and this can include chronic cough.
- Bordetella pertussis is an underrecognized cause of chronic cough that can last weeks to months. It is characterized by its barking cough and is diagnosed via culture or PCR.

- Interstitial lung disease can present with chronic cough, although it typically also presents with progressive shortness of breath and abnormal chest imaging.
- Malignancy, including lung cancer, may present with cough, though typically are associated with other symptoms that would raise suspicion for malignancy such as weight loss, hemoptysis, and abnormal chest imaging.
- Lesions that compromise the upper airway, including arteriovenous malformations, retrotracheal masses, and broncholiths can cause cough.
- Rare causes include:
  - Sarcoidosis, tracheobronchomalacia, mycobacterial disease, irritation of external auditory canal, tracheal diverticuli, occult cystic fibrosis, recurrent aspiration, hyperthyroidism, carcinoid syndrome.
  - Psychogenic cough is a diagnosis of exclusion, occurring less frequently in adults than in children. Many patients with this condition do not cough during sleep, are not awakened by cough, and do not cough when otherwise occupied (working or playing).

Etiology

The etiologies of cough can best be approached within their specific classification as specified above.

Pathophysiology

- Cough receptors exist in the epithelium of the upper and lower respiratory tracts, pericardium, stomach, esophagus, and diaphragm.
  - Afferent receptors are located within the sensory distribution of the trigeminal, glossopharyngeal, superior laryngeal, and vagus nerves.
  - Efferent receptors located in the recurrent laryngeal and spinal nerves respond to signals from a *"cough center"* in the medulla.
- Irritation of the cough receptors by smoke, dust, or fumes leads to stimulation of a complex reflex arc.
  - Once stimulated, an impulse is sent to the cough center.
  - After a series of muscle contractions, an increase in intrathoracic pressure develops, leading to increased airflow through the trachea.
  - These shearing forces help to eliminate mucus and foreign materials.

DIAGNOSIS

The diagnosis can be narrowed down by a careful review of the patient's history and physical exam. Focusing on the three most common causes of chronic cough (postnasal drip, asthma, and GERD) is helpful in limiting the need for extensive evaluation.

Clinical Presentation

History
- A complete history provides important clues in the patient presenting with cough complaints, with close attention to timing of onset as well as alleviating and aggravating factors.
- Concerning symptoms that should prompt immediate evaluation would include hemoptysis, weight loss, night sweats, fevers, and associated shortness of breath.

- Patients should be questioned about medications, especially beta blockers and ACE inhibitors, environmental exposures, and recent respiratory tract infections within the past 3 months.
- It is also important to establish tuberculosis (TB) risk factors, and when appropriate, to determine when the last purified protein derivative (PPD) skin test was completed.
- The medical history should focus on any underlying conditions that may predispose a patient to aspiration, congestive heart failure, and interstitial lung disease.
- Social history should include a detailed history of use of alcohol and tobacco as well as use of vaping devices. A detailed occupational history should be obtained, including past and present exposure to asbestos, silica, coal dust, and fumes.
- Family history should include information regarding asthma, cystic fibrosis, and pulmonary fibrosis.

Physical Examination
- The patient should be observed for any signs of labored breathing.
- Frontal and maxillary sinuses should be palpated for tenderness.
- The nose should be examined with attention to boggy turbinates, mucopurulent secretions, and polyps.
- Cobblestone appearance of the oropharynx suggests postnasal drip.
- Lung auscultation is a key component of the exam, and one must pay special attention to breath sounds, wheezes, and crackles.
- Remember to inspect the extremities for clubbing and peripheral edema. Clubbing may occur with interstitial lung disease, cystic fibrosis, and lung cancer.

Diagnostic Criteria: Sputum Production
- For patients with chronic bronchitis, sputum production is usually insidious.
- It is often worse in the morning, and the appearance is whitish to gray.
- During exacerbations, the sputum may become more profuse and more purulent.
- Cigarette smokers are often used to their baseline productive cough and are less likely to present to their physician unless there is a change in their respiratory status or the character of their sputum.

Differential Diagnosis
- **Upper airway cough syndrome**
  - Absence of symptoms does not exclude the diagnosis of upper airway cough syndrome.
  - Patients may have "silent" postnasal drip and still have a favorable response to combination therapy with an antihistamine, nasal decongestant, and/or nasal steroids.
- **Gastroesophageal reflux disease**
  - The patient may complain of heartburn, regurgitation, a sour taste in their mouth, or dysphagia.
  - Symptoms may be worse at night, when lying flat.
- **Asthma**
  - The classic triad of cough, shortness of breath, and wheezing does not occur in every patient.
  - Chronic cough may be the sole presenting symptom of cough variant asthma.
  - Asthma triggers such as viral infections or seasonal changes may be a clue to cough variant asthma being the etiology of cough.

Diagnostic Testing
- **Chest x-ray (CXR)**
  - CXR can be helpful in establishing an initial diagnosis in chronic cough cases for which there is low clinical suspicion of postnasal drip, asthma, or GERD.
  - A normal radiograph in an immunocompetent host makes a diagnosis such as sarcoidosis, interstitial lung disease, tuberculosis, or bronchiectasis less likely.
  - If there is concern for malignancy, a computed tomography (CT) chest should be performed.
- **Sinus CT scan**
  - Limited sinus CT is the usual test of choice in selected cases with suspected sinus disease.
  - A CT scan should be obtained if a patient has not had improvement in symptoms with one or two courses of appropriate antibiotic therapy for sinusitis.
  - Nasal endoscopy is generally not indicated except in cases in which resistant or unusual organisms are suspected.
- **Pulmonary function tests**
  - Methacholine challenge testing should be performed in patients with a history and physical exam suggestive of asthma.
  - A negative test result essentially eliminates cough-variant asthma as the cause of chronic cough. In patients with a positive response to methacholine challenge, a lack of improvement with bronchodilators may indicate a false-positive test, and further workup should be initiated.
- **Gastrointestinal evaluation**
  - Diagnostic testing for suspected gastroesophageal disease is not routinely recommended.
  - 24-hour esophageal pH monitoring is the single most sensitive and specific test for reflux disease, but it is inconvenient and may not be readily available in some practices.
  - When postnasal drip and asthma have been ruled out, a 4-week trial of antireflux therapy can be initiated.
  - If an inadequate response to a proton pump inhibitor, pH monitoring may be performed. The study should be performed while the patient is on the antireflux therapy to document the efficacy of the medication.
- **Additional testing**
  - If the history, physical exam, lab tests, and plain radiograph data do not provide a diagnosis, referral to a specialist should be considered.
  - A high-resolution chest CT can be performed to rule out rare causes of chronic cough such as bronchiectasis or interstitial lung disease. If the high-resolution CT scan is negative, then more invasive studies can be considered.
  - Echocardiography can be performed to rule out left ventricular dysfunction.
  - Other tests that may be performed include a sweat chloride test for cystic fibrosis (if indicated) and quantitative immunoglobulins to evaluate for rare immunodeficiencies.

TREATMENT

The first step is establishing the underlying etiology. A systematic approach to the evaluation of persistent cough and treatment aimed at the underlying disorder is successful in most cases.

- **Chronic bronchitis**
  - Chronic bronchitis is managed with smoking cessation and bronchodilator therapy.
  - Cough will improve in the majority of patients with cessation of smoking.
  - In patients who continue to smoke, medical therapy may still be helpful.
- **Upper airway cough syndrome**
  - Upper airway cough syndrome may be due to allergic, perennial nonallergic, or vasomotor rhinitis.
  - Removal of the offending environmental precipitant (if possible) is the treatment of choice.
  - Nasal steroids (i.e., fluticasone nasal spray, two sprays per nostril daily) can also be helpful.
  - Nonspecific therapy for any form of rhinitis includes antihistamines and topical decongestants in combination, and ipratropium nasal spray (0.03% nasal solution, two sprays each nostril two to three times daily).
  - First-generation antihistamines have been shown to be more effective in the treatment of cough than the newer, nonsedating agents.
  - Improvement can be expected within 7 days.
- **Asthma**
  - The treatment of cough-variant asthma is identical to that of atopic asthma.
  - Inhaled bronchodilators and inhaled corticosteroids are the mainstays of therapy.
  - Patients may require a brief course of prednisone to improve flares of their asthma.
- **Gastroesophageal reflux disease**
  - GERD is treated with both behavioral modification and medication.
  - Patients should avoid eating for 3 hours before bedtime, and specifically, avoid reflux inducing foods (i.e., fatty foods, chocolate, and alcohol).
  - Patients should elevate the head of their bed with foam wedges or use a mechanized bed.
  - Treatment with a proton pump inhibitor should be instituted, especially in patients who do not respond to behavioral therapy, or in those patients with severe symptoms.
- **Sinusitis**
  - Most mild cases of mild sinusitis respond to topical or oral decongestants.
  - In more severe cases, or in recurrent infections, an antihistamine in combination with a decongestant may be more effective.
  - Bacterial sinusitis can be treated with an appropriate antibiotic (amoxicillin-clavulanate, 500 mg/125 mg by mouth tid, or clarithromycin, 500 mg by mouth bid) for a 10–14-day course.
- **Medication-induced cough**
  - Discontinuation of the offending ACE inhibitors or beta blockers often results in relief of symptoms within 1–4 days, but may take several weeks.
  - Substitutions of alternate drugs within the same class are unlikely to be effective, although alternatives such as ARBs may be useful substitutes.
- **Nonasthmatic eosinophilic bronchitis**
  - Most often treated with a trial of inhaled corticosteroids.

- In one study, inhaled budesonide, 400 μg twice daily for 4 weeks, markedly improved airway inflammation and cough sensitivity in patients with eosinophilic bronchitis.[1]
- Optimal duration of therapy is not clear.
- **Bronchiectasis**
  - Antibiotics directed against the most frequently encountered pathogens (*H. influenza, Pseudomonas aeruginosa, and S. pneumonia*) help to reduce cough and sputum production.
  - Patients generally require a minimum of 7 days of therapy.
  - Airway clearance therapy is an essential aspect of management of bronchiectasis, with the use of airway clearance devices as well as nebulized bronchodilators and hypertonic saline used to improve chronic cough and clear out mucous from underlying bronchiectasis.
- **Interstitial lung disease:** Treatment is directed at the underlying lung disease.
- **Lung cancer**
  - For non–small-cell lung cancer, resection, if possible, is the treatment of choice.
  - Treatment for nonresectable malignancy involves chemotherapy and/or radiation therapy.
- **Congestive heart failure:** Treatment is directed at the underlying disorder.
- **Somatic cough disorder (psychogenic cough)**
  - Removal of psychological stressors and behavioral modification therapy are probably the best treatment modalities for psychogenic cough.
  - Antitussives have little or no proven role in the therapy of psychogenic cough.
  - Gabapentin has been used with some success in the treatment of refractory cough believed secondary to psychogenic causes.
  - Speech therapy for paradoxical vocal fold motion has been effective.

SPECIAL CONSIDERATIONS

- An acute cough is defined as lasting <3 weeks, whereas a chronic cough is defined as lasting >3 weeks.
- Cough receptors exist in the epithelium of the upper and lower respiratory tracts, pericardium, stomach, esophagus, and diaphragm. Afferent receptors are located within the sensory distribution of the trigeminal, glossopharyngeal, superior pharyngeal, and vagus nerves.
- Irritation of the cough receptors leads to stimulation of a complex reflex arc.
- Viral infections of the upper respiratory tract are the most common cause of acute cough.
- Upper airway cough syndrome is the most common cause of persistent cough in nonsmokers.
- The first step in the management of a patient with a chronic cough is establishing the etiology (see Table 7-1).

REFERENCE

1. Brightling CE, Ward R, Wardlaw AJ, Pavord ID. Airway inflammation, airway responsiveness and cough before and after inhaled budesonide in patients with eosinophilic bronchitis. *Eur Respir J*. 2000; 15(4):682–686.

Asthma

8

Jonah Graves, Tri Pham, and James G. Krings

GENERAL PRINCIPLES

- Asthma is a disease characterized by chronic airway inflammation and airway hyperreactivity to a wide variety of stimuli (or triggers).
- Airway hyperreactivity can result in airflow obstruction and respiratory symptoms, including cough, dyspnea, chest tightness, and wheezing.
- Asthma is episodic in nature with exacerbations (or attacks) often separated by symptom-free intervals.
- Asthma exacerbations are characterized by an increasing symptom burden caused by increased airway reactivity and unstable lung function. Exacerbations are often triggered by exposure to irritants, allergens, or infections.
- The symptoms of asthma overlap with other mimicking syndromes including vocal cord dysfunction, subglottic stenosis, tracheobronchomalacia, heart failure, and chronic obstructive pulmonary disease (COPD), which are important to consider and, at times, exclude prior to making a diagnosis of asthma.
- Asthma affects patients of all ages and management strategies differ between the pediatric and adult populations. This text will focus on the management of adolescent and adult patients (age ≥12 years).
- Asthma is prevalent in the US, and affects approximately 25 million people, or 8% of the US population.[1]
- Asthma morbidity and mortality are inversely associated with socioeconomic status with the burdens of asthma disproportionately affecting non-White and lower socioeconomic status populations. In childhood, asthma disproportionately affects males; in adulthood, asthma disproportionately affects females.[2]
- The total direct and indirect cost of asthma in the US, stemming from health care expenditures, work and school absenteeism, and mortality, amounts to approximately $80 billion US dollars annually.[3]

DIAGNOSIS

Clinical Presentation

History
- Patients with asthma frequently present to clinicians after experiencing episodic symptoms, including dyspnea, cough, wheezing, and chest tightness.

- Patients often report worsening symptoms with specific exposures (e.g., smoke, volatile cleaning products, gasoline fumes, allergens, dust, etc.).
- Patients may only experience symptoms during or after exercise, which is termed exercise-induced asthma.
- A subset of patients reports worsening asthma symptoms and hypersensitivity to aspirin (and other nonsteroidal anti-inflammatory drugs [NSAIDs]) and typically have comorbid rhinitis and nasal polyposis. This syndrome is referred to as aspirin-exacerbated respiratory disease.

Physical Examination
- The physical examination for a patient with asthma is often normal in asymptomatic periods.
- Auscultation of the lungs may reveal wheezing when a patient with asthma is symptomatic.
- Extrapulmonary exam findings suggestive of allergic disease are pertinent, including atopic dermatitis, rhinosinusitis, and nasal polyps.

Diagnostic Testing
- The diagnosis of asthma can be elusive and should begin with a detailed history and physical exam to ensure the presentation is compatible with asthma.
- **Pulmonary function testing** (PFT) is essential in making a diagnosis of asthma; however, normal testing is frequently encountered in patients with asthma and should not exclude the diagnosis. Characteristic PFT findings of asthma include reversible airflow obstruction, lung hyperinflation, and air trapping.
  - Airflow obstruction is confirmed with **spirometry**:
    - Traditionally, a reduction in the forced expiratory volume over 1 second (FEV_1) over forced vital capacity (FVC) ratio resulting in an FEV_1/FVC <70% predicted defines obstructive lung disease.
    - The 2021 American Thoracic Society (ATS)/European Respiratory Society (ERS) technical standards now recommend using an FEV_1/FVC <5th percentile (i.e., the lower limit of normal) to define airflow obstruction. The severity of airflow obstruction can then be defined based on the FEV_1 using z-scores (or FEV_1 cutoffs).[4]
    - Note that the ATS/ERS now recommends using race-neutral reference equations when interpreting PFTs.
  - Reversible airflow obstruction is indicated by an increase in either the FEV_1 or FVC by >10% of the predicted value following administration of a short-acting bronchodilator.[4]
  - Severe asthma can ultimately result in severe airway remodeling with airflow obstruction becoming irreversible (i.e., fixed airflow obstruction).
  - Lung hyperinflation and air trapping are confirmed with **plethysmography** by an increased total lung capacity and residual volume, respectively.
  - In patients with otherwise normal PFTs, **bronchoprovocation testing** can be performed with methacholine, exercise, or eucapnic voluntary hyperventilation to evaluate airway hyperresponsiveness. Bronchoprovocation testing is most helpful in excluding a diagnosis of asthma by the absence of hyperresponsiveness.

- Measurement of the **fractional exhaled nitric oxide (FeNO)** should be considered in patients suspected of having asthma, and in particular those who are being considered for biologic treatment.[5]
  - FeNO levels are generally increased in the setting of type 2 (T2) inflammation, which affects the majority of patients with asthma.
  - FeNO levels can be used to guide the escalation and de-escalation of asthma treatment, and FeNO levels directly correlate with the frequency of asthma exacerbations and a positive response to corticosteroids.[5]
- **Imaging** with a CXR should be considered to rule out other causes of dyspnea, cough, or wheezing in patients being evaluated for asthma. Quantitative CT, hyperpolarized MRI, and calculation of mucus plug scores are being studied in the research setting. These advanced imaging modalities may be increasingly used in the clinical setting in the future.[6]

TREATMENT

Medications

- In general, asthma therapies should be started and adjusted in a stepwise fashion, as delineated by the Global Initiative for Asthma (GINA).[7] If symptoms are insufficiently controlled, therapy should be stepped up every 2–3 months. Once sufficiently controlled for a minimum of 3 months, a step down in therapy should be considered.
- If previously untreated, the initial treatment step should be chosen based on symptom severity.[7]

GINA Steps 1–2 (i.e., Mild Asthma)
- **Preferred therapies**
  - **Anti-inflammatory reliever (AIR)** therapy with combination low-dose inhaled corticosteroid (ICS) and formoterol is the GINA preferred regimen for patients with mild asthma. AIR has been shown in multiple large, randomized trials to be superior to as-needed short-acting beta-agonist (SABA) monotherapy and noninferior (or superior) to maintenance ICS plus as-needed SABA therapy at preventing severe asthma exacerbations.[8]
  - Formoterol is a particular rapid-onset, long-acting beta-agonist (LABA) that provides a similar quick-onset relief of asthma symptoms as SABAs. ICS-formoterol inhalers are the only combination therapies that should be used for AIR.
  - Budesonide-formoterol 160/4.5 μg one puff as needed via a dry powder inhaler (DPI) (maximum 12 puffs in 24 hours) has the most supportive data among ICS-formoterol inhalers for AIR.
  - ICS-formoterol can be taken prior to exercise in patients with exercise-induced symptoms.
- **Nonpreferred alternative therapies**
  - ICS taken concurrently with an as-needed SABA (GINA step 1) when symptoms occur or scheduled maintenance low-dose ICS with an as-needed SABA (GINA step 2) are alternative asthma regimens to be considered.
  - Combination ICS-albuterol is now commercially available in the US but the evidence for its efficacy and safety in mild asthma is limited to a single, 6-month study.[9]

- **Monotherapy with as-needed SABA is no longer recommended by GINA.** SABA overuse is associated with an increased risk of asthma-associated morbidity and mortality.[7,10]

GINA Steps 3–4 (i.e., Moderate-to-Severe Asthma)
- **Preferred therapies**
  - **Single maintenance and reliever therapy (SMART)** with low-dose ICS-formoterol is the preferred regimen in patients with uncontrolled symptoms despite good adherence and technique to GINA steps 1 and 2 therapies.
    - SMART is superior to fixed-dose ICS-containing combination inhalers plus as-needed SABA and its use decreases a patient's risk of a severe asthma exacerbation, hospitalization, and ED visit.[11]
    - In addition to GINA, the National Asthma Education and Prevention Program (NAEPP) similarly strongly recommends SMART for patients with moderate-to-severe asthma.[12]
  - Available regimens include Budesonide-formoterol 160–4.5 μg one to two puffs one to two times daily and one puff as needed has the most supportive data among ICS-formoterol regimens for SMART.
- **Nonpreferred alternative therapies**
  - For patients who are symptomatically stable on traditional inhaler regimens, or for whom SMART is not feasible, maintenance ICS-LABA can be used with an as-needed SABA or as-needed ICS-albuterol.
  - A recent landmark trial found that as-needed use of ICS-albuterol was superior to as-needed use of albuterol, when used with a standard maintenance inhaler.[13]

GINA Step 5 (i.e., Severe Asthma)
- **Preferred therapies**
  - Patients with uncontrolled symptoms despite good adherence and technique with GINA step 4 therapies should be referred to a specialist for phenotyping and further consideration of add-on therapies (listed below).
  - GINA recommends SMART with budesonide-formoterol 160/4.5 μg two puffs twice daily and one puff as needed.
- **Nonpreferred alternative therapies:** Maintenance ICS-LABA can be used with an as-needed SABA or as-needed ICS-albuterol if SMART is not feasible.

Pharmacologic Add-On Therapies
- **Biologic therapies** with monoclonal antibody–targeting pathways involving immunoglobulin (Ig)-E, interleukin (IL)-5, IL-4, IL13, and thymic stromal lymphopoietin (TSLP) are highly effective and should be considered in patients with severe asthma (GINA step 5). There are no head-to-head trials comparing biologic agents; thus, therapies are selected based on drug- and patient-specific considerations, including asthma phenotype. Current FDA-approved biologic therapies are listed in Table 8-1.
  - An **allergic phenotype** is suggested by a history of atopy and an elevated total and allergen-specific IgE. Monoclonal antibody–targeting IgE (omalizumab) should be considered in this population.

TABLE 8-1 BIOLOGIC THERAPIES FOR TREATMENT OF ASTHMA

Drug	Target	Indication(s)	Dosing
Omalizumab	IgE	Moderate-to-severe allergic asthma and exacerbation in the last year with IgE level of 30–700 IU/mL and positive skin testing or IgE to specific perennial allergen	SC every 2–4 wk; dosing based on body weight and pretreatment IgE
Mepolizumab	IL-5 ligand	Severe T2-high asthma and severe asthma exacerbation(s) in the last year with serum AEC ≥150–300 cells/μL	SC every 4 wk; fixed dose
Reslizumab	IL-5 ligand	Severe T2-high asthma and severe exacerbation(s) in the last year with serum AEC ≥150–300 cells/μL	IV every 4 wk; weight-based dosing
Benralizumab	IL-5 receptor alpha	Severe T2-high asthma and severe exacerbation(s) in the last year with serum AEC ≥150–300 cells/μL	SC every 4 wk for the first three doses, then every 8 wk; fixed dose

TABLE 8-1	BIOLOGIC THERAPIES FOR TREATMENT OF ASTHMA (Continued)			
Drug		**Target**	**Indication(s)**	**Dosing**
Dupilumab		IL-4 receptor alpha	Moderate-to-severe T2-high asthma and severe exacerbation(s) in the last year with serum AEC 150–1,500 cells/μL and/or FeNO ≥25 ppb; or, oral steroid dependent	SC every 2 wk; available in two doses with higher dose preferred for steroid-dependent asthma or concomitant severe atopic dermatitis
Tezepelumab		TSLP	Severe asthma and severe exacerbation(s) in the last year	SC every 4 wk

AEC, absolute eosinophil count; FeNO, fractional exhaled nitric oxide; Ig, immunoglobulin; IL, interleukin; IV, intravenous; SC, subcutaneous; TSLP, thymic stromal lymphopoietin.

- ○ An **eosinophilic (T2-high) phenotype** is suggested by an elevated FeNO and peripheral/sputum eosinophilia. Monoclonal antibody–targeting IL-5 (mepolizumab, reslizumanb), IL-5 receptor alpha (benralizumab), and the IL-4 receptor alpha (dupilumb) should be considered in this population.
- ○ Monoclonal antibody–targeting TSLP (tezepelumab) is approved for all patients with severe asthma and can be used in patients **with or without a T2-high phenotype**.
- **Antileukotriene agents** can be used for adjunctive control in patients with mild, moderate, or severe asthma and should be especially considered in patients with aspirin-exacerbated respiratory disease and/or concurrent allergic rhinitis.
  - ○ There are two available classes of agents targeting the leukotriene pathway: leukotriene receptor antagonists (montelukast, zafirlukast) and the 5-lipoxygenase enzyme antagonist (zileuton).
  - ○ Some patients have a dramatic response to antileukotriene agents, while other patients derive little or no benefit.
  - ○ Antileukotriene agents can be considered in patients who cannot use ICS inhalers, though they are less effective than ICSs at preventing exacerbations and should not be considered as first line.[14]

- **Sublingual immunotherapy** can be considered in patients with asthma and comorbid allergic rhinitis with persistent asthma symptoms.[7]
- **Long-acting muscarinic antagonists (LAMAs)** can be added on as an adjunctive agent for patients uncontrolled on GINA steps 4–5. Available LAMA inhalers specifically approved for use in asthma include tiotropium and combination fluticasone furoate-umeclidium-vilanterol.
- **Azithromycin** dosed three times weekly on a chronic basis (at least 6 months) can be considered in patients with severe asthma (GINA step 5) and has been shown to reduce exacerbations requiring systemic steroids.[15]
- **Chronic corticosteroids** can be considered as a last resort in patients with refractory asthma despite high-dose ICS and trial of other add-on therapies (GINA step 5).
- **Methylxanthines** were historically used in the management of chronic, severe asthma; however, in light of their side-effect profile in contrast to other newer therapies, they are generally not recommended.

Nonpharmacologic Therapies
- **Bronchial thermoplasty (BT)** is an outpatient procedural-based therapy for patients with severe asthma that has been shown to improve asthma-related quality of life and reduce exacerbation frequency.[16]
- BT is performed by advancing a radiofrequency catheter through a bronchoscope to deliver a fixed duration and intensity of thermal energy to small airways, reducing their surrounding smooth muscle mass and ultimately reducing airway hyperreactivity.
- The procedure is performed during three bronchoscopies approximately 3 weeks apart and is associated with an increased risk of exacerbation requiring hospitalization during the procedure period.[16]
- BT should be exclusively performed at centers with experience in complex bronchoscopy and severe asthma management and should ideally be performed only as part of a clinical registry. Access to BT may be increasingly limited based on manufacturing of ablation probes.

Lifestyle Modification and Multimorbidity Management
- **Smoking cessation** and **avoidance of environmental irritants and allergens** should be assessed and encouraged in all patients with asthma.
- **Gastroesophageal reflux disease (GERD)** is a common comorbidity in patients with asthma and can worsen asthma severity. GERD treatment has been shown to improve asthma outcomes in patients with symptomatic GERD (but not those without symptoms of GERD).[17]
- **Obesity** is a risk factor for asthma and is associated with worse asthma severity.[18] Weight reduction should be encouraged in patients with comorbid asthma and obesity. Research interest in glucagon-like peptide-1 (GLP-1) agonists as part of asthma management is increasing.
- **Allergic rhinitis** is commonly comorbid with asthma and treatment with intranasal corticosteroids has been shown to improve lung function and asthma symptoms in select patients.[19]

- **Paroxysmal vocal fold motion disorder (PVFMD)** is a common comorbidity and mimicker of asthma. PVFMD symptoms overlap with asthma and can be a cause of difficult-to-control symptoms that are not responsive to asthma therapies. Patients with refractory asthma symptoms or upper airway symptoms, including impaired voice quality or throat tightness, should be referred for endoscopic evaluation.

ACUTE ASTHMA EXACERBATIONS

Clinical Presentation

History
- Patients with an acute asthma exacerbation present with worsening shortness of breath, wheezing, chest tightness, and/or cough.
- Risk factors for severe asthma exacerbations include recurrent need for oral corticosteroids for asthma, hospitalization(s) or emergency care visit(s) for asthma within the past year, use of more than one canister per month of SABAs, and poor adherence to maintenance ICS-containing medications.

Physical Examination
- In the acute setting, an initial, rapid exam is necessary to identify patients with severe airflow obstruction needing immediate resuscitation. Severe airflow obstruction is indicated by the use of accessory, respiratory muscles, nasal alar flaring, inability to speak in full sentences, tachycardia, tachypnea, pulsus paradoxus (a drop in inspiratory systolic pressure >10 mm Hg), and a peak expiratory flow (PEF) rate <200 L/min.
- Other findings that should prompt immediate intervention include:
  - Reduced mental status should warrant consideration of endotracheal intubation.
  - Depressed respiratory effort and paradoxical diaphragmatic movement may indicate respiratory muscle fatigue and impending respiratory failure.
  - Absent or diminished breath sounds may indicate air trapping and insufficient airflow to generate a wheeze.
- Up to half of patients with severe airflow obstruction do not manifest the above findings.

Diagnostic Testing
- PEF assessment is a portable, quick, and safe method for evaluating asthma exacerbation severity. PEF may be particularly beneficial in pediatrics or in patients who have difficulty recognizing their symptoms.
  - Normal PEF values are predicted using age, sex, and height.
  - PEF rate <70% of the patient's predicted (or personal best) is indicative of an asthma exacerbation and <50% indicates a severe exacerbation.
  - Serial PEF measurements are effective for assessing a patient's response to therapy in the acute setting.

- **Peripheral oxygen saturation (SpO_2) measurement**
  - PEF is a poor predictor of hypoxemia; thus, measurement of SpO_2 with transcutaneous pulse oximetry is necessary in the acute setting.
  - Generally, asthma is not associated with significant hypoxemia. If significant hypoxemia is present, alternative diagnoses (e.g., pulmonary embolism, or pneumonia) should be considered.
- **Arterial blood gas** (ABG) analyses
  - PEF is a useful predictor of hypercapnia, which typically develops when PEF <25% of predicted (or personal best).
  - Most patients with an acute asthma exacerbation will have a low $PaCO_2$ resulting from hyperventilation.
  - A normal or elevated $PaCO_2$ is indicative of increasing physiologic dead space and/or respiratory muscle fatigue.
  - A rising $PaCO_2$ indicates a risk of impending respiratory failure and should prompt consideration of careful utilization of noninvasive ventilation or endotracheal intubation.
- **CXR**
  - The CXR is of limited diagnostic utility in acute asthma exacerbations. However, CXRs can help evaluate for alternative etiologies of respiratory failure such as pneumonia or pneumothorax.
  - Hyperinflation is the most common radiographic abnormality in acute asthma exacerbations.

Management of Asthma Exacerbations
Level-of-Care Considerations
- Depending on severity, asthma exacerbations can be self-managed at home or require evaluation and management in the ambulatory, hospital, or intensive care setting.
- All patients should have a personalized asthma action plan that outlines necessary steps to take if they experience worsening symptoms and/or a reduction in their PEF.
- Self-management at home may be appropriate for patients who have mildly worsening symptoms and/or reduction in PEF.
- The decision to admit or discharge a patient from the emergency department should depend on the patient's initial response to treatment (after 60 minutes or three treatments with short-acting bronchodilator) and the patient's level of social support and ability to obtain follow-up care.
  - Initial response to therapy is a better predictor of the need for hospitalization than severity of airflow obstruction on presentation.[20]
  If posttreatment PEF is >60% predicted (or 40–60% in patients with few risk factors for severe exacerbation and close follow-up), discharge from the emergency department may be appropriate. If posttreatment PEF is <40% (or if pretreatment PEF is <25%), then admission is generally warranted.[7]
- Admission to an intensive care unit should be considered for patients with exam findings of severe airflow obstruction, marked hypoxemia, hypercapnia, or need (or potential need) for noninvasive or invasive mechanical ventilation (IMV).

- The remainder of this section will focus on the management of asthma exacerbations in the emergency department and inpatient settings.

Medications
- **First line**
  - **Inhaled SABAs** are the mainstay of bronchodilator therapy in the acute setting. Albuterol is dosed 2.5–5 mg by continuous-flow (updraft) nebulization until improvement or toxicity. Alternatively, albuterol can be administered in a metered-dose inhaler (MDI) via spacer, at regular dosing intervals.
  - **Systemic corticosteroids** speed resolution of asthma exacerbations and should be administered to all patients with moderate or severe exacerbations. The ideal dose and duration of systemic corticosteroids is not well defined.[21]
  - In most cases, **oral corticosteroids,** given as an equivalent of **prednisone** 40–60 mg daily, are effective.
  - In life-threatening exacerbations, intravenous **methylprednisolone** 40–60 mg every 6 hours is often given initially, although data supporting this dosing is limited.
    - Tapering should not begin until there is objective evidence of clinical improvement, usually at 24–48 hours.
    - Tapering is often prescribed over 7–14 days.
    - ICS should generally be continued if previously prescribed and started in ICS-naïve patients in the setting of an exacerbation.
- **Second line**
  - Inhaled short-acting antimuscarinic medications can be used in combination with SABAs in patients with severe or refractory asthma exacerbations and have been shown to modestly reduce the need for hospitalization if used in the emergency department setting.[22] Ipratropium is dosed as 0.5 mg by continuous-flow nebulization or MDI concomitantly with SABAs until improvement.
  - **Magnesium sulfate** can be given in severe exacerbations and may modestly reduce the need for hospital admission and improve lung function if used in the emergency department setting.[23] Magnesium sulfate is dosed as 2 g IV infused over 20 minutes.
  - **Parenteral bronchodilators,** including **epinephrine** and **terbutaline,** may be utilized in last-case scenarios with refractory airflow obstruction in patients who are too unstable for inhaled bronchodilators, but their use should be extremely uncommon.
  - **Methylxanthines** including theophylline or aminophylline are available; however, they have a narrow therapeutic window with a prohibitive side-effect profile. Accordingly, routine use is not recommended.[7]
  - **Antibiotics** are not recommended for the treatment of asthma exacerbations unless there is evidence of a concurrent pneumonia or other comorbid infection.

Nonpharmacologic Therapies
- **Heliox** is a blend of helium and oxygen with a lower density than air that decreases turbulent airflow in airways. Heliox (70:30 or 80:20 helium:oxygen

mixture) can be considered in patients with severe asthma exacerbation who do not respond to initial therapy.
- **Noninvasive positive pressure ventilation (NPPV)** improves alveolar ventilation and reduces work of breathing. Data supporting the use of NPPV during COPD exacerbations is robust, compared with asthma. However, recent retrospective data demonstrated that careful use of NPPV during asthma exacerbations may reduce endotracheal intubation rates and even improve in-hospital mortality.[24]
  - NPPV should generally only be utilized in the emergency department or intensive care unit setting and managed by providers experienced in the use of NPPV.
  - Sedatives should generally not be used to facilitate NPPV adherence as this may precipitate worsening respiratory failure.
- **Invasive mechanical ventilation (IMV)** should be considered in anyone with refractory or worsening respiratory failure despite the use of NPPV or in patients with altered mental status with an unstable airway for whom use of NPPV is contraindicated.
  - IMV in patients with severe asthma exacerbations can be a high-risk procedure. Caution and diligent ventilator management is necessary to avoid dynamic hyperinflation and barotrauma.
  - Patients receiving IMV may need additional salvage therapies, including inhaled anesthetics, ketamine, and paralytics.[25]
  - In patients with near fatal asthma receiving IMV, use of venovenous extracorporeal membrane oxygenation (VV-ECMO) is an option, and its use has had favorable outcomes reported in retrospective cohort studies.[26,27]

REFERENCES

1. Most Recent National Asthma Data. 2023. Accessed December 30, 2023. https://www.cdc.gov/asthma/most_recent_national_asthma_data.htm
2. Pate CA, Zahran HS, Qin X, Johnson C, Hummelman E, Malilay J. Asthma surveillance—United States, 2006–2018. *MMWR Surveill Summ.* 2021;70(5):1–32.
3. Nurmagambetov T, Kuwahara R, Garbe P. The economic burden of asthma in the United States, 2008–2013. *Ann Am Thorac Soc.* 2018;15(3):348–356.
4. Stanojevic S, Kaminsky DA, Miller MR, et al. ERS/ATS technical standard on interpretive strategies for routine lung function tests. *Eur Respir J.* 2022;60(1):2101499.
5. Khatri SB, Iaccarino JM, Barochia A, et al. Use of fractional exhaled nitric oxide to guide the treatment of asthma: An Official American Thoracic Society Clinical Practice Guideline. *Am J Respir Crit Care Med.* 2021;204(10):e97–e109.
6. Krings JG, Wenzel SE, Castro M. The emerging role of quantitative imaging in asthma. *Br J Radiol.* 2022;95(1132):20201133.
7. Global Initiative for Asthma. Global Strategy for Asthma Management and Prevention, 2023. Updated July 2023. Accessed December 15, 2023. www.ginasthma.org
8. Crossingham I, Turner S, Ramakrishnan S, et al. Combination fixed-dose beta agonist and steroid inhaler as required for adults or children with mild asthma. *Cochrane Database Syst Rev.* 2021;5(5):CD013518.

9. Papi A, Canonica GW, Maestrelli P, et al. Rescue use of beclomethasone and albuterol in a single inhaler for mild asthma. *N Engl J Med.* 2007;356(20):2040–2052.
10. Nwaru BI, Ekström M, Hasvold P, Wiklund F, Telg G, Janson C. Overuse of short-acting β2-agonists in asthma is associated with increased risk of exacerbation and mortality: a nationwide cohort study of the global SABINA programme. *Eur Respir J.* 2020;55(4):1901872.
11. Kew KM, Karner C, Mindus SM, Ferrara G. Combination formoterol and budesonide as maintenance and reliever therapy versus combination inhaler maintenance for chronic asthma in adults and children. *Cochrane Database Syst Rev.* 2013;2013(12):CD009019.
12. Cloutier MM, Baptist AP, Blake KV, et al. 2020 Focused updates to the asthma management guidelines: a report from the National Asthma Education and Prevention Program Coordinating Committee Expert Panel Working Group. *J Allergy Clin Immunol.* 2020;146(6):1217–1270.
13. Papi A, Chipps BE, Beasley R, et al. Albuterol–budesonide fixed-dose combination rescue inhaler for asthma. *N Engl J Med.* 2022;386(22):2071–2083.
14. Chauhan BF, Ducharme FM. Anti-leukotriene agents compared to inhaled corticosteroids in the management of recurrent and/or chronic asthma in adults and children. *Cochrane Database Syst Rev.* 2012;2012(5):CD002314.
15. Hiles SA, McDonald VM, Guilhermino M, Brusselle GG, Gibson PG. Does maintenance azithromycin reduce asthma exacerbations? An individual participant data meta-analysis. *Eur Respir J.* 2019;54(5):1901381.
16. Torrego A, Solà I, Munoz AM, et al. Bronchial thermoplasty for moderate or severe persistent asthma in adults. *Cochrane Database Syst Rev.* 2014;2014(3):CD009910.
17. Chan WW, Chiou E, Obstein KL, Tignor AS, Whitlock TL. The efficacy of proton pump inhibitors for the treatment of asthma in adults: a meta-analysis. *Arch Intern Med.* 2011;171(7):620–629.
18. Peters U, Dixon AE, Forno E. Obesity and asthma. *J Allergy Clin Immunol.* 2018;141(4):1169–1179.
19. Lohia S, Schlosser RJ, Soler ZM. Impact of intranasal corticosteroids on asthma outcomes in allergic rhinitis: a meta-analysis. *Allergy.* 2013;68(5):569–579.
20. Wilson MM, Irwin RS, Connolly AE, Linden C, Manno MM. A prospective evaluation of the 1-hour decision point for admission versus discharge in acute asthma. *J Intensive Care Med.* 2003;18(5):275–285.
21. Normansell R, Kew KM, Mansour G. Different oral corticosteroid regimens for acute asthma. *Cochrane Database Syst Rev.* 2016;2016(5):CD011801.
22. Kirkland SW, Vandenberghe C, Voaklander B, Nikel T, Campbell S, Rowe BH. Combined inhaled beta-agonist and anticholinergic agents for emergency management in adults with asthma. *Cochrane Database Syst Rev.* 2017;1(1):CD001284.
23. Kew KM, Kirtchuk L, Michell CI. Intravenous magnesium sulfate for treating adults with acute asthma in the emergency department. *Cochrane Database Syst Rev.* 2014;2014(5):CD010909.
24. Althoff MD, Holguin F, Yang F, et al. Noninvasive ventilation use in critically ill patients with acute asthma exacerbations. *Am J Respir Crit Care Med.* 2020;202(11):1520–1530.
25. Leatherman J. Mechanical ventilation for severe asthma. *Chest.* 2015;147(6):1671–1680.

26. Zakrajsek JK, Min SJ, Ho PM, et al. Extracorporeal membrane oxygenation for refractory asthma exacerbations with respiratory failure. *Chest.* 2023;163(1): 38–51.
27. Yeo HJ, Kim D, Jeon D, Kim YS, Rycus P, Cho WH. Extracorporeal membrane oxygenation for life-threatening asthma refractory to mechanical ventilation: analysis of the Extracorporeal Life Support Organization registry. *Crit Care.* 2017; 21(1):297.

Chronic Obstructive Pulmonary Disease

Francisco Novoa, Roger D. Yusen, and Rodrigo Vazquez Guillamet

GENERAL PRINCIPLES

Definition
- Chronic obstructive pulmonary disease (COPD) is a common, preventable, treatable, and usually progressive condition characterized by persistent airflow limitation (i.e., not fully reversible) and an enhanced chronic inflammatory response to noxious particles or gases.
- Patients with COPD have emphysema and/or airways disease (e.g., chronic bronchitis).
  - Emphysema, defined pathologically, consists of nonuniform distal airway enlargement associated with destruction of the acini, loss of lung elasticity, and absence of significant parenchymal fibrosis.
  - Chronic bronchitis is defined clinically as cough productive of (e.g., at least two tablespoons of) sputum on most days of 3 consecutive months in 2 consecutive years, in the absence of other lung diseases.
  - COPD has characteristics that overlap with asthma, and both conditions may occur in the same patient.
  - Although asthma, bronchiectasis, obliterative bronchiolitis, and sarcoidosis often have associated expiratory airflow obstruction, they do not fall within the classification of COPD.

Classification
- The Global Obstructive Lung Disease 2024 (GOLD) classification of COPD bases its assessment on the patient's level of symptoms, exacerbation history, spirometric abnormality, and identification of comorbidities.[1]
- Postbronchodilator spirometric pulmonary function tests determine the grade of airflow limitation (Table 9-1).[1] Height, weight, gender, and sometimes race determine predicted normal values for the forced expiratory volume in 1 second (FEV1) and forced vital capacity (FVC).
- An FEV1/FVC ratio of <0.7 is required for diagnosis.

Epidemiology
- COPD is frequently misdiagnosed.
- In the US, ~5% of the population has COPD
- While age-adjusted prevalence has remained stable among US adults over the last decade, death rates have experienced a continued slow decline.
- Death rates continue to rise among women in small metropolitan areas and the Midwest.[2]

TABLE 9-1: 2024 GOLD SEVERITY GRADE OF AIRFLOW LIMITATION FOR PATIENTS THAT HAVE COPD[a]

Stage	Characteristics
GOLD 1: mild	• FEV_1/FVC <70% • FEV_1 ≥80% predicted
GOLD 2: moderate	• FEV_1/FVC <70% • 50% ≤FEV_1 <80% predicted
GOLD 3: severe	• FEV_1/FVC <70% • 30% ≤FEV_1 <50% predicted
GOLD 4: very severe	• FEV_1/FVC <70% • FEV_1 <30% predicted

[a]Based on postbronchodilator FEV1.

GOLD, Global Initiative for Obstructive Lung Disease; COPD, chronic obstructive lung disease; FEV1, forced expiratory volume in 1 second; FVC, forced vital capacity.

Reproduced with permission from Global Initiative for Chronic Obstructive Lung Disease (GOLD). Global strategy for the diagnosis, management and prevention of COPD (2024 Report). © Global Initiative for Chronic Obstructive Lung Disease (GOLD). https://goldcopd.org/2024-gold-report/

Pathophysiology
- Inhaled particles that cause lung inflammation may induce parenchymal tissue destruction (e.g., emphysema) and cause airway disease (e.g., airway fibrosis) through the disruption of normal repair and defense mechanisms.
- Increased mucus production from goblet cell hyperplasia.
- Genetic disorders may create a predisposition to developing COPD (e.g., SERPINA 1 gene mutations).[3]
- Role of airway infections in COPD
  - Defective innate immune responses promote persistent airway bacterial colonization and recurrent airway infections.
  - Acute airway infections often lead to acute exacerbations and subsequently worsened lung function.
  - Viral infections (e.g., influenza, rhinovirus, and adenovirus) and bacterial infection (e.g., *Haemophilus influenzae*, *Streptococcus pneumoniae*, *Moraxella catarrhalis*, and *Mycoplasma pneumoniae*) cause most exacerbations.

Risk Factors
- The risk of developing COPD correlates with the total lifetime burden of exposure to inhaled toxins.
  - The most important risk factor for the development of COPD is cigarette smoking, which is associated with the majority of cases. However, only a minority of smokers develop clinically significant COPD, suggesting that genetic predisposition and other environmental factors may be required for its development.
  - Cigar and pipe smokers are also at increased risk of developing COPD.
  - One in four individuals with COPD are never smokers.
  - Occupational exposure and indoor air pollution may lead to COPD.
  - Approximately 50% of COPD cases develop due to abnormal lung growth and development.[4]

- Genetic disorders may lead to the development of COPD. α1-Antitrypsin deficiency (A1ATD) contributes to <1% of COPD cases.
  - α1-Antitrypsin inhibits neutrophil-derived elastase, an enzyme responsible for the destruction of lung parenchyma in emphysema.
  - Patients with A1ATD carry a genetic polymorphism that leads to decreased α1-antitrypsin serum levels.
  - A1ATD should be considered in every patient with COPD but especially in patients with emphysema who have:
    - COPD and a minimal smoking history.
    - Early-onset COPD (<45 years).[1]
    - Family history of COPD.
    - Predominance of lower lobe emphysema seen on imaging studies.[1]

Associated Conditions

A number of extrapulmonary comorbidities have been identified in those with COPD such as cardiovascular disease, lung cancer, osteoporosis, skeletal muscle dysfunction, depression, and metabolic syndrome.

DIAGNOSIS

- Symptoms of dyspnea or chronic cough should lead to an evaluation.
- History of heavy smoking should prompt further evaluation in the appropriate clinical setting.
- Spirometry is required to make the diagnosis of COPD.
- Radiographic diagnosis of emphysema in a computed tomography should prompt complete evaluation.

Clinical Presentation

Symptoms of COPD typically consist of increased dyspnea with exertion, decreased exercise tolerance, and increased sputum production.

History

- Chronic cough and sputum production may precede the development of COPD by many years.
- COPD may develop without chronic cough or sputum production.
- Dyspnea from COPD typically develops after the FEV1 has significantly decreased (e.g., <60% of the predicted normal value) over many years.
- Clinicians should perform a thorough medical history assessment, and question patients regarding symptoms, risk factors, clinical course, comorbidities, medications, and family history.

Physical Examination

Physical examination findings suggestive of COPD do not become apparent until after COPD has significantly progressed and include:

- Accessory muscle use, pursed lip breathing, and Hoover sign.
- Hyperinflation of the lungs associated with hyperresonant chest percussion.
- Decreased breath and heart sounds.
- Expiratory wheezes variably occur.
- Clubbing of the fingers not expected.

- Symptoms of cor pulmonale occur less commonly:
  - Elevated jugular venous pressure (JVP).
  - Lower extremity edema.
  - Right ventricular precordial heave, increased S2 and P2 strength, right-sided S3, and tricuspid regurgitation.

Diagnostic Criteria
- Spirometry is used to diagnose COPD, and the FEV1 determines the severity of the expiratory airflow obstruction based on the GOLD stages, see Table 9-1 for classification schema.[1]
- Peak expiratory flow measurement has high sensitivity but low specificity.
- Symptoms and examination findings assist with diagnosis.
- Imaging studies provide evidence of the presence or absence of emphysema.

Differential Diagnosis
- Asthma
- Bronchiectasis
- Reactive airways dysfunction syndrome
- Bronchiolitis obliterans
- Lymphangioleiomyomatosis (LAM)
- Sarcoidosis
- Langerhans cell histiocytosis
- Panbronchiolitis
- Fixed or variable airway obstruction in the upper airways
- Vocal cord dysfunction
- Congestive heart failure (will not cause expiratory airflow obstruction)
- Tuberculosis (TB)

Diagnostic Testing
Laboratory Testing
- We suggest obtaining an arterial blood gas (ABG) if the patient has a low SpO_2 (e.g., <92%), FEV1 very low (e.g., <35%), or signs of respiratory or right heart failure occur.
- Complete blood count (CBC), to look for polycythemia and presence of eosinophilia.
- Complete metabolic panel, to look for elevated bicarbonate level.
- α1-Antitrypsin screening.[1]

Imaging
- CXR posteroanterior and lateral to assess for emphysema or other conditions that could produce similar signs or symptoms.
- CT chest for those meeting criteria for lung cancer screening, frequent exacerbations, or candidates for lung volume reduction procedures.

Diagnostic Procedures
- Pulmonary function tests
  - Spirometry: pre- and postbronchodilator (FEV1/FVC <0.70 and scooping of the expiratory limb of the flow–volume curve).
  - Lung volumes (e.g., air trapping [elevated residual volume (RV)] and thoracic hyperinflation [e.g., elevated total lung capacity (TLC)]).

○ Diffusing capacity (e.g., reduced diffusing capacity of the lung for carbon monoxide [DLCO]).
- Pulse oximetry assessment at rest, with exercise, and possibly during sleep.
- Cardiac testing, when appropriate, to assist with a dyspnea evaluation.

TREATMENT

Acute Exacerbations

- COPD exacerbations are diagnosed clinically based on a worsening in respiratory symptoms beyond the expected day-to-day variation.
- COPD exacerbations typically increase (compared to baseline) one or more of the following:
  ○ Dyspnea
  ○ Cough and sputum production
  ○ Sputum purulence
- The first step taken when encountering a patient with an acute exacerbation should be a quick assessment to determine the need for hospitalization or intensive care unit (ICU) admission for impending respiratory failure (Table 9-2).[5]
- Indications for inpatient admission include:
  ○ Marked dyspnea
  ○ New physical findings such as cyanosis or peripheral edema
  ○ New or worsened hypoxemia/hypercapnia
  ○ Lack of adequate response to initial medical management
  ○ Consider hospital admission for those with advanced age or significant comorbidities
- Initial assessment should include CXR, ECG, ABG, CBC, chemistry panel, brain natriuretic peptide (BNP), and cardiac enzymes. ABG provides important information about alveolar gas exchange and acid–base status not obtained by pulse oximetry. ABGs can differentiate between acute and chronic respiratory acidosis and may indicate a need for assisted ventilation and ICU admission.
- Additional testing
  ○ Consider chest CT to evaluate for pulmonary embolism
  ○ Spirometry is not recommended during an exacerbation

TABLE 9-2 INDICATIONS FOR ICU ADMISSION
Severe dyspnea that does not adequately respond to initial therapy
Mental status deterioration (e.g., confusion, coma, lethargy)
Persistently worse or worsening hypercapnia or respiratory acidosis
Persistently worse or worsening hypoxemia
Lack of adequate response to supplemental oxygen and/or noninvasive positive pressure ventilation

Data from Steer J, Gibson J, Bourke SC. The DECAF Score: predicting hospital mortality in exacerbations of chronic obstructive pulmonary disease. *Thorax*. 2012; 67(11):970–976.

Medications

- General considerations regarding **bronchodilator therapy**
  - First-line therapy for symptomatic management of a COPD exacerbation.
  - Multiple randomized controlled trials have demonstrated the similar efficacy of short-acting β2-agonists (SABA) and short-acting anticholinergic (SAAC) agents for rapidly improving symptoms during an acute COPD exacerbation.
  - Combination therapy using a SABA/SAAC has added benefits beyond either agent alone (reduction in hospital length of stay duration and increase in FEV_1).
  - Combination therapy with SABA/SAAC may also have a more rapid onset of action, longer duration of action, and fewer side effects (owing to smaller doses of each individual agent) than use of higher doses of a single agent.
  - Long-acting agents are typically not recommended for the management of acute exacerbations of COPD because of the risk of side effects in combination with high-dose short-acting bronchodilator therapy and a lack of demonstrated efficacy and safety in this setting. Long-acting agents should typically be initiated prior to hospital discharge.
- **Inhaled SABA**
  - Albuterol may be administered q30–60min as tolerated. Subsequent treatment frequency can be decreased, eventually to q4–6h, as the acute exacerbation begins to resolve.
  - β2-Agonists may cause tremor, nervousness, tachycardia, tachyarrhythmias, and hypokalemia.
- **Inhaled SAACs**
  - Ipratropium may be dosed at 4–8 puffs or nebulized q4–6h for a COPD exacerbation.
  - Ipratropium is generally well tolerated and tends to produce fewer of the other side effects characteristic of β2-agonist agents.
  - Anticholinergic agents may cause dry mouth, dry eyes, bladder outlet obstruction/urinary retention, and acute angle glaucoma exacerbation.
- **Corticosteroids**
  - Systemic administration of corticosteroids is recommended during acute exacerbations of COPD requiring hospitalization.
  - Corticosteroids minimize recovery time, decrease hospital length of stay, reduce the incidence of relapse, and improve lung function toward baseline.
  - A randomized trial of patients hospitalized for COPD exacerbations found that oral systemic corticosteroids were noninferior to IV corticosteroids.[6]
  - The most common adverse effect of systemic corticosteroid administration is hyperglycemia, but other acute adverse effects include but are not limited to systemic hypertension, insomnia, and mood changes.
  - A typical steroid regimen is 40 mg PO for 5 days;[7] some patients may require a taper over 10–14 days.
  - Outpatient management
    - Short courses of oral steroids in patients with moderate to severe COPD can improve the outcomes of patients with exacerbations discharged from the emergency department (ED).
    - Inhaled steroids currently do not have a role in the treatment of acute COPD exacerbations.

- **Antibiotics**
  - Current methods do not reliably differentiate bacteria-caused exacerbations from those produced by viruses.
  - Commonly implicated bacterial pathogens: *S. pneumoniae,* nontypeable *H. influenzae* and *Haemophilus parainfluenzae, Chlamydia pneumoniae,* and *M. catarrhalis.*
  - Sputum cultures in the absence of pneumonia or bronchiectasis are likely of little benefit.
  - Antibiotics (usually for 5–10 days) are recommended during a COPD exacerbation for those with[1]:
    - Increased sputum purulence and sputum volume and increased dyspnea **OR**
    - Have increased sputum purulence with only one other cardinal symptom **OR**
    - Requiring mechanical ventilation.
  - Because of rampant antibiotic resistance, particularly in *S. pneumoniae*, broader-spectrum antibiotic coverage is commonly recommended for acute exacerbations, using one of the following:
    - Amoxicillin/clavulanate
    - Respiratory fluoroquinolone (e.g., levofloxacin or moxifloxacin)
    - Macrolide antibiotic (e.g., azithromycin, erythromycin, or clarithromycin)
- **Methylxanthines**
  - The role of parenteral or oral methylxanthines (e.g., theophylline) during an acute exacerbation is unclear.
  - Considered third-line agents due to their narrow therapeutic window and potential for severe side effects.

Other Nonpharmacologic Therapies

- **Oxygen**
  - Oxygen should be administered to achieve a PaO_2 of >55–60 mm Hg (≥89–90% oxyhemoglobin saturation on pulse oximetry).
  - Worsening hypercapnia may occur with oxygen administration in patients with baseline hypercapnia, and ABG should be checked ~30–60 minutes after starting oxygen therapy.
  - An increased or new requirement for supplemental oxygen may indicate the presence of a complicating condition such as pulmonary embolism, pneumonia, pneumothorax, or heart failure.
- **Noninvasive ventilation**
  - Noninvasive positive-pressure ventilation (NIPPV) is useful for improving oxygenation, decreasing hypercapnia, and relieving work of breathing in patients with acute COPD exacerbation and acute respiratory failure.
  - NIPPV decreases intubation and mortality rates.[8]
  - Methods of NIPPV
    - Continuous positive airway pressure ventilation (CPAP) improves oxygenation and work of breathing.
    - Bilevel positive airway pressure ventilation (BiPAP) is the preferred method for treatment of respiratory failure associated with acute respiratory acidosis. The larger the gradient between high-, and low-pressure settings, the greater the ventilatory support (improvement in PCO_2) provided by NIPPV.

TABLE 9-3 CRITERIA FOR NONINVASIVE POSITIVE PRESSURE VENTILATION

Inclusion Criteria
Severe dyspnea, with signs of respiratory muscle fatigue or increased work of breathing (e.g., use of accessory muscles, paradoxical abdominal motion), or
pH 7.30–7.35 and $PaCO_2$ >45 mm Hg

Exclusion Criteria
Altered mental status
Respiratory arrest
Cardiovascular instability
High aspiration risk
Recent facial or gastroesophageal surgery
Nasopharyngeal abnormalities
Extreme obesity

- Most patients tolerate NIPPV, which has been shown to decrease mortality, the need for endotracheal intubation, and length of hospitalization.
- To be effective, patients must be awake and cooperative with NIPPV. See inclusion and exclusion criteria for NIPPV in Table 9-3.
- **Follow-up:** For patients hospitalized for a COPD exacerbation, discharge plans should include reinforcement of smoking cessation, review of home medication regimen, assessment of metered dose inhaled (MDI) technique and training when needed, vaccination updates, education, oxygen assessment, outpatient pulmonary rehabilitation, and health care provider follow-up.

CHRONIC COPD TREATMENT

Long-term management of COPD should aim to reduce symptoms and decrease risk for the frequency and severity of acute exacerbations, progression of disease, morbidity, side effects of therapy, and mortality.

Of the medical therapies, randomized controlled trials have demonstrated that smoking cessation and the correction of hypoxemia with supplemental oxygen improve survival. There is also a potential for improved survival in carefully selected individuals undergoing lung volume reduction surgery (LVRS) and lung transplantation. Recent trials also suggest an improvement in survival for highly symptomatic individuals with at least moderate obstruction with the combination of an inhaled corticosteroid, long-acting anticholinergic, and long-acting β-agonist.

Medications

- General considerations regarding **bronchodilator therapy**
  - Bronchodilator therapy may control symptoms, increase exercise tolerance, improve lung function, and decrease the frequency and severity of exacerbations.
  - Recent studies suggest decreased mortality and slower lung function decline associated with the combination of long-acting β2-agonist (LABA),

long-acting anticholinergics (LAACs), and inhaled corticosteroids (ICS) in moderate to severe, symptomatic COPD.[9,10]
- Clinicians should prescribe scheduled and on-demand bronchodilators.
- Short-acting bronchodilators (SABA and/or SAAC) are preferred for those with mild symptoms, mild airflow obstruction, and low risk of exacerbation.
- Long-acting agents are recommended for those with more severe disease.
- MDIs are preferred over nebulizers for outpatient management. However, for those with severe dyspnea, weakness, or poor coordination, nebulizers may be preferred.
- Respiratory societies promote LAMA–LABA combination as first-line treatment for those requiring scheduled bronchodilators and consideration of LABA-LAMA-ICS for those with high burden of symptoms and blood eosinophils >300 cells/microL.[1]

- **Anticholinergic agents**
  - Ipratropium is effective as initial bronchodilator therapy.
  - It has a longer duration of action and less toxicity than available β2-agonists such as albuterol.
  - The usual dosage of 2 puffs q4–6h can be doubled or tripled to achieve maximal bronchodilation.
- **β2-Agonists**
  - Albuterol is the mainstay β2-agonist.
  - Titrate up to the standard albuterol dose of 2 puffs q4–6h for symptomatic relief.
- **Combination therapy**
  - Combination therapy with a β2-agonist and an anticholinergic provides a greater benefit in terms of symptoms and bronchodilation (FEV1) than does either agent alone.
  - It is also convenient to have both drugs in a single MDI.
  - Patients often benefit from the use of combination short-acting therapy with a simultaneous LABA.
- **Long-acting inhaled medical therapy**
  - LABAs and LAACs can reduce exacerbations and improve dyspnea in patients with moderate to severe disease.
  - LABAs
    - Improve respiratory symptoms
    - Increase morning peak expiratory flows
    - Decrease the use of rescue bronchodilator therapy
  - Oral formulations of β2-agonists should be avoided, as they provide similar efficacy to inhaled agents with a higher risk of toxic side effects.
  - A recent randomized controlled trial in patients with moderate to severe COPD found that tiotropium (an LAAC agent) had greater efficacy than salmeterol for preventing COPD exacerbations.[11]
- **Inhaled corticosteroids**
  - Inhaled maintenance corticosteroid (ICS) therapy increases the FEV1 and decreases the frequency and severity of exacerbations in patients with moderate to severe disease.
  - ICS is associated with an increased risk of pneumonia.
  - The use of ICS in isolation is not recommended in COPD.

- LABA–LAMA–ICS should be considered in the initial management of patients with eosinophilia (>300 cells*ml-1) and high burden of symptoms
- Inhaled steroids should be administered after inhaled bronchodilator treatment, and patients should rinse the mouth and spit after each use to avoid thrush and hoarseness.
- **Systemic corticosteroids:** the use of oral corticosteroids in chronic stable COPD is generally discouraged due to their numerous side effects.
- **Methylxanthines**
  - Theophylline is a long-acting phosphodiesterase (PDE) inhibitor from the methylxanthine class and has demonstrated efficacy in the long-term management of COPD.[12] However, the risks of toxicity may outweigh the benefits and are not generally recommended.
  - A common starting dose of long-acting theophylline for an average-sized patient is 200 mg PO q12h, with the usual therapeutic dose being between 400 and 900 mg/d.
  - Serum levels should be checked 1–2 weeks after each dose adjustment, aiming for a level of 10 ± 2 μg/mL checked 4 hours after dosing, and monitored at least twice yearly.
  - Continued inhalation of tobacco smoke lowers theophylline levels.
  - Withdrawal of theophylline may lead to exacerbations of right heart failure.
  - Clinicians should be aware of multiple potential drug interactions.
- **Vaccines**
  - Influenza vaccination decreases morbidity and mortality and should be administered annually to all patients who have COPD.
  - According to the Advisory Committee on Immunization Practices, all patients with COPD should receive the pneumococcal vaccine.[13] It is important to note that different formulations exist. A single revaccination can be given if the patient received the vaccine >5 years earlier and was aged <65 years at the time of primary vaccination.
  - COVID-19 vaccines are recommended for patients with COPD.
  - Vaccination against *B. pertussis*, tetanus, and diphtheria should be provided if not received during adolescence.
  - Respiratory syncytial virus vaccination is approved and recommended for individuals over 60 years of age with COPD.
- **PDE4 selective inhibitors**
  - The selective inhibition of PDE4 by more recently available medications (e.g., cilomilast and roflumilast) decreases bronchial constriction and inflammation and improves FEV1 without the significant side effects associated with the nonselective PDE inhibitor theophylline.
  - Common side effects from PDE4 inhibitors include headache, nausea, and weight loss.
  - A recent randomized trial demonstrated that roflumilast, a PDE4 inhibitor, reduced exacerbations, and improved lung function in patients with moderate to severe COPD.[12]
- **Chronic antibiotic treatment**
  - The macrolide class of antibiotics (azithromycin, erythromycin, and clarithromycin) has increasingly been studied in lung disease for both its antimicrobial and immune regulatory function.

- A randomized trial demonstrated that addition of a macrolide antibiotic to inhaled medical therapy reduced the number of COPD exacerbations.[13]
- Side effects of chronic macrolide therapy include QTc prolongation, hearing loss, and a theoretical risk of developing resistant infections.
- **Mucolytics, antioxidant agents, and vasodilators** have not been shown to be of benefit in COPD.
- **Nedocromil and leukotriene modifiers,** used frequently for the treatment of asthma, have not been adequately tested for the treatment of COPD and are therefore not recommended at this time.
- **Antitussives are not specifically recommended** in COPD because of the protective role of coughing in clearing secretions.

Other Nonpharmacologic Therapies
- **Oxygen therapy**
  - Long-term supplemental oxygen therapy (>15 h/d) decreases mortality and improves physical and mental function in hypoxemic patients who have COPD.[14]
  - Oxygen therapy reduces the sensation of dyspnea and increases oxygen delivery to the heart, skeletal muscles, and the brain.
  - Experimental evidence suggests that hyperoxemia induces cellular oxidative stress via imbalance in oxidants and antioxidants, and it may hasten airway dysfunction and parenchymal destruction.
  - Thus, supplemental oxygen therapy should only be used in a goal-targeted fashion.
  - Assessment for oxygen therapy
    - A baseline room-air ABG should be performed routinely in patients with an FEV1 <40% or clinical signs suggesting respiratory failure and/or right heart failure.
    - A monitored exercise oxygen assessment may identify increased needs of supplemental oxygen with activity.
    - Patients with evidence of sleep-disordered breathing, and possibly those with severe to very severe COPD not using supplemental oxygen at rest, should undergo evaluation of oxygenation during sleep.
    - Patients receiving long-term oxygen therapy should undergo routine reevaluation at least once yearly, and more frequently in the setting of changing clinical conditions (e.g., during an exacerbation and about a month after an exacerbation).
  - Supplemental oxygen is prescribed based on PaO_2 or SpO_2 at rest, during sleep, and with exertion (Table 9-4).
    - Desaturation is more common during sleep in patients with COPD, and patients requiring supplemental oxygen during exertion often need it during sleep.
    - While the exact amount required nocturnally might be measured with home overnight pulse oximetry, it is reasonable to set the oxygen to be delivered during sleep as 1 L/min greater than that required during rest when awake.
  - The use of oxygen for patients who have isolated nocturnal or isolated exercise-induced desaturation remains controversial, with a lack of benefit in most studies.[15]

TABLE 9-4 INDICATIONS FOR LONG-TERM SUPPLEMENTAL OXYGEN ADMINISTRATION

Continuous Administration
Resting PaO_2 ≤55 mm Hg or arterial oxygen saturation (SaO_2) ≤88%
Resting PaO_2 of 56–59 mm Hg or SaO_2 ≤89%, if patient has polycythemia (Hct ≥55%) or evidence of cor pulmonale

Noncontinuous Administration (criteria for oxygen supplementation at rest not met)
PaO_2 ≤55 mm Hg or SaO_2 ≤88% during exertion[a]
PaO_2 ≤55 mm Hg or SaO_2 ≤88% during sleep[a]

[a]Use in this population has not been consistently associated with clinical benefit.

- Oxygen delivery systems
  - Continuous flow, dual-prong nasal cannula serves most patients regardless of activity level. Patients rarely require higher concentrations of oxygen, and in these cases, the use of a reservoir system with an oxymizer or high-flow nasal cannula may be most cost-effective.
  - In all cases, whenever an oxygen prescription is written, it should state the delivery system required (liquid, compressed gas, or concentrator), the delivery device required (e.g., nasal cannula), the required oxygen flow rates (liters per minute), and settings for rest, sleep, and exercise.
- **Pulmonary rehabilitation**
  - Exercise training is the foundation of pulmonary rehabilitation, and an exercise program may return a patient to a more functional and satisfactory life.
  - Pulmonary rehabilitation (as defined by the American Thoracic Society) is a multidisciplinary program of care for patients with chronic respiratory impairment that is individually tailored and designed to optimize physical and social performance and autonomy.
  - Patients with COPD who should be referred to a comprehensive rehabilitation program include those who have severe dyspnea despite optimal medical management, have reduced exercise tolerance, and experience a restriction in activities.
  - Pulmonary rehabilitation[16]
    - Improves exercise tolerance
    - Improves dyspnea
    - Improves quality of life
  - Pulmonary rehabilitation components include medical therapy, supplemental oxygen, exercise, education, psychosocial/behavioral intervention, and outcome assessment.
  - A cautious approach toward exercise is required for patients with conditions such as coronary artery disease or pulmonary hypertension.

Surgical Management
- Surgical options for the treatment of COPD include bullectomy, LVRS, and lung transplantation.

- **Bullectomy** in carefully selected patients with giant bullous disease may improve lung function and decrease symptoms.[17] Generally, patients with bullae that occupy at least 50% of the hemithorax with other areas of relatively preserved lung are the best candidates for bullectomy.
  - A chest CT scan helps to determine the location and the extent of emphysema.
- **LVRS** performed by experienced surgeons in appropriately selected patients can improve functioning and quality of life, and increase survival.[18]
  - Patients with predominantly upper lobe disease achieve the best results.
  - Target areas for resection consist of focal areas of emphysematous lung that are accessible to surgical resection.
  - Poor candidates for LVRS include patients with an FEV1 ≤20%, and either a very low DLCO or homogeneously distributed disease (without target areas).
  - **Endoscopic lung volume reductions via devices, biologic agents, or other approaches** continue to undergo evaluation, but surgical approach (i.e., LVRS) has shown the greatest efficacy.
- **Lung transplantation** may improve quality of life in patients and may confer a survival benefit in patients with very severe COPD.[19]
  - The International Society of Heart and Lung Transplantation (ISHLT) provides guidance regarding indications for lung transplantation.[20]
  - Patients with COPD and BODE (BMI, airway Obstruction by FEV1, Dyspnea by the Medical Research Council Dyspnea scale, and Exercise capacity by 6-minute walk distance) score of 7–10, low FEV1 (e.g., <25%), hypercapnia, pulmonary arterial hypertension, and severe clinical course may be appropriate for a transplant evaluation.
  - Lung transplantation is typically not an option for elderly patients (age >70–75 years) or those with significant comorbidities.

Lifestyle/Risk Modification

Smoking Cessation should be discussed with all smokers during every office visit and during hospitalizations (see Chapter 10, for details).

PROGNOSIS

- COPD causes significant morbidity and mortality.
- Worsened expiratory airflow obstruction has an increased risk of exacerbations and death.
- Previously treated exacerbations predict recurrent exacerbations.
- The BODE score[21] and other validated scoring systems classify COPD severity and predict mortality and other adverse outcomes.

REFERENCES

1. Global Initiative for Chronic Obstructive Lung Disease (GOLD). Global strategy for the diagnosis, management and prevention of COPD, updated 2024. Accessed April 8, 2024. https://goldcopd.org/2024-gold-report/
2. Carlson SA, Wheaton AG, Watson KB, Liu Y, Croft JB, Greenlund KJ. Geographic differences in sex-specific chronic obstructive pulmonary disease mortality rate trends among adults aged ≥25 years—United States, 1999–2019. *MMWR.* 2022;71:613–618.

3. Larsson C. Natural history and life expectancy in severe alpha1-antitrypsin deficiency, Pi Z. *Acta Medica Scandinavica.* 1978;204(5):345–351.
4. Lange P, Celli B, Agustí A, et al. Lung-function trajectories leading to chronic obstructive pulmonary disease. *NEJM.* 2015;373:111–122.
5. Steer J, Gibson J, Bourke SC. The DECAF Score: predicting hospital mortality in exacerbations of chronic obstructive pulmonary disease. *Thorax.* 2012;67:970–976.
6. de Jong YP, Uil SM, Grotjohan HP, Postma DS, Kerstjens HAM, van den Berg JWK. Oral or IV prednisolone in the treatment of COPD exacerbations: a randomized, controlled, double-blind study. *Chest.* 2007;132:1741–1747.
7. Leuppi JD, Schuetz P, Bingisser R, et al. Short-term vs conventional glucocorticoid therapy in acute exacerbations of chronic obstructive pulmonary disease: the REDUCE Randomized Clinical Trial. *JAMA.* 2013;309:2223–2231.
8. Murciano D, Auclair MH, Pariente R, Aubier M. A randomized, controlled trial of theophylline in patients with severe chronic obstructive pulmonary disease. *NEJM.* 1989;320(23):1521–1525.
9. Rabe KF, Martinez FJ, Ferguson GT, et al. Triple inhaled therapy at two glucocorticoid doses in moderate-to-very-severe COPD. *NEJM.* 2020;383:35–48.
10. Lipson DA, Barnhart F, Brealey N, et al. Once-daily single-inhaler triple versus dual therapy in patients with COPD. *NEJM.* 2018;378:1671–1680.
11. Kim DK, Bridges CB, Harriman KH. Advisory committee on immunization practices recommended immunization schedule for adults aged 19 years or older—United States, 2015. *MMWR.* 2015;64:91–92.
12. Rabe KF, Bateman ED, O'Donnell D, Witte S, Bredenbröker D, Bethke TD. Roflumilast—an oral anti-inflammatory treatment for chronic obstructive pulmonary disease: a randomised controlled trial. *Lancet.* 2005;366:563–571.
13. Seemungal TAR, Wilkinson TMA, Hurst JR, Perera WR, Sapsford RJ, Wedzicha JA. Long-term erythromycin therapy is associated with decreased chronic obstructive pulmonary disease exacerbations. *Am J Respir Crit Care Med.* 2008;178:1139–1147.
14. Long term domiciliary oxygen therapy in chronic hypoxic cor pulmonale complicating chronic bronchitis and emphysema. Report of the Medical Research Council Working Party. *Lancet.* 1981;1:681–686.
15. Albert RK, Au DH, Blackford AL, et al. A randomized trial of long-term oxygen for COPD with moderate desaturation. *NEJM.* 2016;375:1617–1627.
16. Casaburi R, ZuWallack R. Pulmonary rehabilitation for management of chronic obstructive pulmonary disease. *NEJM.* 2009;360:1329–1335.
17. Palla A, Desideri M, Rossi G, et al. Elective surgery for giant bullous emphysema: a 5-year clinical and functional follow-up. *Chest.* 2005;128:2043–2050.
18. Naunheim KS, Wood DE, Mohsenifar Z, et al. Long-term follow-up of patients receiving lung-volume-reduction surgery versus medical therapy for severe emphysema by the National Emphysema Treatment Trial Research Group. *Ann Thorac Surg.* 2006;82:431–443.
19. Lahzami S, Bridevaux PO, Soccal PM, et al. Survival impact of lung transplantation for COPD. *Eur Respir J.* 2010;36:74–80.
20. Leard LE, Holm AM, Valapour M, et al. Consensus document for the selection of lung transplant candidates: An update from the International Society for Heart and Lung Transplantation. *J Heart Lung Transplant.* 2021;40:1349–1379.
21. Celli BR, Cote CG, Marin JM, et al. The body-mass index, airflow obstruction, dyspnea, and exercise capacity index in chronic obstructive pulmonary disease. *NEJM.* 2004;350:1005–1012.

Tobacco and Inhalational Abuse

10

Zachary Lonjers

GENERAL PRINCIPLES

Epidemiology
- The prevalence of cigarette smoking exceeds 1 billion individuals worldwide and accounts for greater than 7 million deaths annually, including more than 400,000 deaths in the US.[1,2]
- In 2022, 22.7% of people in the US aged 12 and older reported using tobacco products or vaped nicotine in the month prior to being surveyed. This included more than 40 million individuals who smoked cigarettes and 23 million individuals who vaped nicotine.[3]
- Rates of smoking vary based on ethnicity, region, socioeconomic status, and education. Smoking rates are also higher among people with disabilities, substance use problems, mental health disorders, people with HIV/AIDS, and people insured by Medicaid.[4]
- Second- and third-hand smoke represent an underappreciated and definite risk to the household members of smokers and the general public.

Pathophysiology
- Nicotine stimulates acetylcholine receptors in the brain and activates the sympathetic nervous system, leading to elevated circulating levels of norepinephrine, epinephrine, vasopressin, growth hormone, cortisol, and endorphins. Nicotine also stimulates specific dopaminergic reward centers in the brain leading to its psychological addiction.[2] These result in increases in heart rate, blood pressure, cardiac stroke volume, and coronary blood flow.
- Other effects of nicotine use include arousal early in the day, relaxation during stressful situations, and an increased metabolic rate with reduced hunger leading to body weight reduction.
- Nicotine is addictive, and people become physiologically (and psychologically) dependent on its effects. People who quit experience withdrawal symptoms with the peak varying from 24 hours to 4 weeks after quitting. Withdrawal symptoms include anxiety, impatience, restlessness, irritability, hostility, difficulty concentrating, nicotine cravings, headaches, insomnia, depression, dysphoria, and hunger. Patients with a previous history of major depression, bipolar disorder, or alcohol and drug abuse may be especially susceptible to withdrawal and relapse.
- Psychological addiction can continue for months to years following quitting. Daily activities related to smoking such as eating, drinking, sex, being around other smokers, and driving can act as triggers for nicotine cravings.

Associated Conditions

- There are multiple known carcinogens in cigarette smoke, resulting in a high risk of lung, oral, esophageal, laryngeal, and urothelial cancers.[2]
- The risk of lung cancer increases in relation to the amount an individual smokes and the age at which he or she started smoking.
- Cigarette smoking alters immunity in the lung as well as the structure and function of the airways. Smokers have a lower forced expiratory volume over 1 second (FEV_1) and an accelerated rate of FEV_1 decline when compared with nonsmokers. Cigarette smoking has resulted in a high prevalence of chronic obstructive pulmonary disease (COPD). It is also an important trigger for asthma exacerbations.
- There is evidence that smoking contributes to vascular endothelial damage, coronary vasospasm, and increased platelet aggregation. Cigarette smoking is a known risk factor for coronary artery disease, hypertension, and stroke. Smoking also alters the senses of taste and smell.
- Smoking cessation mitigates some of these risks but does not decrease the risk to that of a lifelong nonsmoker.
- E-cigarette or vaping product use-associated lung injury (EVALI) was identified in 2019 as an emerging cause of acute lung injury. While the majority of cases were eventually associated with tetrahydrocannabinol (THC) and vitamin E acetate additives, it remains possible that nicotine or other compounds may be responsible or contributing.[5] The incidence has declined in subsequent years.

DIAGNOSIS

- Studies have shown that physicians often do not address tobacco use with their patients.[6,7] A variety of factors leading to this have been identified, including perceived lack of training and awareness of resources, frustration that patients continue to smoke despite the development of pulmonary disease, low expectations that patients will actually quit, and low reimbursements for time spent discussing smoking cessation.
- Clinicians can use the Modified Fagerström Test for Nicotine Dependence to grade patient's dependence.[8] Patients should be considered highly dependent on nicotine if they smoke >20 cigarettes per day, smoke their first cigarette of the day within 30 minutes of awakening, or if during a previous quit attempt, they developed strong cravings or withdrawal symptoms. Because nicotine is an addictive substance, patients can be expected to cycle through multiple periods of relapse and remission. Physicians should support each quit attempt as they would for patients in alcohol or drug rehabilitation.

Diagnostic Criteria

- The following steps, initially developed by the National Cancer Institute as the "Four A's" program, can be used in most outpatient settings to identify smokers and aid quitting. The Four A's have been expanded to the Five A's by the Clinical Practice Guidelines for Treating Tobacco Use and Dependence.[9]
- **Ask: Systematically identify all tobacco users at every visit.** Ask at every visit about smoking: *Do you smoke? Have you considered quitting? Are you ready to*

quit? What can I do to help you quit? Consider expanding documentation of vital signs to include tobacco use.
- **Advise: Strongly urge all tobacco users to quit** at every visit. The goal is to present compelling evidence about the importance of quitting and to educate the patient about methods for quitting and the help available. Clear, strong, and personalized advice based on the patient's health and his or her social situation works best. For example, tie tobacco use to current illness or if the patient lives with children, the adverse effects of smoking on children.
- **Assess: Determine willingness to make a quit attempt** by asking the patient to make a quit attempt at this time. If he or she is willing to try quitting, provide assistance and further information. Schedule a return visit to prepare a plan for smoking cessation. If the patient is not ready to quit, continue to educate him or her about the risks of smoking and offer to schedule a follow-up visit to continue the discussion. However, even among smokers who report no plans to quit, pharmacotherapy use has been associated with increased quit attempts, fewer cigarettes smoked, and greater abstinence rates.[6,10]
- **Assist: Aid the patient in quitting** with the development of a quit plan. Give consideration to drawing up a contract for the patient to sign in a similar fashion to a narcotics contract or asthma management plan. Discuss the patient's motivation for quitting and the benefits and drawbacks of quitting. Identify roadblocks to quitting and discuss strategies for overcoming these. Encourage the patient to discuss the plan with family and friends and enlist their support. Suggest the patient remove all tobacco-related products from the house as the quit date approaches.
  - The smoker may also want to avoid alcohol because it is a cue for many patients to smoke.
  - Initiating an exercise plan should be encouraged, with the goal being twofold: (a) occupying the patient's free time, leaving less time to smoke, and (b) helping avoid the weight gain associated with nicotine withdrawal. The average weight gain with smoking cessation is 2–3 kg, and it may be delayed by the use of pharmacologic agents.
  - Provide pharmacologic therapy after assessment of the individual's dependence and risk factors. Patients also benefit from counseling and/or scheduled follow-up. Most states have free telephone quit lines that patients can call for information and help with quitting. Encourage total abstinence as the ultimate goal but acknowledge that even cutting down the number of cigarettes by 50% has some benefits and may improve later quit success. Similarly, nicotine replacement, even for long periods, is considered safer than smoking.
  - With patients who have had previous failed quit attempts, the discussion should center on the reasons for the failure and developing strategies to cope with these problems. Common reasons for failure include withdrawal, cravings, stress, illness, and situational factors.
- **Arrange: Arrange follow-up visits** to confirm and maintain abstinence. The physician, a counselor, or even office staff can perform the follow-up. Focus on positive health benefits of cessation and congratulate the patient on quitting. Assess and treat withdrawal symptoms as needed. Educate patients about the numerous resources available to them to help them stay abstinent. If patients relapse, offer encouragement, discuss reasons for failure, and offer continued support.

TREATMENT

- Achieving smoking cessation centers around a combination of counseling and behavior modification, strong social support, a knowledgeable and motivated patient, and pharmacologic therapies.
- Although the medication labels and inserts caution against using multiple nicotine products concurrently, research has shown that agents can be used in combination safely and with greater efficacy.[11]
- While results of the best single or combination of agents have varied across meta-analyses and trials, recent clinical practice guidelines recommend the use of varenicline or a combination of nicotine replacement products (e.g., patch and a short-acting agent) for initial therapy.[6,12,13]
- Additional recommendations were recently published by the American Thoracic Society including[6]:
  - Use varenicline rather than a nicotine patch in isolation.
  - Use varenicline rather than bupropion.
  - Use varenicline rather than a nicotine patch in adults with a comorbid psychiatric condition.
  - Use varenicline and a nicotine patch in combination rather than varenicline alone.

Medications

Nicotine Replacement Therapy

- Nicotine replacement therapy (NRT) works via direct absorption into the circulation through the buccal mucosa, nasal mucosa, or skin. NRT should be considered for any smoker attempting cessation, though there is theoretical risk for use in individuals with unstable angina or at the time of an acute coronary event. There is, however, no significant increased cardiovascular risk in patients with clinically stable cardiovascular disease.[12]
- It has not been approved for use during pregnancy, but because circulatory levels are similar to or lower than those achieved by actual cigarette smoking, NRT should be safer than continued smoking.
- NRT may be used in a step-down method, but doing so may prolong the total duration of therapy. There is a low potential for dependence because blood nicotine levels achieved with any method of NRT are lower than levels achieved through cigarette smoking. NRT also does not produce tar or carbon monoxide, which are other substances linked to the ill effects of smoking.
- Underuse (not overuse) of NRT is a substantial problem that hinders quit success, and some research shows that smokers are more concerned about nicotine addiction than the harms of smoking. Health care professionals should inform patients of the relative harms.
- The recommended course of treatment varies by NRT product, but some people (especially heavy smokers) may benefit from longer periods and combinations of NRT until they are confident they will not relapse.
- In general, it is advised that patients start NRT on their quit date and not smoke while on NRT. However, some studies have shown positive effects of starting the patch prior to the quit date.[13] Patients using NRT should be encouraged not to give up if they relapse and have a cigarette. In these cases, the patient may benefit from a higher dose of NRT or a combination of products.

- Nicotine patch
    - There are two types of nicotine patches available: a 24-hour release form and a 16-hour release form. They are applied to the skin and changed every day over a total period of about 8–10 weeks. The maximum strength of the 24-hour patch is 21 mg, whereas the maximum strength of the 16-hour patch is 15 mg. Peak action is within 2–9 hours of application. The 21-mg patches are frequently used for 4–6 weeks followed by a short taper (14 mg/d for 2–4 weeks, then 7 mg/d for 2–4 weeks) to wean the patient off of the patches completely.
    - Advantages of the patch include convenience and a minimal need for instruction.
    - Disadvantages include pruritus or erythema at the application site and possible allergy to the adhesive. Alternative delivery methods should be considered in patients with eczema or skin conditions. Some patients also develop sleep disturbances, anxiety, appetite disturbances, rash, headache, nausea, vertigo, or dyspepsia.
    - The 24-hour patch is believed to be more effective against early morning urges but has also been associated with a greater incidence of sleep disturbances. Some of the side effects can be mitigated by removing the patch at bedtime or lowering the dose.
    - Six-month quit rates with the patch range from 22% to 42%, whereas permanent cessation rates range from 5–28%.
- **Nicotine gum and lozenges**
    - Nicotine gum was the first NRT approved for use in the US and is readily available over the counter. The gum is chewed briefly until a tingling sensation is noted, then is "parked" in the mouth against the buccal mucosa. The location of parked gum should be rotated regularly. Each piece of gum is used for about 30 minutes and the effects of the absorbed nicotine peak within 20–40 minutes. Individuals who smoke their first cigarette within 30 minutes of waking are recommended to use the 4 mg gum strength, and others should use the 2 mg strength. Maximum dosing recommendations are 24 pieces of either dose per day. It is suggested that patients start with a fixed dose (e.g., 1 piece every 1–2 hours while awake) for up to 6 weeks followed by a taper over the next 6 weeks, though extended use (e.g., greater than 12 weeks) is often used for a more durable effect.
    - The most obvious advantage of this method is that gum chewing is socially acceptable in most settings and the gum can be chewed whenever a patient has a craving.
    - The disadvantages include a higher level of instruction for proper use and difficulty of use for people with temporomandibular joint problems or dentures, or those who are edentulous. Other disadvantages include air swallowing, hiccups, indigestion, nausea, stomachache, burning sensation in the throat, and a sore jaw. The gum has also been noted to have a bad taste.
    - Because absorption of the nicotine is based on pH in the oral cavity, ingestion of coffee and carbonated beverages before use may lead to poor absorption. Food intake can also disrupt the absorption. Oftentimes people do not use the correct dosage or amount of the gum during the day to stave off cravings.

- Nicotine lozenges have a similar nicotine delivery system as the gum and dosing is similar. The lozenge should require less instruction than the gum, but has similar efficacy. Patients should not chew or swallow the lozenge, but allow it to dissolve completely in the mouth, which takes about 20–30 minutes. As with the gum, patients should move the lozenge around their mouth and "park" it occasionally.
- **Nicotine inhaler**
  - A nicotine inhaler consists of nicotine plugs inside hollow cigarette-like rods (a long cartridge). The nicotine levels peak in 10–15 minutes after inhalation. Although it is called an inhaler, 95% of the nicotine is absorbed in the mouth and esophagus, not in the lung. The usual dosing is 6–16 nicotine cartridges per day. One cartridge (10-mg nicotine) is used up after about 20 minutes of active puffing. The recommended initial duration of treatment is up to 12 weeks followed by a taper over 6–12 weeks.
  - This form of NRT may be especially effective for cravings because of the faster onset of action. It also satisfies the hand-to-mouth ritual of cigarette smoking.
  - Disadvantages of this method include awkwardness of using an inhaler in certain social settings, cough, and throat irritation.
  - Nicotine inhalers are currently available by prescription only.
- **Nicotine nasal spray**
  - The nasal spray most closely resembles the effects of actual cigarette smoking because of the high peak blood levels obtained and the rapid onset of action in 5–7 minutes. The levels of nicotine in the blood obtained with this method, although higher than other forms of NRT, are still lower than levels achieved with cigarette smoking. Dosing is 1 spray per nostril up to 2 times per hour, not to exceed 40 times per day. The recommended initial treatment is up to 12 weeks followed by a taper over 4–6 weeks.
  - The advantage of the nasal spray is that users are able to satisfy cravings rapidly.
  - The disadvantages include local irritation of the nose, eyes, and throat, as well as headache, burning sensation, sneezing, and watery eyes. Some patients are also embarrassed to use the spray in public. Rhinitis or nasal congestion may negatively affect absorption. Nicotine nasal spray should be avoided in patients with asthma.
  - Nicotine nasal sprays are currently available by prescription only.
- **Electronic cigarettes**
  - Electronic cigarettes are battery-powered devices that aerosolize nicotine for inhalation, either as a self-contained disposable device or with replaceable cartridges. They have not been approved by the Food and Drug Administration (FDA) for use as a smoking cessation aid and potential long-term risks of use are uncertain.
  - There have been limited studies assessing the efficacy of electronic cigarette use as pharmacologic therapy to assist with smoking cessation.[7] The current quality of evidence is uncertain, though some data suggest that varenicline may be more effective.
  - Other studies have shown increased abstinence rates with electronic cigarettes compared with the use of nicotine patches, but many individuals continued to use electronic cigarettes following the completion of these studies, reflecting a phenomenon of substitution rather than nicotine cessation.

Non-Nicotine Pharmacotherapies
- Varenicline and bupropion are considered first-line therapies, and both require a prescription and close physician monitoring.
  - **Varenicline**
    - Varenicline is a partial agonist of the nicotinic acetylcholine receptor. It helps reduce nicotine withdrawal symptoms, but also blocks nicotine binding, reducing the effects of exogenous nicotine that lead to the pleasurable effects of smoking and dependence.
    - A meta-analysis demonstrated that varenicline was associated with greater abstinence compared to bupropion or NRT alone, with similar outcomes compared to combination NRT.[14]
    - The starting dose of varenicline is 0.5 mg daily, increased to 0.5 mg twice daily on days 4–7, and finally increased to 1 mg twice daily until the end of treatment (generally 12 weeks, but can be extended up to 1 year).
    - Individuals may choose a fixed quit date, for example, on day 8 of therapy, or alternative approaches such as a flexible quit date after day 8 or with a plan for gradual reduction in smoking with a goal of cessation before 12 weeks.
    - Side effects include nausea, abnormal dreams, and insomnia. Prior concern for increased neuropsychiatric effects including suicidal ideation and behaviors were not observed with increased frequency in a postmarketing trial,[15] leading the FDA to remove its boxed warning in 2016. Similarly, concerns for increased cardiovascular events have not been substantiated in subsequent studies, with continued smoking likely outweighing risks in individuals with high-risk cardiovascular disease.[12]
    - Current guidelines recommend the use of varenicline in combination with NRT.[6]
    - Varenicline is FDA pregnancy category C and not recommended for use in pregnant patients.
  - **Bupropion**
    - The effectiveness of bupropion in smoking cessation is believed to be related to the dopaminergic and noradrenergic effects of the drug. The noradrenergic modifications may limit nicotine withdrawal symptoms, while the dopaminergic modulation may affect areas of the brain that are involved with the reinforcing properties of addictive drugs such as nicotine.
    - Bupropion has been shown to be an effective agent to assist with smoking cessation, but studies have shown it to be inferior to varenicline or combination NRT.[6]
    - The starting dose is 150 mg daily for 3 days and then increased to 150 mg twice daily, with a quit date the following week. It is generally used for 12 weeks but may be extended for up to 1 year. Although approved at higher doses for use as an antidepressant, 300 mg daily is the maximum dose indicated for smoking cessation.
    - Side effects include insomnia, dry mouth, nervousness, difficulty concentrating, rash, and constipation.
    - It is contraindicated in patients with a seizure history, as it lowers the seizure threshold, and it should not be used by patients with anorexia nervosa or bulimia nervosa, patients undergoing alcohol withdrawal, or patients who have used an monoamine oxidase inhibitors (MAOI) in the previous 2 weeks.

- There were previous concerns for neuropsychiatric side effects observed in postmarketing case reports, but this risk was not substantiated in the same randomized trial described above with varenicline, and its boxed warning was removed.[15]
- Bupropion is in pregnancy category B, and while efficacy studies are limited, it can be used to assist with smoking cessation during pregnancy.
- Other therapies include:
  - **Tricyclic antidepressants** have been investigated and have shown modest results. Side effects include dry mouth and sedation. Currently, bupropion remains the only antidepressant that has been approved for smoking cessation, however.
  - **Anxiolytics** such as **benzodiazepines and buspirone** have been used in patients with increased anxiety symptoms during smoking cessation attempts. Although there is no proven benefit for the use of these drugs in smoking cessation, they may be helpful in selected individuals.
  - Some physicians have tried to diminish withdrawal symptoms with **clonidine**. There is little evidence to support this use, however.
  - There is no convincing evidence that **naloxone or naltrexone** is effective in smoking cessation.

Other Nonpharmacologic Therapies

- **Behavioral counseling**
  - Nonpharmacologic therapies are a helpful adjunct to medical therapy, and there is ample evidence that counseling improves a patient's chance of quitting.[2] Most studies of smoking cessation have a counseling component or, at the very minimum, regular appointments with counselors or clinicians to reinforce and remind patients of their goal to quit.
  - Counseling and support are now available through a variety of media and locations based on patient preference.
  - Any amount of counseling is known to be effective, even if it is simply a physician advising a smoker to quit. Brief interventions by physicians, often no longer than 3–10 minutes, can increase cessation rates.
  - There is a dose–response relationship between counseling intensity and effectiveness. High-intensity counseling lasting greater than 20 minutes or at more than 2 visits is more effective than brief interventions.
  - The components of successful smoking cessation counseling are variable and center mostly on cognitive behavioral therapy. This includes self-monitoring and awareness of personal cues and patterns that encourage smoking and how to avoid them. Relapse prevention can also be important. For example, some patients may need to avoid going to bars or drinking alcoholic beverages if such activities trigger a relapse to smoking. Avoiding other smokers may also be helpful.
  - Smoking cessation groups are often organized by hospitals or workplaces with the assistance of the American Lung Association. They allow smokers to share their difficulties in a group setting. Most states have telephone quit lines that patients can call at any time to obtain assistance with quitting.
  - Several web-based resources are available including www.becomeanex.org,[16] www.freedomfromsmoking.org,[17] and www.smokefree.gov.[18]

- Telephone quit lines are another established option, with 1-800-QUITNOW functioning as a national portal to state-specific resources.
- Hospitalized smokers provide a unique opportunity for aggressive inpatient counseling by medical personnel. Most US medical campuses are now smoke-free. Patients can be closely monitored for nicotine withdrawal side effects. NRT can be instrumental in the hospital and should be offered to patients by admitting physicians.
- **Alternative therapies**
  - Other aids that are used commercially, but are unproven, include hypnosis, auricular therapy, acupuncture or acupressure, biofeedback, relaxation or meditation, herbal remedies, teas, or supplements.
  - Nicotine fading involves gradual decreases in the amount of tobacco used or switching to lower nicotine cigarettes. This may be beneficial to some individuals, including prior to a more firm quit date.

MONITORING/FOLLOW-UP

- Nicotine affects the metabolism of several medications including warfarin, heparin, antipsychotics, and theophylline, and physicians should carefully review the medication list of patients who are quitting or have recently quit.
- For previous smokers who quit in the distant past, no further intervention is needed. Individuals should, however, be congratulated on their achievements.
- For smokers who quit within the past year, reinforcement is given along with reeducation on the benefits of having quit. Discuss any problems that they may have encountered and possible solutions. Again, congratulations are in order.

PROGNOSIS

- Many of the health risks of tobacco use are reduced upon cessation.
- The risk of smoking relapse remains high and physicians should understand about relapses. Physicians and patients need to evaluate the causes for relapse and reinforce the importance of trying to quit again.

REFERENCES

1. GBD 2019 Tobacco Collaborators. Spatial, temporal, and demographic patterns in prevalence of smoking tobacco use and attributable disease burden in 204 countries and territories, 1990–2019: a systematic analysis from the Global Burden of Disease Study 2019. *Lancet.* 2021;397:2337–2360.
2. U.S. Department of Health and Human Services. *Smoking Cessation. A Report of the Surgeon General.* U.S. Department of Health and Human Services, Centers for Disease Control and Prevention, National Center for Chronic Disease Prevention and Health Promotion, Office on Smoking and Health; 2020.
3. Substance Abuse and Mental Health Services Administration. *Key Substance Use and Mental Health Indicators in the United States: Results from the 2022 National Survey on Drug Use and Health.* Center for Behavioral Health Statistics and Quality, Substance Abuse and Mental Health Services Administration; 2023.
4. Brossart L, Moreland-Russell S, Andersen S, et al. *Best Practices User Guides: Health Equity in Tobacco Prevention and Control.* Center for Public Health Systems Science; 2015. Last accessed May 31, 2024. https://www.cdc.gov/tobacco/stateandcommunity/guides/pdfs/bp-health-equity.pdf

5. Layden JE, Ghinai I, Pray I, et al. Pulmonary illness related to E-cigarette use in Illinois and Wisconsin—final report. *N Engl J Med.* 2020;382:903–916.
6. Leone FT, Zhang Y, Evers-Casey S, et al. Initiating pharmacologic treatment in tobacco-dependent adults: an Official American Thoracic Society Clinical Practice Guideline. *Am J Respir Crit Care Med.* 2020;202:e5–e31.
7. van Eerd EAM, Bech Risør M, Spigt M, et al. Why do physicians lack engagement with smoking cessation treatment in their COPD patients? A multinational qualitative study. *NPJ Prim Care Respir Med.* 2017;27:41.
8. Heatherton TF, Kozlowski LT, Frecker RC, Fagerström KO. The Fagerström test for nicotine dependence: a revision of the Fagerström Tolerance Questionnaire. *Br J Addict.* 1991;86:1119–1127.
9. Fiore MC, Bailey WC, Cohen SJ, et al. *Treating Tobacco Use and Dependence. Quick Reference Guide for Clinicians.* US Department of Health and Human Services; 2000.
10. Hughes JR, Rennard SI, Fingar JR, Talbot SK, Callas PW, Fagerstrom KO. Efficacy of varenicline to prompt quit attempts in smokers not currently trying to quit: a randomized placebo-controlled trial. *Nicotine Tob Res.* 2011;13:955–964.
11. Zapawa LM, Hughes JR, Benowitz NL, Rigotti NA, Shiffman S. Cautions and warnings on the US OTC label for nicotine replacement: what's a doctor to do? *Addict Behav.* 2011;36:327–332.
12. Barua RS, Rigotti NA, Benowitz NL, et al. 2018 ACC Expert consensus decision pathway on tobacco cessation treatment: a report of the American College of Cardiology Task Force on Clinical Expert Consensus Documents. *J Am Coll Cardiol.* 2018;72:3332–3365.
13. Theodoulou A, Chepkin SC, Ye W, et al. Different doses, durations and modes of delivery of nicotine replacement therapy for smoking cessation. *Cochrane Database Syst Rev.* 2023;6:CD013308.
14. Livingstone-Banks J, Fanshawe TR, Thomas KH, et al. Nicotine receptor partial agonists for smoking cessation. *Cochrane Database Syst Rev.* 2023;5:CD006103.
15. Anthenelli RM, Benowitz NL, West R, et al. Neuropsychiatric safety and efficacy of varenicline, bupropion, and nicotine patch in smokers with and without psychiatric disorders (EAGLES): a double-blind, randomised, placebo-controlled clinical trial. *Lancet.* 2016;387:2507–2520.
16. EX. The Go-To Guide on Your Quitting Journey. 2024. Accessed May 31, 2024. www.becomeanex.org
17. American Lung Association. 2023. Accessed May 31, 2024. www.freedomfromsmoking.org
18. National Cancer Institute. Accessed May 31, 2024. www.smokefree.gov

Community-Acquired Pneumonia

11

Samuel Windham

GENERAL PRINCIPLES

- Community-acquired pneumonia (CAP) is a significant cause of morbidity and mortality in the US.
- CAP is estimated to cause over 1.5 million hospitalizations annually.[1]
  - Although dependent on patient setting and patient comorbidities, CAP is associated with ~100,000 deaths during hospitalization annually.
  - One in three patients admitted for CAP will die within 1 year of admission.
- Administration of appropriate antimicrobials and management for severe pneumonia have a significant benefit on patient survival.
  - ~50% of CAP will have no causative organism identified.
  - Resistance to antimicrobials is common.
- The most widely recognized guidelines for the treatment of CAP include those of the American Thoracic Society (ATS), the Infectious Diseases Society of America (IDSA), the Canadian Infectious Disease Society, and Canadian Thoracic Society.

Definition

- CAP is a primary infection of lung parenchyma. Bacterial or viral invasion causes inflammation and alveolar infiltration that result in focal consolidation.
- CAP is distinctive from hospital-acquired pneumonia (HAP) in that the infection is acquired in the community. The term health care–associated pneumonia (HCAP) is no longer used due to lack of association with outcomes or presence of resistant organisms.

Classification

- Typical bacterial: *Streptococcus pneumoniae, Staphylococcus aureus, Haemophilus influenzae,* Group A streptococci, *Moraxella catarrhalis,* mixed anaerobes (aspiration), and aerobic gram-negative organisms.
- Atypical bacterial: *Legionella pneumophila, Mycoplasma pneumoniae, Chlamydophila pneumoniae.*
- Viral: Influenza A and B, respiratory syncytial virus (RSV), severe acute respiratory syndrome coronavirus 2 (SARS-CoV-2) adenovirus, rhinoviruses, rubeola, varicella.

Epidemiology

- Pneumonia and influenza combine to be the ninth leading cause of death in the US in 2019.
- In 2019, there were over 49,000 deaths due to pneumonia and influenza. The rate of deaths due to pneumonia is decreasing.

- Pneumonia is more common in the winter months and in the elderly population.
- Men and African Americans are slightly more affected than women and Caucasians.[2]

Etiology
- The most common etiology for CAP is *S. pneumoniae*, followed by *H. influenzae*, then influenza virus.
- Frequently, pneumonia is preceded by an upper airway infection or viral illness.
- The two most frequently encountered resistant organisms requiring targeted therapy in CAP are methicillin-resistant *Staphylococcus aureus* (MRSA) and *Pseudomonas aeruginosa* (PsA).

Pathophysiology
- Lobar pneumonia is characterized by consolidation of a large portion of lung. Consolidation of airspaces is caused by host inflammatory infiltration in response to bacterial infection of lung tissue.
- Bronchopneumonia similarly involves acute inflammation, but the consolidated areas are patchy and often multilobar or bilateral. This pattern is more common to atypical viral pneumonias or mycoplasma pneumonias.

Risk Factors
- Predisposing comorbid conditions: chronic obstructive pulmonary disease (COPD), heart failure, chronic renal disease.
- Host factors: advanced age, tobacco use, prior history of pneumonia, recent viral respiratory infection.
- Immunosuppressed states: HIV infection, chemotherapy, solid organ and stem cell transplant recipients.
- Mechanical: dysphagia, lung cancer, mechanical obstruction of bronchus, hiatal hernia, radiation esophagitis.
- Aspiration risk factors: alcoholism and drug intoxication, altered mental status, seizure disorder, stroke, procedural sedation, and anesthesia.
- Mucus clearance: cystic fibrosis, Kartagener syndrome, immotile cilia syndrome.

Prevention
Prevention should include major risk factor modifications such as smoking cessation, vaccination against influenza and pneumococcus, and maintaining oral health.

DIAGNOSIS

The gold standard for diagnosis of pneumonia is a two-view (posteroanterior and lateral) CXR demonstrating a new pulmonary opacity. Clinical signs and symptoms should correlate with active infection and pulmonic consolidation.

Clinical Presentation
- Patients may experience fever, chills, productive cough, shortness of breath, and chest pain.
- Physical examination findings may include fever, tachypnea, tachycardia, abnormal breath sounds including rhonchi or crackles, increased tactile fremitus, dullness to percussion, and reduced chest movement.

Differential Diagnosis
- The differential diagnosis for pneumonia includes pathology that causes radiographic consolidations that can mimic pneumonia. These include acute heart failure exacerbation and other causes of pulmonary edema, malignancy, pulmonary embolism (PE) with infarct, septic embolism, and foreign body aspiration with lobar collapse.
- Multiple different bacteria, viruses, and fungi can cause acute pneumonia.

Diagnostic Testing
- Previously, the primary objective of diagnostic testing was to identify a causative agent.
- More recent literature has shown that only certain subpopulations of CAP patients may benefit from undergoing testing to identify a causative organism.[3]
- Current guidelines recommend evaluating for causative organisms via respiratory secretion culture and/or blood cultures in only select subpopulations of CAP.
  - IDSA/ATS severe CAP criteria (see Table 11-1).[3]
  - Patients with a history of hospitalization and receipt of parenteral antibiotics in the last 90 days.
  - Patients with a history of previously positive culture or polymerase chain reaction (PCR) for MRSA or PsA.
  - Patients who are being treated empirically for MRSA or PsA to potentially de-escalate therapy.

TABLE 11-1 INFECTIOUS DISEASES SOCIETY OF AMERICA/AMERICAN THORACIC SOCIETY CRITERIA FOR DEFINING SEVERE COMMUNITY-ACQUIRED PNEUMONIA

Criteria for Determining Severity of CAP (ICU Admit is Recommended for Patients with ≥1 Major Criteria or ≥3 Minor Criteria)

Major criteria
Invasive mechanical ventilation
Septic shock with the need for vasopressors

Minor criteria
Respiratory rate ≥30 breaths/min
PaO_2/FiO_2 ratio ≤250
Multilobar infiltrates
Confusion/disorientation
Uremia (BUN >20 mg/dL)
Leukopenia (white blood cell [WBC] count <4,000 cells/mm^3)
Thrombocytopenia (platelet count <100,000 cells/mm^3)
Hypothermia (core temperature <36 °C)
Hypotension requiring aggressive fluid resuscitation

Reproduced with permission from Metlay JP, Waterer GW, Long AC, et al. Diagnosis and treatment of adults with community-acquired pneumonia. An Official Clinical Practice Guideline of the American Thoracic Society and Infectious Diseases Society of America. *Am J Respir Crit Care Med.* 2019;200:e45–e67.

Laboratories
- Initial inpatient and outpatient studies should include complete blood count (CBC) with differential, basic metabolic profile (BMP), and liver function tests (LFTs).
- Blood cultures are positive in ~9% of hospitalized patients.[3]
- Blood cultures and sputum cultures are recommended by guidelines only in the subpopulations listed above.
- HIV testing should be considered.
- Urine studies such as urine pneumococcal and *Legionella* antigen assays can assist in microbe identification but have not been shown to influence outcomes and are recommended only in severe CAP.
- For patients with suspected influenza or COVID-19, nasopharyngeal viral culture and immunofluorescence, or PCR should be obtained. For *M. pneumonia*, PCR or serology can aid in diagnosis.
- The appropriate use of procalcitonin remains controversial. It is not recommended to utilize procalcitonin as it has not been consistently shown to be reliable indicator of bacterial infection.

Imaging
- Two-view CXR is the imaging study of choice. Pneumonic infiltrates can develop after volume resuscitation in volume-depleted patients.
- CT is not required for the diagnosis of pneumonia.
- CT should be performed when clinical symptoms do not suggest infection as the cause of radiographic infiltrate (e.g., malignancy). CT can also be used to evaluate empyema, cavitary disease, interstitial lung disease, and in patients who fail to respond to antibiotics.

Diagnostic Procedures
- Invasive diagnostic procedures such as bronchoscopy and bronchoalveolar lavage are rarely required but can be of use in nonresponders, critically ill patients, or immunocompromised hosts.
- Diagnostic thoracentesis should be performed for pleural effusions with adequate ultrasound windows. Sampling of fluid helps rule out empyema, which would require tube thoracostomy. Pleural fluid testing should include cell count and differential, protein, lactate dehydrogenase, pH, glucose, Gram stain, and culture.
- Tracheal aspiration should be performed on patients requiring intubation.

TREATMENT

- Care should be triaged to inpatient versus outpatient treatment. Patients should also be evaluated for severity of illness, for example, patients requiring ICU admission versus admission to a medical floor.
- The Pneumonia Severity Index (PSI or PORT Score) is preferred over CURB-65.[4]
- Medical and psychosocial issues like poor oral intake, cognitive impairment, or impaired functional status should also play a role in determining inpatient versus outpatient therapy.

Medications
- **Outpatient, previously healthy**[3]
  - Amoxicillin 1 g PO tid PLUS
  - Doxycycline 100 mg PO bid OR
  - Macrolide (NOTE: Do not use if local pneumococcal macrolide resistance rates >25%)
    - Azithromycin 500 mg PO × 1, then 250 mg PO daily × 4 days
    - Clarithromycin 500 mg PO bid or clarithromycin XL 1000 mg PO daily
    - Erythromycin 250–500 mg PO q6h
- **Outpatient with comorbidities**[3] (e.g., heart/lung/liver/renal disease, diabetes, alcoholism, malignancy, asplenia, immunosuppressed, prior use of antibiotics)
  - Respiratory quinolone (any of the following) **OR**
    - Levofloxacin 750 mg PO daily
    - Moxifloxacin 400 mg PO daily
  - β-Lactam (any of the following) **PLUS** macrolide **OR** doxycycline
    - Amoxicillin 1 g PO tid
    - Amoxicillin-clavulanate 875 mg/125 mg PO bid
    - Cefpodoxime 200 mg PO bid
    - Cefuroxime 500 mg PO bid
- **Inpatient therapy nonsevere**[3] (see Figure 11-1)
  - Respiratory quinolone (any of the following) **OR**
    - Levofloxacin 750 mg IV daily
    - Moxifloxacin 400 mg IV daily

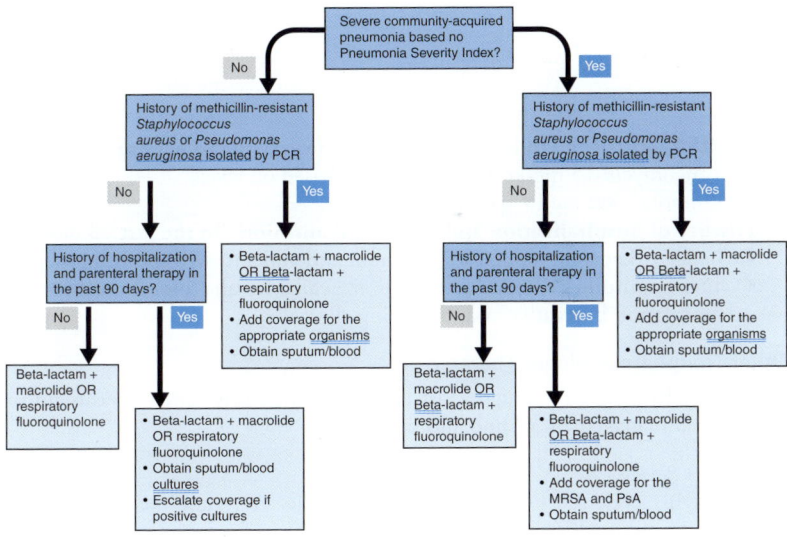

Figure 11-1 Empiric therapy for inpatient community-acquired pneumonia.

- β-Lactam (any of the following) **PLUS** macrolide (e.g., azithromycin 500 mg IV daily) **OR** doxycycline 100–200 mg IV bid
  - Cefotaxime 1 g IV q8h
  - Ceftriaxone 1 g IV q24h
  - Ampicillin/sulbactam 3 g IV q6h
  - Ertapenem 1 g IV q24h
- **History of MRSA or PsA isolated by PCR or culture:**
  - **PsA (any of the following):**
    - Piperacillin-tazobactam 4.5 g IV q6h
    - Cefepime 2 g IV q8h
    - Ceftazidime 2 g IV q8h
    - Imipenem 500 mg IV q6h
    - Meropenem 1 g IV q8h
    - Aztreonam 2 g IV q8h
  - **MRSA (any of the following):**
    - Vancomycin 15 mg/kg IV q12 h, adjust based on levels
    - Linezolid 600 mg IV q12h
- **History of hospitalization and parenteral antibiotic in the last 90 days**
  - Obtain sputum, MRSA nares PCR if available, and blood cultures.
  - Escalate to above mentioned targeted therapy if cultures are positive.
- **Inpatient therapy severe**[3] (see Figure 11-1)
  - IV β-lactam **PLUS**
  - IV respiratory quinolone **OR** IV azithromycin
  - **History of MRSA or PsA isolated by PCR or culture**
    - **PsA (any of the following) in place of other β-Lactam**
      - Piperacillin-tazobactam 4.5 g IV q6h
      - Cefepime 2 g IV q8h
      - Ceftazidime 2 g IV q8h
      - Imipenem 500 mg IV q6h
      - Meropenem 1 g IV q8h
      - Aztreonam 2 g IV q8h
    - **MRSA (any of the following) in conjunction with β-Lactam:**
      - Vancomycin 15 mg/kg IV q12h, adjust based on levels
      - Linezolid 600 mg IV q12h
  - **History of hospitalization and parenteral antibiotic in the last 90 days**
    - Change β-Lactam to anti-PsA β-Lactam and add anti-MRSA antibiotic.
    - Obtain sputum, MRSA nares PCR if available, and blood cultures for de-escalation if negative and improving clinically.

Other Nonpharmacologic Therapies

Pulmonary hygiene with cough assist devices or chest physiotherapy can aid in the medical management of pneumonia.

Steroids for Severe CAP
- Steroids in severe CAP is a controversial topic. A recent meta-analysis of 16 trials found no difference in all-cause mortality with corticosteroids though did find a significantly lower risk for progression to need for mechanical ventilation.[5]

- A subsequent randomized controlled trial of hydrocortisone in severe CAP showed a significant decrease in 28-day mortality in the hydrocortisone group.[6] There were no significant differences in hospital-acquired infections or gastrointestinal bleeding in the treatment arm.
- Given that the meta-analysis showed a plausible mechanism for decreasing mortality, a decreased need for intubation, and the mortality benefit seen in the RCT, the use of hydrocortisone should be considered in severe CAP.
- **Steroids for severe CAP**
  - Hydrocortisone 200 mg daily divided in two or four doses.
  - Duration of 4 days that can be extended to 7 days if no clinical improvement.
  - Taper steroids for total of 8–14 days.

Duration of Antimicrobial Therapy

- Minimum duration should be 5 days with current recommendations for 7 days for suspected or proven MRSA or PsA.
- Antibiotics should not be tapered until the patient has been afebrile for 48–72 hours, symptoms are improving, and the white blood cell (WBC) count is decreasing.
- Patients may be switched to oral antibiotics once improvement is noted clinically and they are stable enough to take oral medicines.

Surgical Management

- If present, an empyema should be drained with thoracostomy tube placement.
- Drainage of lung abscess is controversial. Chest physiotherapy should be used to promote natural expectoration. Complications of percutaneous or surgical drainage can include bronchopleural fistula and pneumothorax.

MONITORING/FOLLOW-UP

- Infiltrate on CXR will persist longer than clinical symptoms of pneumonia.
- Routine follow-up CXR is not recommended. However, there is evidence to suggest that follow-up radiography in select groups (e.g., >50 years old, tobacco users) may reveal other diagnoses including malignancy.[7,8]

OUTCOME/PROGNOSIS

- Treatment failure
  - Occurs in 10–15% of cases, and mortality is increased nearly fivefold in some studies.[9]
  - It is important to distinguish clinical deterioration from failure in symptomatic improvement.
- Clinical deterioration
  - Within 72 hours: typically resistant organisms, alternate diagnosis (consider PE, acute respiratory distress syndrome [ARDS], pulmonary vasculitis syndromes, polymicrobial infection due to aspiration), severe illness, and natural progression of disease to respiratory and/or multiorgan failure.
  - After 72 hours: nosocomial infections, severe comorbid conditions, PE, myocardial infarction (MI), renal failure.

- Failure in symptomatic improvement
  - Within 72 hours: typically normal response.
  - After 72 hours: resistant organisms or inappropriate antibiotic selection, local complications (parapneumonic effusion or empyema), alternate diagnosis (pulmonary edema, malignancy, vasculitis, PE), drug fevers.
- Patients with CAP that do not improve with standard-of-care therapy or with recurrent episodes of CAP should be tested for dimorphic fungi (*blastomyces*, *histoplasma*, and *coccidioides*) via urine antigen regardless of geographic location, as global warming and travel have changed the epidemiology of these organisms.[10]
- Overall mortality from pneumonia ranges based on severity of disease and host factors. In one meta-analysis, mortality ranged from 5.1% in hospitalized and ambulatory patients to 36.5% in patients requiring ICU care.[11]

REFERENCES

1. Ramirez JA, Wiemken TL, Peyrani P, et al; University of Louisville Pneumonia Study Group. Adults hospitalized with pneumonia in the United States: incidence, epidemiology, and mortality. *Clin Infect Dis.* 2017;65:1806–1812.
2. Xu J, Murphy SL, Kochanek KD, Arias E. Deaths: final data for 2019. *Natl Vital Stat Rep.* 2021. Accessed August 27, 2024. https://www.cdc.gov/nchs/data/nvsr70/nvsr70-08-508.pdf
3. Metlay JP, Waterer GW, Long AC, et al. Diagnosis and treatment of adults with community-acquired pneumonia. An official clinical practice guideline of the American Thoracic Society and Infectious Diseases Society of America. *Am J Respir Crit Care Med.* 2019;200:e45–e67.
4. Aujesky D, Auble TE, Yealy DM, et al. Prospective comparison of three validated prediction rules for prognosis in community-acquired pneumonia. *Am J Med.* 2005;118:384–392.
5. Saleem N, Kulkarni A, Snow TAC, Ambler G, Singer M, Arulkumaran N. Effect of corticosteroids on mortality and clinical cure in community-acquired pneumonia: a systematic review, meta-analysis, and meta-regression of randomized controlled trials. *Chest.* 2023;163:484–497.
6. Dequin PF, Meziani F, Quenot JP, et al; CRICS-TriGGERSep Network. Hydrocortisone in severe community-acquired pneumonia. *N Engl J Med.* 2023;388:1931–1941.
7. Tang KL, Eurich DT, Minhas-Sandhu JK, Marrie TJ, Majumdar SR. Incidence, correlates, and chest radiographic yield of new lung cancer diagnosis in 3398 patients with pneumonia. *Arch Intern Med.* 2011;171:1193–1198.
8. Little BP, Gilman MD, Humphrey KL, et al. Outcome of recommendations for radiographic follow-up of pneumonia on outpatient chest radiography. *Am J Roentgenol.* 2014;202:54–59.
9. Menendez R, Torres A. Treatment failure in community-acquired pneumonia. *Chest.* 2007;132:1348–1355.
10. Mazi PB, Sahrmann JM, Olsen MA, et al. The Geographic distribution of dimorphic mycoses in the United States for the modern era. *Clin Infect Dis.* 2023;76:1295–1301.
11. Fine MJ, Smith MA, Carson CA. Prognosis and outcomes of patients with community acquired pneumonia: a meta-analysis. *JAMA.* 1996;275:134–141.

Nosocomial Pneumonia

M. Cristina Vazquez Guillamet and Marin H. Kollef

GENERAL PRINCIPLES

Definition
- Nosocomial pneumonia (NP) occurs in patients in the hospital and those with recent contact with the health care system.[1,2]
- Patients with NP are at risk for infection with different organisms than those presenting with community-acquired pneumonia (CAP).

Classification
Patients with NP are classified as:

- **Hospital-acquired pneumonia (HAP)** is pneumonia occurring greater than 48 hours after admission to the hospital.
- **Ventilated hospital–acquired pneumonia (vHAP)** is HAP that decompensates requiring tracheal intubation and mechanical ventilation.
- **Ventilator-acquired pneumonia (VAP)** is pneumonia occurring greater than 48 hours after intubation of the trachea and initiation of mechanical ventilation.
- **Health care–associated pneumonia (HCAP)** is pneumonia in patients presenting from the community with the following risk factors:
  - **Original criteria derived from risk factors for health care–associated bacteremia with a resistant pathogen:**
    - Hospitalization for 2 or more days in an acute care facility within 90 days of infection
    - Presentation from a nursing home or long-term care facility
    - Attending a hospital or hemodialysis clinic
    - Receiving intravenous antibiotic therapy, chemotherapy, or wound care within 30 days of infection
    - Family member with multidrug-resistant pathogen
  - **Pneumonia–specific risk factors**
    - Recent hospitalization (within 90 days) for ≥2 days or recent antibiotic use
    - Immunosuppression
    - Nonambulatory status
    - Tube feeds
    - Use of gastric acid–suppressive agents
  - Although the term HCAP is controversial and some guidelines recommend against its use as it may lead to overly broad antibiotic use, it helps to highlight community-onset patients with pneumonia who may be at risk for infection with more antibiotic-resistant nosocomial pathogens. Understanding local risk factors for presence of infection with such pathogens is crucial in clinical decision making.[3]

Epidemiology

- NP is the most clinically significant hospital-acquired infection and the leading cause of death from all nosocomial infections.
- There has been a rise in hospital-associated infections, including NP, due to antibiotic-resistant bacteria resulting in greater patient morbidity and mortality.
- Inappropriate initial antibiotic treatment (i.e., antimicrobial regimens not active against the offending pathogens) of NP increases the risk of hospital mortality and may also predispose to the emergence of antibiotic-resistant bacteria.
- Patients with **HAP** and **HCAP** have mortality rates of 15–20%, which is significantly worse than patients with CAP.[4–6]
- **VAP** appears to be an independent determinant of mortality in critically ill patients requiring mechanical ventilation, and mortality rates range from 25–50% in different series.[4–6]
- **vHAP** is associated with a greater mortality compared to both **HAP** and **VAP**. This may partly be related to delays in the administration of effective antibiotic therapy for patients with **HAP** that transitions to **vHAP**.[7,8]
- However, patients who develop VAP have a higher severity of illness and have longer ICU and hospital stays.[6]
- In an analysis of 4,479 patients from a multicenter database, using a model taking into account severity of illness and other confounding factors, the 30-day attributable mortality for VAP was 4.4%.[9]
- More importantly, emerging clinical data suggest that the application of new management strategies for the prevention and treatment of VAP could result in improved patient outcomes.
- However, the recent SARS-CoV-2 pandemic saw higher rates of all NPs largely due to more prolonged durations of mechanical ventilation and greater patient exposure to empiric courses of broad-spectrum antibiotics.

Etiology

- Infectious organisms that commonly result in NP are generally different from those that are most commonly associated with CAP.
- HAP can be divided into early- and late-onset infections. However, this distinction may not be clinically relevant in areas where significant numbers of patients enter the hospital already having risk factors for infection with antibiotic-resistant bacteria. Understanding local pathogen predominance and patient mix is crucial to ensure that early appropriate antibiotic therapy is administered in a timely manner.
- **Early-onset HAP** occurs between days 2–4 of hospitalization.
  - These infections are more often due to common community-acquired pathogens such as *Streptococcus pneumoniae*, methicillin-sensitive *Staphylococcus aureus*, and *Haemophilus influenza*, unless the patient has risk factor for antibiotic resistance or local epidemiology indicates otherwise.
  - Specific risk factors have been associated with certain pathogens. Aspiration has been associated with mouth anaerobes, gram-negative enteric bacilli, and *S. aureus*.
- **Late-onset HAP** occurs after **4 days** of hospitalization. It is associated with more antibiotic-resistant and potentially more virulent organisms such as methicillin-resistant *S. aureus*, *Pseudomonas aeruginosa*, and *Acinetobacter* species.[10]

- In certain areas of the world, including Asia and parts of Europe, antimicrobial resistance is common and increasing, including in the community setting.
- In one large, international study of HAP and VAP, multidrug-resistance rates for *Acinetobacter* species and *P. aeruginosa* were 82.0% and 42.8% respectively. Extensively drug-resistance rates were 51.1% and 4.9%.[11]
- Patients with HCAP may be at risk for infection with the same organisms that are responsible for late-onset HAP depending on local epidemiology.

Pathophysiology
- The pathogenesis of HAP and VAP is linked to two separate but related processes:
  - **Colonization of the aerodigestive tract** with pathogenic organisms, and
  - **Aspiration** of contaminated secretions.
- The most common **sources of NP pathogens** are:
  - Microaspiration of oropharyngeal secretions
  - Aspiration of esophageal/gastric contents
  - Inhalation of infected aerosols
  - Hematogenous spread from distant infection
  - Exogenous penetration from the pleural space
  - Direct inoculation (e.g., resulting from intubation)
- Bacterial colonization of the oropharynx is universal, and *S. pneumoniae,* various anaerobes, and, occasionally, *H. influenzae* are found in the oropharynx of normal subjects.
- However, colonization with gram-negative bacilli, notably virulent organisms such as *P. aeruginosa* and *Acinetobacter* species, is rare in healthy individuals.
- It is known that oropharyngeal and tracheal colonization with *P. aeruginosa* and enteric gram-negative bacilli increases with length of hospital stay, antibiotic exposure, and severity of illness.
- **Aspiration** of oropharyngeal secretions is common, even in healthy individuals.
- However, the rate of aspiration is higher in patients with impaired levels of consciousness and inability to adequately protect their airway.
- **Factors promoting aspiration** include:
  - Reduced levels of consciousness
  - Blunted gag reflex
  - Abnormal swallowing for any reason
  - Delayed gastric emptying
  - Decreased gastrointestinal (GI) motility
  - Supine positioning
- Reflux and aspiration of nonsterile gastric contents (especially when antiacids are used) is also a possible mechanism of pathogen entry into the lungs, although its role is generally less significant than that of oropharyngeal microbial colonization.
- The stomach has been implicated, particularly in late-onset VAP, as a potential reservoir for the aspiration of contaminated secretions.

Risk Factors
- A number of risk factors for the development of NP have been described.[12–15]
- These risk factors generally promote either **aspiration** or **colonization** of the aerodigestive tract with pathogenic bacteria (Table 12-1).

TABLE 12-1 RISK FACTORS FOR NOSOCOMIAL PNEUMONIA

Aspiration	Colonization of the Aerodigestive Tract
Witnessed aspiration	COPD
Supine positioning	Use of histamine type 2 antagonists
Coma	Tracheostomy
Enteral nutrition	Prior antibiotic exposure
Reintubation	Age >60 y
Tracheostomy	ARDS
ARDS	
Head trauma	
Intracranial pressure monitoring	

ARDS, acute respiratory distress syndrome; COPD, chronic obstructive pulmonary disease.

Prevention
- A number of pharmacologic and nonpharmacologic interventions have been studied as modalities to minimize NP, especially VAP.
- The strategies with best clinical evidence include those in Table 12-2.

DIAGNOSIS

Clinical Presentation
- **HAP or VAP is suspected** when a patient develops:
  - A new or progressive pulmonary infiltrate
  - Fever
  - Leukocytosis
  - Purulent tracheobronchial secretions

TABLE 12-2 EFFECTIVE STRATEGIES FOR PREVENTING NOSOCOMIAL PNEUMONIA

Effective hand washing by hospital personnel
Protective gowns and gloves
Avoiding large gastric volumes
Oral (nonnasal) intubation
Stress ulcer prophylaxis using non–pH-lowering agents in intubated patients
Avoiding unnecessary antibiotics
Elevation of the head of the bed
Appropriate initial empiric antibiotic therapy
Shortening the duration of intubation and mechanical ventilation (promoting effective awakening trials and weaning trials)

- However, a number of noninfectious causes of fever and pulmonary infiltrates can also occur in these patients, making clinical criteria nonspecific for the diagnosis of NP, and a number of studies have demonstrated the limitations of using clinical parameters alone for establishing the diagnosis of VAP.[16]
- Autopsy results in a series of patients with acute lung injury demonstrated that clinical criteria alone had a sensitivity of 69% and a specificity of 75%.[17]
- Noninfectious causes of fever and pulmonary infiltrates that can mimic NP include:
  - Chemical aspiration without infection
  - Atelectasis
  - Pulmonary embolism (PE) with pulmonary infarction
  - Acute respiratory distress syndrome (ARDS)
  - Pulmonary hemorrhage
  - Lung contusion
  - Infiltrative tumor
  - Radiation pneumonitis
  - Drug or hypersensitivity reactions
- However, the conclusion that clinical diagnosis of VAP is markedly inferior to other methods has not been universal.
- Clinical criteria for the diagnosis of VAP have also been used to manage antibiotic therapy more effectively.
- One group of investigators used the Clinical Pulmonary Infection Score to limit the duration of antibiotic therapy for patients at low risk for VAP.[18]
- The **Clinical Pulmonary Infection Score** is a simple scoring system evaluating temperature, blood leukocyte count, tracheal secretions, oxygenation, and pulmonary infiltrates.[18]
- Such a strategy may allow improved use of empiric antibiotics for patients with suspected VAP; however, a subsequent study failed to confirm the diagnostic accuracy of this approach.[19]

Diagnostic Testing

- The limitations and inaccuracies in clinical decision making have been the motivation for using other techniques to diagnose VAP.
- These techniques include a variety of methods for sampling material from the airways and alveoli, including bronchoscopic and nonbronchoscopic techniques.[20–27]
- **Bronchoscopic sampling of the lower airways,** using either a protected specimen brush or bronchoalveolar lavage (BAL), is currently accepted as the most accurate method of diagnosing VAP, short of direct tissue examination.
  - Quantitative or semiquantitative cultures are usually performed on the bronchoscopic specimens, with the diagnosis of VAP being made when some appropriate threshold is exceeded.
  - From a practical standpoint, quantitative cultures between 100 and 1,000 cfu/mL for **protected brush specimens** and between 1000 and 10,000 cfu/mL for **BAL specimens** should probably be considered positive.
  - It is important to note that few studies have shown that lower airway specimens obtained with bronchoscopic sampling meaningfully influence patient outcomes.
  - Additionally, BAL specimens allow assessment of the percent neutrophils in a cytospin specimen of lavage fluid. Greater than 50% neutrophils supports a diagnosis of VAP in nonneutropenic patients.

- **Tracheal aspirates** can be obtained with ease from endotracheal tubes (ETT), making them an attractive alternative diagnostic technique for patients with suspected VAP.
  - However, tracheal aspirates are nonspecific for establishing the diagnosis of VAP, because tracheobronchial bacterial colonization is common in critically ill patients as a consequence of biofilm formation on the surface of ETTs.
  - As a result, tracheal aspirates have been of limited utility because of the increased accuracy of specimens obtained by bronchoscopy.
  - Nevertheless, tracheal aspirate specimens have good overall sensitivity for the identification of pathogens associated with VAP.
  - The availability of commercial multiplex polymerase chain reaction (PCR) methods for assessing the presence of pathogens in BAL fluid and tracheal aspirate specimens has the potential to improve upon the overall appropriateness of antibiotic therapy as demonstrated by a recent trial.[28,29]

TREATMENT

Medications

- There are two overriding principles that make up the strategy of antibiotic treatment of HAP:
  - The first is to **provide an appropriate initial antimicrobial regimen** that is likely to be active against the pathogen(s) causing infection.[30-34]
  - The second is to **limit the unnecessary use of antibiotics**.
- **De-escalation** is a strategy that attempts to unify these two principles into a single strategy that optimizes patient outcomes while minimizing the emergence of antibiotic resistance.
  - The **first goal of antibiotic de-escalation** requires the administration of an appropriate empiric regimen to patients with suspected NP.
    - Decisions regarding antibiotic selection often occur in the absence of identified pathogens. However, molecular methods such as multiplex PCR can provide rapid pathogen and resistance gene identification increasing the rapidity with which de-escalation can occur.
    - It is imperative that clinicians be aware of both the microorganisms likely to be associated with infection and appropriate antimicrobial options in their patient population.
    - The most common pathogens associated with the administration of **inappropriate** antimicrobial treatment in patients with HAP include potentially antibiotic-resistant **gram-negative bacteria** (*P. aeruginosa*, *Acinetobacter* species, *Klebsiella pneumoniae*, and *Enterobacter* species) and ***S. aureus***, especially strains with methicillin resistance.[35-37]
    - It is important to recognize that the predominant pathogens associated with hospital-associated infections may **vary between hospitals** as well as **between specialized units within individual hospitals**.
    - Therefore, clinicians should be aware of the prevailing bacterial pathogens in their hospitals and their associated antimicrobial susceptibilities.
    - This awareness should help in the selection of empiric antibiotic regimens that are less likely to provide inappropriate treatment for hospital-associated infections.
    - Recommended therapies are summarized in Table 12-3.

TABLE 12-3   THERAPY FOR NOSOCOMIAL PNEUMONIA

Early-onset NP, no specific risk factors
Organisms: Enteric gram negatives, including *Enterobacter* spp., *Escherichia coli*, *Klebsiella* spp., *Proteus* spp., *Serratia marcescens*. Also *Streptococcus pneumoniae*, *Haemophilus influenzae*, and methicillin-sensitive *Staphylococcus aureus*.

Therapy:
Nonpseudomonal third-generation cephalosporin (ceftriaxone) or β-lactam–β-lactamase inhibitor combination (ampicillin/sulbactam).
For penicillin-allergic patients, fluoroquinolone or clindamycin plus aztreonam.

Late-onset NP
Organisms: Any of the above organisms plus *Pseudomonas aeruginosa*, *Acinetobacter baumanii*, methicillin-resistant *S. aureus*.

Therapy:
Antipseudomonal β-lactam plus aminoglycoside or antipseudomonal fluoroquinolone (ciprofloxacin) ± vancomycin or linezolid.
For *A. baumanii*, consider inhaled or IV colistin ± minocycline in addition to a carbapenem.
When infection with MDR bacterial is suspected, especially, carbapenem-resistant isolates, consider the use of the following newer agents based on local epidemiology and antibiotic susceptibility patterns:
Ceftolozane-tazobactam
Ceftazidime-avibactam
Imipenem-cilastatin-relebactam
Cefiderocol
Plazomicin
Eravacycline
Sulbactam-durlobactam
Meropenem-vaborbactam

MDR, multidrug resistant; NP, nosocomial pneumonia.

- The **second goal of antibiotic de-escalation** is to avoid the unnecessary administration of antibiotics.
  - Physicians practicing in the hospital setting are frequently faced with the dilemma of caring for acutely ill patients with suspected nosocomial infection owing to the presence of nonspecific clinical findings (fever, leukocytosis, hemodynamic instability).
  - Failure to provide treatment with an appropriate initial antimicrobial regimen may result in greater morbidity, whereas unnecessary antibiotic treatment can lead to colonization or infection with antibiotic-resistant pathogens. Original

criteria to identify patients at risk for HCAP caused by resistant pathogens proved to be too inclusive thus leading to antibiotic overuse and worse outcomes. Recently developed pneumonia-specific risk factors may allow for a more accurate stratification.[5]

- The **third goal of antibiotic de-escalation** is tailoring therapy based on the patient's culture results.
  - Tailoring therapy will help to avoid unnecessary broad-spectrum antibiotic usage and is a strategy to help to decrease the incidence of antibiotic-resistant organisms.
  - In patients with HCAP, those with negative culture results have a lower severity of illness and mortality than culture-positive patients, and one study has shown it is safe to de-escalate therapy to usual CAP regimens in these patients.

Duration of Therapy

- Despite the thoroughness of many guidelines, durations of therapy remain an imprecise science.
- Treatment for 7–10 days has been advocated for treatment of *S. aureus* or *H. influenzae* infection.
- Longer courses of antibiotics have been proposed for gram-negative necrotizing pneumonias or with isolation of *Pseudomonas* spp.
- The results of a large, randomized trial comparing 8 days of appropriate antibiotic therapy for VAP to 15 days of treatment showed similar efficacy. A recent study showed similar findings for pneumonia caused by *Pseudomonas* spp.[38,39]
- However, longer courses of antibiotic therapy have been associated with statistically greater emergence of multiply resistant bacteria.
- In a study of patients with serious infections in the intensive care unit, the antibiotic course for those with VAP was safely shortened to 7.2 days using a procalcitonin-based discontinuation protocol. However, procalcitonin assays are not currently in widespread clinical use.[40]

REFERENCES

1. Bergin SP, Calvert SB, Farley J, et al. PROPHETIC EU: prospective identification of pneumonia in hospitalized patients in the intensive care unit in European and United States cohorts. *Open Forum Infect Dis.* 2022;9:ofac231.
2. Bergin SP, Coles A, Calvert SB, et al. PROPHETIC: prospective identification of pneumonia in hospitalized patients in the ICU. *Chest.* 2020;158:2370–2380.
3. Kollef MH, Shorr A, Tabak YP, Gupta V, Liu LZ, Johannes RS. Epidemiology and outcomes of health care-associated pneumonia: results from a large US database of culture-positive pneumonia. *Chest.* 2005;128:3854–3862.
4. Chastre J, Fagon JY. Ventilator-associated pneumonia. *Am J Respir Crit Care Med.* 2002;165:867–903.
5. Kalil AC, Metersky ML, Klompas M, et al. Management of adults with hospital-acquired and ventilator-associated pneumonia: 2016 clinical practice guidelines by the Infectious Diseases Society of America and the American Thoracic Society. *Clin Infect Dis.* 2016;63:e61–e111.
6. Zilberberg MD, Nathanson BH, Puzniak LA, Shorr AF. Descriptive epidemiology and outcomes of nonventilated hospital-acquired, ventilated hospital-acquired, and

ventilator-associated bacterial pneumonia in the United States, 2012–2019. *Crit Care Med.* 2022;50:460–468.
7. Micek ST, Chew B, Hampton N, Kollef MH. A case-control study assessing the impact of nonventilated hospital-acquired pneumonia on patient outcomes. *Chest.* 2016;150:1008–1014.
8. Motowski H, Ilges D, Hampton N, Kollef MH, Micek ST. Determinants of mortality for ventilated hospital-acquired pneumonia and ventilator-associated pneumonia. *Crit Care Explor.* 2023;5:e0867.
9. Bekaert M, Timsit JF, Vansteelandt S, et al; Outcomerea Study Group. Attributable mortality of ventilator-associated pneumonia: a reappraisal using casual analysis. *Am J Respir Crit Care Med.* 2011;184:1133–1139.
10. Shindo Y, Ito R, Kobayashi D, et al. Risk factors for drug-resistant pathogens in community-acquired and healthcare-associated pneumonia. *Am J Respir Crit Care Med.* 2013;188:985–995.
11. Chung DR, Song JH, Kim SH, et al. High prevalence of multidrug-resistant nonfermenters in hospital-acquired pneumonia in Asia. *Am J Respir Crit Care Med.* 2011;184:1409–1417.
12. Cook DJ, Kollef MH. Risk factors for ICU-acquired pneumonia. *JAMA.* 1998;279:1605–1606.
13. Kollef MH. Epidemiology and risk factors for nosocomial pneumonia. *Clin Chest Med.* 1999;20:653–670.
14. Lynch JP III. Hospital-acquired pneumonia: risk factors, microbiology, and treatment. *Chest.* 2001;119:373S–384S.
15. Prod'hom G, Leuenberger P, Koerfer J, et al. Nosocomial pneumonia in mechanically ventilated patients receiving antacid, ranitidine, or sucralfate as prophylaxis for stress ulcer. A randomized controlled trial. *Ann Intern Med.* 1994;120:653–662.
16. Meduri GU. Diagnosis and differential diagnosis of ventilator-associated pneumonia. *Clin Chest Med.* 1995;16:61–93.
17. Fabregas N, Ewig S, Torres A, et al. Clinical diagnosis of ventilator associated pneumonia revisited: comparative validation using immediate post-mortem lung biopsies. *Thorax.* 1999;54:867–873.
18. Singh N, Rogers P, Atwood CW, Wagener MM, Yu VL. Short-course empiric antibiotic therapy for patients with pulmonary infiltrates in the intensive care unit. A proposed solution for indiscriminate antibiotic prescription. *Am J Respir Crit Care Med.* 2000;162:505–511.
19. Fagon JY, Chastre J, Hance AJ, Domart Y, Trouillet JL, Gibert C. Evaluation of clinical judgment in the identification and treatment of nosocomial pneumonia in ventilated patients. *Chest.* 1993;103:547–553.
20. Andrews CP, Coalson JJ, Smith JD, Johanson WG Jr. Diagnosis of nosocomial bacterial pneumonia in acute, diffuse lung injury. *Chest.* 1981;80:254–258.
21. Fagon JY, Chastre J, Hance AJ, et al. Detection of nosocomial lung infection in ventilated patients. Use of a protected specimen brush and quantitative culture techniques in 147 patients. *Am Rev Respir Dis.* 1988;138:110–116.
22. Fagon JY, Chastre J, Wolff M, et al. Invasive and noninvasive strategies for management of suspected ventilator-associated pneumonia. A randomized trial. *Ann Intern Med.* 2000;132:621–630.
23. Fartoukh M, Maitre B, Honoré S, Cerf C, Zahar JR, Brun-Buisson C. Diagnosing pneumonia during mechanical ventilation: the clinical pulmonary infection score revisited. *Am J Respir Crit Care Med.* 2003;168:173–179.
24. Heyland DK, Cook DJ, Marshall J, et al. The clinical utility of invasive diagnostic techniques in the setting of ventilator-associated pneumonia. Canadian Critical Care Trials Group. *Chest.* 1999;115:1076–1084.

25. Kirtland SH, Corley DE, Winterbauer RH, et al. The diagnosis of ventilator-associated pneumonia: a comparison of histologic, microbiologic, and clinical criteria. *Chest.* 1997;112:445–457.
26. Niederman MS, Torres A, Summer W. Invasive diagnostic testing is not needed routinely to manage suspected ventilator-associated pneumonia. *Am J Respir Crit Care Med.* 1994;150:565–569.
27. Torres A, Niederman MS, Chastre J, et al. Summary of the international clinical guidelines for the management of hospital-acquired and ventilator-acquired pneumonia. *ERJ Open Res.* 2018;4:00028–2018.
28. Darie AM, Khanna N, Jahn K, et al. Fast multiplex bacterial PCR of bronchoalveolar lavage for antibiotic stewardship in hospitalised patients with pneumonia at risk of Gram-negative bacterial infection (Flagship II): a multicentre, randomised controlled trial. *Respir Med.* 2022;10:877–887.
29. Renaud C, Kollef MH. Classical and molecular techniques to diagnose HAP/VAP. *Semin Respir Crit Care Med.* 2022;43:219–228.
30. Attridge RT, Frei CR, Restrepo MI, et al. Guideline-concordant therapy and outcomes in healthcare-associated pneumonia. *Eur Respir J.* 2011;38:878–887.
31. Cross JT Jr, Campbell GD Jr. Therapy of nosocomial pneumonia. *Med Clin North Am.* 2001;85:1583–1594.
32. Kollef MH, Sherman G, Ward S, Fraser VJ. Inadequate antimicrobial treatment of infections. a risk factor for hospital mortality among critically ill patients. *Chest.* 1999;115:462–474.
33. Martin-Loeches I, Torres A, Nagavci B, et al. ERS/ESICM/ESCMID/ALAT guidelines for the management of severe community-acquired pneumonia. *Eur Respir J.* 2023;61:2200735.
34. Miwa T, Lizza B, Burnham J, Honda H, Kollef M. How to use new antibiotics in the therapy of ventilator-associated pneumonia. *Curr Opin Infect Dis.* 2022;35:140–148.
35. Reynolds D, Burnham JP, Vazquez Guillamet C, et al. The threat of multidrug-resistant/extensively drug-resistant Gram-negative respiratory infections: another pandemic. *Eur Respir Rev.* 2022;31:220068.
36. Vincent JL, Sakr Y, Singer M, et al; EPIC III Investigators. Prevalence and outcomes of infection among patients in intensive care units in 2017. *JAMA.* 2020;323:1478–1487.
37. Zaragoza R, Vidal-Cortés P, Aguilar G, et al. Update of the treatment of nosocomial pneumonia in the ICU. *Crit Care.* 2020;24:383.
38. Bougle A, Tuffet S, Federici L, et al; iDIAPASON Trial Investigators. Comparison of 8 versus 15 days of antibiotic therapy for Pseudomonas aeruginosa ventilator-associated pneumonia in adults: a randomized, controlled, open-label trial. *Intensive Care Med.* 2022;48:841–849.
39. Chastre J, Wolff M, Fagon JY, et al; PneumA Trial Group. Comparison of two durations of antibiotic therapy to treat ventilator-associated pneumonia (VAP). *Am J Respir Crit Care Med.* 2003;167:A21.
40. Bouadma L, Luyt CE, Tubach F, et al; PRORATA Trial Group. Use of procalcitonin to reduce patient's exposure to antibiotics in intensive care units (PRORATA trial): a multicenter randomized controlled trial. *Lancet.* 2010;375:463–474.

Mycobacterial Pulmonary Disease

13

Shail Mehta

GENERAL PRINCIPLES

- Mycobacterial pulmonary disease is composed of two entities:
  - Pulmonary tuberculosis (TB)
  - Nontuberculous mycobacterial (NTM) pulmonary disease
- Pulmonary TB can be divided into two groups[1]:
  - Latent (inactive) TB, also known as tuberculosis infection (TBI).
  - Active TB, aka secondary TB, which is now known as tuberculosis disease

Latent TB/TBI

GENERAL PRINCIPLES

- TBI affects about one-quarter of the world's population.[2]
- Recommended treatment is about 80–90% successful in preventing active disease.[3]
- In general, testing should only be performed if treatment of TBI is indicated. In order to diagnose TBI, TB disease must be ruled out.
- Whom to test[4]:
  - Those at risk of new infection (close contacts of persons with active TB, health care workers with high rates of occupational exposure, and residents of correctional facilities and homeless shelters) should be considered for testing.
  - Persons at high risk of reactivation (progression to active disease) should be tested and treated (Table 13-1).
  - Persons at moderate or slightly increased risk of reactivation who live in an area where TB is prevalent should be considered for testing (Table 13-1).

DIAGNOSIS[5]

- There are two major types of tests for the diagnosis of TBI—tuberculin skin test (TST) and interferon-gamma release assay (IGRA) blood test. IGRA is more specific than the TST.
- IGRA is preferred in persons with low–moderate risk of reactivation. However, in resource-limited settings using the TST is acceptable. IGRA should be used in those with prior Bacillus Calmette–Guérin (BCG) vaccination as they may have a false-positive TST due to vaccination.
- In persons with high risk of reactivation, either the TST or IGRA is acceptable.
- In persons with a history of NTM infection, IGRA is preferred as NTM infection may be associated with a false-positive TST.
- Criteria for positive TST (size, in mm) varies based on the individual's risk of reactivation, please see Table 13-2.[6]

TABLE 13-1 RISK OF TB REACTIVATION

High risk of reactivation of TB	HIV, chemotherapy, transplant recipient, lymphoma/leukemia, head and neck cancer, abnormal CXR with apical fibronodular changes or granulomas, silicosis, renal failure requiring dialysis, treatment with TNF-α inhibitors
Moderate risk of reactivation of TB	Diabetes mellitus (type I or II) Chronic use of glucocorticoids (≥15 mg prednisone/d for ≥1 mo)
Slightly increased risk of reactivation of TB	Underweight, 1 pack/d or greater smoking, CXR with solitary granuloma, individuals born in or residing in countries with high rates of TB

TB, tuberculosis; TNF-α, tissue necrosis factor alpha.

TABLE 13-2 CRITERIA FOR POSITIVE TST

TST Induration Size	Groups in Which Considered Positive
>5 mm	HIV Recent contact of person with TB disease Chest radiograph with evidence of prior TB Immunocompromised patients with organ transplants, on chronic glucocorticoids - Organ transplant recipients - Other immunosuppressed people (patients on prolonged therapy with ≥15 mg/d of prednisone or taking TNF-α inhibitors)
>10 mm	People born in endemic areas, persons who abuse drugs, mycobacteriology lab workers, residents of high-risk congregate settings, people with silicosis, DM, CKD, head and neck cancer, leukemia/lymphoma; low body weight; children younger than 5; infants, children, and adolescents exposed to high-risk adults
>15 mm	People with no risk factors for TB

CKD, chronic kidney disease; DM, diabetes mellitus; TB, tuberculosis; TNF-α, tissue necrosis factor alpha; TST, tuberculin skin test.

- Repeat testing is considered in special circumstances (e.g., ongoing or repeated exposure with prior negative TST or IGRA).

TREATMENT

- Active TB must be ruled out prior to diagnosing and treating TBI. Patients should be asked about symptoms such as cough, weight loss, fevers/chills/night sweats. Sputum cultures and CXR or CT should be obtained if symptomatic.
- Although no regimen is superior, currently guidelines favor a rifamycin-based regimen in the US.[7] Isoniazid (INH)-based regimens have a higher risk of hepatotoxicity.
- Typical rifamycin-based regimens include daily rifampin (RIF) for 4 months, daily INH/RIF for 3 months, and weekly INH/rifapentine for 3 months (3HP).[7]
- If a rifamycin-based regimen cannot be used, INH daily for 9 months can be used.[7] Due to a risk of neuropathy with INH, all patients should be given pyridoxine supplementation.

Active Pulmonary TB/Tuberculosis Disease

DIAGNOSIS

- The diagnosis of pulmonary TB is suspected based on clinical symptoms, history of exposure, and known latent TB/TBI, either treated or untreated.
- Typical symptoms include cough for greater than 3 weeks, fever/chills, night sweats, hemoptysis, weight loss, and lymphadenopathy. As these are nonspecific, other diseases should also be considered.
- The diagnosis of pulmonary TB requires sampling.[5] Most commonly, this is performed by obtaining three sputum samples with at least one morning specimen for acid fast bacilli (AFB) smear and culture. If patients cannot produce sputa, samples may be induced with hypertonic saline.
- Pulmonary TB may also be diagnosed via bronchoscopic washing/lavage, as well as sampling of pleural fluid, or a lung or pleural biopsy.
- A definitive diagnosis of TB is made on the basis of recovery of TB from AFB culture, or more rapidly via nucleic acid amplification (NAA) test.[5] A positive AFB smear is helpful although not confirmatory. Chest radiograph or CT is also useful for supporting the diagnosis.
- IGRA and TST may be helpful but cannot differentiate between TBI and active TB.
- HIV status, if not already known, should be determined in all patients with TB.

SPECIAL CONSIDERATIONS

- There are special public health and infection prevention considerations for patients with active pulmonary TB.

- Patients who are hospitalized with suspected pulmonary TB should be placed in airborne infection isolation[8] until determined to be at low risk of transmission, typically by three consecutive AFB smear-negative sputa or negative NAA testing.[9]
- Once a person is confirmed to have active TB, a contact investigation should take place with public health officials, and contacts should be tested for active or latent TB in order to limit spread of infection.[10]

TREATMENT

- A traditional treatment regimen[11] consists of RIF, INH, pyrazinamide (PZA), and ethambutol (EMB) for 2 months (intensive phase), followed by RIF and INH alone for an additional 4 months (continuation phase) or 6 months total. If testing is available prior to 2 months confirming that the isolate is susceptible to RIF/INH/PZA, EMB may be stopped earlier.
- Therapy is usually given daily to start but at the treating clinician's discretion may be given three times weekly after clinical improvement.
- In some cases (cavitary disease or persistently positive sputum cultures at 2 months), the continuation phase may be extended to 7 months.
- Sputa are typically obtained every month until two consecutive negative samples are obtained.
- The Centers for Disease Control and Prevention (CDC)/Word Health Organization (WHO) approved a 4-month alternative regimen in which rifapentine is substituted for RIF, and moxifloxacin for EMB, in 2022.[12] This is only approved for nonpregnant patients greater than 40 kg with drug-susceptible TB. Treatment consists of daily rifapentine, INH, PZA, and moxifloxacin for 8 weeks, followed by daily rifapentine, INH, and moxifloxacin for 9 more weeks.
- The treatment of pulmonary TB in HIV patients and drug-resistant TB is more complex and out of the scope of this text.

Nontuberculous Pulmonary Disease

GENERAL PRINCIPLES

- In the US, NTM pulmonary infection is now more common than pulmonary TB.[13]
- Over the last several decades, the incidence of pulmonary NTM has risen in the US and worldwide, particularly in women and older patients.[13] The reasons for this are unclear but may be due to increased awareness and diagnosis of the infection, as well as increased use of immunosuppressive medications.
- NTM are ubiquitous in the environment, existing in soil, water, household surfaces, animals, milk, and food. They can inhabit body surfaces and cavities without causing disease. Eliminating all exposure is practically impossible. There is no clear evidence of person-to-person transmission.
- Epidemiologic investigations of healthy patients in the US using a skin test with a mycobacterium avium complex (MAC) antigen have demonstrated sensitivity indicating prior exposure/infection in 30–40% of patients, and more common in southern states.[14]

- There are several known host risk factors for the development of NTM infections.[15] Genetic and acquired immunodeficiency syndromes associated with NTM disease include defects in interferon-gamma and STAT1 signaling, CD4 lymphopenia (often due to HIV), and medications such as TNF-α inhibitors and glucocorticoids. A group of genetic immunodeficiency syndromes termed "Mendelian susceptibility to mycobacterial disease" is known, but rare, and confers an increased risk of pulmonary and disseminated infection. Patients with structural lung disease such as bronchiectasis (including cystic fibrosis), and chronic obstructive pulmonary disease (COPD) are at higher risk of pulmonary infections.
- The most common NTMs in the US causing pulmonary infection are MAC (slow grower), *Mycobacterium abscessus* (rapid grower), and *Mycobacterium kansasii* (slow grower). Other less common NTM species may also cause pulmonary infection.

DIAGNOSIS

- Unlike TB, there is no distinction between "latent" or inactive disease and active disease/infection. There is no commercial test or treatment for inactive NTM infection given the ubiquitous nature of NTMs and high prevalence of exposure.
- Symptoms of infection are similar to TB and include cough (dry or productive), dyspnea, malaise, fatigue, night sweats, weight loss, and fevers/chills.
- Testing for NTM pulmonary disease should only be performed if infection is suspected.
- The diagnosis is made on the basis of sputum cultures, symptoms, and radiographic findings.[16] Sputa may be obtained spontaneously from patient or induced via hypertonic saline. Two of three sputum for AFB smear/culture should be positive in order to diagnose infection. Alternatively, one positive bronchoscopy culture or lung biopsy/pathology can be used. Alternative diagnoses should be excluded. If a patient meets criteria for positive cultures, has radiographic findings typical of disease (CXR or CT), and symptoms of disease, the diagnosis is made. Not all patients who meet diagnostic criteria require treatment and shared decision making and monitoring off treatment is a reasonable option.
- Identification of NTM from culture is made via Matrix-assisted laser desorption time-of-flight mass spectrometry (MALDI-TOF MS) or high-performance liquid chromatography (HPLC) at some reference laboratories. Other methods of identification include nucleic acid probes, and ribosomal RNA sequencing. Nucleic acid probes and HPLC may not identify individual NTM species, especially *M. abscessus*, which may affect treatment decisions.[17]

TREATMENT

- Per current American Thoracic Society/Infectious Disease Society of America (ATS/IDSA) guidelines, treatment is initiated with three active drugs and continued until sputum cultures are negative for 1 year.[16] A typical duration of treatment is 1.5–3 years.

- For patients with bronchiectasis, airway clearance measures such as hypertonic saline, positive expiratory pressure (PEP) therapy, and vest physiotherapy are recommended to help mobilize and clear sputum.
- Immunosuppression and inhaled steroids should be minimized or discontinued if possible.
- Recurrence/reinfection after treatment of MAC is high and reported at 10–40%.[18] All patients should be monitored after treatment for NTM disease and in the long term for recurrence.

Mycobacterium Avium Complex Lung Disease
- MAC is the most common cause of NTM pulmonary infection in the US.[19]
- "MAC" is an umbrella term encompassing several species including *Mycobacterium avium*, *Mycobacterium intracellulare*, *Mycobacterium chimaera*, and others.
- Two major phenotypes of MAC lung disease exist—a bronchiectatic/nodular phenotype is more common in patients with bronchiectasis or no prior lung disease, and a fibrocavitary phenotype is more common in smokers and those with COPD. The bronchiectatic phenotype is classically associated with lingular and right middle lobe bronchiectasis and tree-in-bud nodules. The fibrocavitary phenotype is associated with upper lobe cavities and volume loss and is generally a more severe form of disease. Patients may not fit neatly into one category.[20]
- The typical treatment of MAC includes three active drugs—azithromycin (or clarithromycin), RIF, and EMB.[16] Three times a week treatment is used for less severe disease, and daily treatment for cavitary or recurrent or refractory disease. For fibrocavitary disease, 8 weeks of IV amikacin is also given initially to improve odds of treatment success in the absence of contraindications (chronic kidney disease, hearing loss, older age).[16] After starting treatment, sputum cultures should be obtained monthly. If sputum cultures remain positive at 6 months, inhaled liposomal amikacin should be added once daily as this will increase the odds of culture conversion.[16]
- Surgical resection may be considered for localized cavitary disease or bronchiectasis which is not responding to antibiotic therapy. Surgery is unlikely to help diffuse disease.
- Treatment is continued until sputum cultures are negative for 1 year.[16] Some patients may not clear sputa even after treatment for 2–3 years. In these patients, shared decision making should be used to determine whether to continue treatment or to monitor off treatment.
- Susceptibility testing is typically performed every 6 months on cultures. Macrolide resistance due to a functional erythromycin resistance methylase (ERM) gene is rare and typically occurs when the treatment of MAC is prolonged or in those with more severe, cavitary disease. Susceptibility testing is only clinically useful for determining macrolide, and IV and inhaled amikacin susceptibility.[16] In cases of macrolide resistance, inhaled liposomal amikacin may be used as a third drug in addition to RIF and EMB.[16] Another option is clofazimine (off-label).[16]

Mycobacterium abscessus
- *M. abscessus* is a rapid grower that can cause both bronchiectatic/nodular disease and cavitary disease.

- *M. abscessus* is inherently drug-resistant, complicating treatment.[17] Susceptibility testing must be performed.[16] There are three primary subspecies of *M. abscessus—massiliense, bolletii,* and *abscessus.* Typically, *abscessus* and *bollettii* have a functional ERM gene that confers macrolide resistance, but this should be confirmed by testing.[17]
- Initial treatment of *M. abscessus* consists of two to three IV drugs for 2 months, and possibly one oral drug. Three active drugs should be used, based on susceptibility testing.[16] Typical IV antibiotics used include imipenem, cefoxitin, amikacin, and tigecycline. A macrolide should always be used as an oral agent initially if resistance is not present.
- When 2 months of IV antibiotics have been completed, an oral/inhaled regimen is continued with three active drugs.[16] Based on susceptibility testing, typical drugs used would include azithromycin, linezolid or tedizolid, inhaled amikacin, omadacycline, clofazimine, and doxycycline. Treatment is given daily. Sputa for AFB smear/culture should be obtained every 1–2 months. Treatment is continued until sputa are negative for 1 year.

Mycobacterium kansasii

- *M. kansasii* is historically more prevalent in the Midwest and Southern US. It classically causes cavitary, upper lobe disease in patients with a history of smoking and COPD, HIV, and alcohol abuse. Radiographically, it may mimic TB and fibro-cavitary MAC. It can also cause milder forms of disease associated with bronchiectasis.[21] *M. kansasii* has been isolated from tap water in endemic areas, suggesting a source of inoculation.[22]
- The usual treatment consists of three times weekly or daily (depending on severity) azithromycin, RIF, and EMB.[16] Susceptibility testing should be performed to evaluate for the presence of macrolide or RIF resistance.[16] INH can be used in place of azithromycin if macrolide resistance is present. Moxifloxacin may be used for RIF resistance.
- Sputum cultures should be obtained every 1–2 months on treatment. Treatment is continued until cultures are clear for 1 year. Susceptibility testing should be performed every 6 months to monitor for the development of resistance. In general, patients respond well to treatment with clearance of sputum cultures and a lower risk of recurrence compared to MAC.

REFERENCES

1. Behr MA, Kaufmann E, Duffin J, Edelstein PH, Ramakrishnan L. Latent tuberculosis: two centuries of confusion. *Am J Respir Crit Care Med.* 2021;204:142–148.
2. World Health Organization. Global Tuberculosis Report 2023. Accessed August 23, 2024. https://www.who.int/teams/global-tuberculosis-programme/tb-reports/global-tuberculosis-report-2023
3. Sterling TR, Villarino ME, Borisov AS, et al; TB Trials Consortium PREVENT TB Study Team. Three months of rifapentine and isoniazid for latent tuberculosis infection. *N Engl J Med.* 2011;365:2155–2166.
4. US Preventive Services Task Force; Mangione CM, Barry MJ, Nicholson WK, et al. Screening for latent tuberculosis infection in adults: US Preventive Services Task Force recommendation statement. *JAMA.* 2023;329:1487–1494.
5. Lewinsohn DM, Leonard MK, LoBue PA, et al. Official ATS/IDSA/CDC clinical practice guidelines: diagnosis of tuberculosis in adults and children. *Clin Infect Dis.* 2017;64:111–115.

6. CDC. Mantoux Tuberculin Skin Testing Fact Sheet. 2024. Accessed August 23, 2024. https://www.cdc.gov/tb/hcp/mantoux/skin-test-fact-sheet.html
7. Sterling TR, Njie G, Zenner D, et al. Guidelines for the treatment of latent tuberculosis infection: recommendations from the National Tuberculosis Controllers Association and CDC, 2020. *MMWR Recomm Rep.* 2020;69:1–11.
8. Moran GJ, Barrett TW, Mower WR, et al; EMERGEncy ID NET Study Group. Decision instrument for the isolation of pneumonia patients with suspected pulmonary tuberculosis admitted through US emergency departments. *Ann Emerg Med.* 2009;53:625–632.
9. Cowan JF, Chandler AS, Kracen E, et al. Clinical impact and cost-effectiveness of Xpert MTB/RIF testing in hospitalized patients with presumptive pulmonary tuberculosis in the United States. *Clin Infect Dis.* 2017;64:482–489.
10. Young KH, Ehman M, Reves R, et al. Tuberculosis contact investigations–United States, 2003–2012. *Morb Mortal Wkly Rep.* 2016;64:1369–1374.
11. Nahid P, Dorman SE, Alipanah N, et al. Official American Thoracic Society/Centers for Disease Control and Prevention/Infectious Diseases Society of America Clinical Practice Guidelines: treatment of drug-susceptible tuberculosis. *Clin Infect Dis.* 2016;63:e147–e195.
12. Dorman SE, Nahid P, Kurbatova EV, et al. Four-month rifapentine regimens with or without moxifloxacin for tuberculosis. *N Engl J Med.* 2021;384:1705–1718.
13. Winthrop KL, Marras TK, Adjemian J, Zhang H, Wang P, Zhang Q. Incidence and prevalence of nontuberculous mycobacterial lung disease in a large U.S. Managed Care Health Plan, 2008–2015. *Ann Am Thorac Soc.* 2020;17:178–185.
14. von Reyn CF, Williams DE, Horsburgh CR Jr, et al. Dual skin testing with Mycobacterium avium sensitin and purified protein derivative to discriminate pulmonary disease due to M. avium complex from pulmonary disease due to Mycobacterium tuberculosis. *J Infect Dis.* 1998;177:730–736.
15. Lake MA, Ambrose LR, Lipman MCI, Lowe DM. "Why me, why now?" Using clinical immunology and epidemiology to explain who gets nontuberculous mycobacterial infection. *BMC Med.* 2016;14:54.
16. Daley CL, Iaccarino JM, Lange C, et al. Treatment of nontuberculous mycobacterial pulmonary disease: an official ATS/ERS/ESCMID/IDSA clinical practice guideline. *Clin Infect Dis.* 2020;71:e1–e36.
17. Griffith DE, Brown-Elliott BA, Benwill JL, Wallace RJ Jr. Mycobacterium abscessus. "Pleased to meet you, hope you guess my name…." *Ann Am Thorac Soc.* 2015; 12:436–439.
18. Koh WJ, Moon SM, Kim SY, et al. Outcomes of *Mycobacterium avium* complex lung disease based on clinical phenotype. *Eur Respir J.* 2017;50:1602503.
19. Griffith DE, Aksamit T, Brown-Elliott BA, et al; ATS Mycobacterial Diseases Subcommittee; American Thoracic Society; Infectious Disease Society of America. An official ATS/IDSA statement: diagnosis, treatment, and prevention of nontuberculous mycobacterial diseases. *Am J Respir Crit Care Med.* 2007;175:367–416.
20. Plotinsky RN, Talbot EA, von Reyn CF. Proposed definitions for epidemiologic and clinical studies of Mycobacterium avium complex pulmonary disease. *PLoS One.* 2013; 8:e77385.
21. Shitrit D, Baum GL, Priess R, et al. Pulmonary Mycobacterium kansasii infection in Israel, 1999–2004: clinical features, drug susceptibility, and outcome. *Chest.* 2006; 129:771–776.
22. Steadham JE. High-catalase strains of Mycobacterium kansasii isolated from water in Texas. *J Clin Microbiol.* 1980;11:496–498.

Fungal Pulmonary Infections

14

Christian Hendrix and
Patrick B. Mazi

GENERAL PRINCIPLES

- This chapter outlines commonly encountered fungal infections of the lung.
- Fungal infections are becoming increasingly prevalent due to a growing population of immunocompromised patients and climate change factors expanding fungal geographic distribution. Due to inhalation of fungal conidia, pulmonary fungal infections are the most common invasive infection and can progress to disseminated disease.
- There are three groups of fungal pathogens that infect the lungs:
  - Molds including *Aspergillus, Fusarium, Scedosporium/Lomentospora,* and the mucormycetes (formerly zygomycetes)—*Mucor, Rhizopus, Rhizomucor, Cunninghamella, Saksenaea, Apophysomyces.*
  - Yeasts including *Cryptococcus* and *Pneumocystis jirovecii. Candida* spp. are yeasts commonly isolated from respiratory samples, though pulmonary infection due to *Candida* is very rare and requires histopathology for accurate diagnosis.
  - Dimorphic fungi exist in two forms: as budding yeast forms in tissue and as mold with hyphae in the environment and when incubated at 25 °C for culture. The most common dimorphic fungal pathogens in North America are *Histoplasma, Blastomyces,* and *Coccidioides.*
- This review of fungal pulmonary infections is not intended to be exhaustive; rather, the most common and emerging fungal infections will be reviewed.

Aspergillosis

- *Aspergillus* spp. are hyaline hyphomycetes with typically parallel septate hyphae and dichotomous 45-degree (acute) angle branching. They are soil-dwelling fungi frequently isolated from food, spices, compost, and dust (e.g., from construction sites).[1]
- *Aspergillus fumigatus* complex is the most common species group isolated from patients with aspergillosis. Other clinically relevant species groups include *A. flavus* complex, *A. niger* complex, and *A. terres* complex.
- Due to their environmental ubiquity, inhalation of *Aspergillus* spores is common but rarely results in clinically relevant infection in immunocompetent patients. However, clinically significant presentations often occur in patients with various forms of immunosuppression.[1–4]

- Risk factors for developing infection include neutropenia, prolonged glucocorticoid exposure, advanced HIV, myeloablative chemotherapy, hematopoietic stem cell transplantation, solid organ transplantation, chronic granulomatous disease, and pre-existing structural lung disease.[1-4]
- Severe pneumonia due to respiratory viruses (e.g., influenza, SARS-CoV-2) has been associated with increased risk of invasive pulmonary aspergillosis (IPA). The strength of this association and its clinical relevance is the subject of ongoing debate.
- *Aspergillus* spp. cause a wide spectrum of clinical syndromes in the lung.[1,5]
  - Pulmonary aspergillosis may be categorized as invasive, chronic, and saprophytic, or allergic per Infectious Diseases Society of America (IDSA) guidelines.[4]
  - IPA develops as a bronchopneumonia or invasive sinusitis. Local invasion of adjacent structures, including blood vessels, often results in hemorrhage/hemoptysis and may lead to disseminated disease.
  - Chronic necrotizing aspergillosis (CNA) or subacute IPA is a more indolent form of invasive infection.
  - Chronic and saprophytic syndromes are another syndrome of *Aspergillus* spp. Aspergilloma typifies the saprophytic processes of the lung.
  - Allergic conditions include allergic bronchopulmonary aspergillosis (ABPA).

Invasive Pulmonary Aspergillosis

GENERAL PRINCIPLES

- IPA is often rapidly progressive, **frequently fatal** disease that occurs **primarily in immunocompromised hosts**.
- It is characterized by **direct tissue invasion** by the fungus, **often with dissemination to other organs**.
- *Aspergillus* has a propensity for vascular invasion, resulting in hemorrhage, thrombosis, infarction, and tissue necrosis. It can also invade into adjacent structures, including the intercostal muscles, ribs, and pericardium.
- Risk factors for IPA include prolonged neutropenia or neutrophil dysfunction, hematopoietic stem cell and solid organ transplantation, prolonged and high-dose corticosteroid therapy, hematologic malignancy, advanced HIV, and cytotoxic chemotherapy.[1-5]

DIAGNOSIS

- IPA should be suspected in immunocompromised hosts with persistent fevers that do not respond to treatment with broad-spectrum antibiotics.
- The most common clinical manifestations include pleuritic pain, hemoptysis, pulmonary hemorrhage, and cavitation.[1-5]
- Diagnosis of IPA is difficult due to its nonspecific clinical manifestations and a high index of suspicion must be present in patients with risk factors. As a result, diagnostic criteria have been proposed, incorporating histologic, microbiologic, and antigenic findings. The criteria are summarized in Table 14-1.[1,2]

TABLE 14-1 DIAGNOSTIC CRITERIA FOR THE DIAGNOSIS OF IPA

Major Criteria	Minor Criteria
Halo sign	Symptoms of lower respiratory tract infection
Air-crescent sign	Pleural rub
Cavity within an area of consolidation	Any new infiltrate not fulfilling major criteria
	Pleural effusion

Diagnosis	Criteria
Proven IPA	Histopathologic examination of lung tissue showing hyphae or biopsy specimen with evidence of associated tissue damage **OR** Positive culture for *Aspergillus* from a sample obtained by sterile procedure from the lung and clinically or radiographically abnormal site consistent with infection
Probable IPA	Host risk factor[a] **AND** Positive *Aspergillus* culture from sputum or BAL, or positive galactomannan assay **AND** One major or two minor criteria
Possible IPA	Host risk factor[a] **AND** Positive *Aspergillus* culture from sputum or BAL or positive galactomannan assay **OR** One major or two minor criteria

[a]Prolonged neutropenia or neutrophil dysfunction, hematopoietic stem cell and solid organ transplantation, prolonged and high-dose corticosteroid therapy, hematologic malignancy, advanced AIDS, and cytotoxic therapy.

IPA, invasive pulmonary aspergillosis; BAL, bronchoalveolar lavage.

With permission from Zmeili OS, Soubani AO. Pulmonary aspergillosis: a clinical update. *Q J Med.* 2007;100:317–334.

DIAGNOSTIC TESTING

- Isolation of *Aspergillus* from the sputum has a positive predictive value of 80–90% in immunosuppressed patients; however, negative sputum studies occur in 70% of patients with confirmed IPA.[2]
- Histopathologic diagnosis of aspergillosis remains the gold standard.
  - Lung tissue obtained from thoracoscopic or open lung biopsy preserves tissue architecture optimizing diagnosis but is often deferred in favor less invasive diagnostics.

- Histologic examination demonstrates tissue, often vascular, invasion by septate, acute-angle–branching hyphae.
- Bronchoscopy with bronchoalveolar lavage (BAL) is particularly helpful in patients with diffuse lung involvement and has a sensitivity and specificity of 50% and 97%, respectively.[1–7]
- Serum and BAL fluid testing for **galactomannan** antigen is available but the operating characteristics of such testing are variable, with specificity being better than sensitivity.[1,3,7–10] However, some medications, including β-lactam antibiotics, may be associated with a false-positive result, and antifungals with activity against *Aspergillus* may be associated with a false-negative result.
- Serum polymerase chain reaction (PCR) testing is not yet recommended for routine use in clinical practice.[4]
- CXR findings are nonspecific but may show patchy infiltrates or nodular opacities.[1,2]
- The imaging modality of choice is **high-resolution CT scanning**. Findings may demonstrate a halo sign with a lung nodule surrounded by a ground glass opacity or an air crescent sign.[1–4]

TREATMENT

- Despite the introduction of new antifungal agents, the mortality of IPA remains high. Therapy should be initiated as soon as there is clinical suspicion of IPA.
- **The current treatment of choice is voriconazole** at 6 mg/kg IV bid on day 1, followed by 4 mg/kg IV daily for an additional 6 days. After 6 days of IV therapy, switching to voriconazole 200 mg PO bid can be considered.[2–5]
  - Voriconazole should be avoided as empiric antimold treatment because it does not have activity against mucormycetes.
  - Empiric treatment with another triazole (posaconazole or isavuconazole) or lipid formulation of amphotericin B is preferred until the diagnosis of aspergillosis is confirmed.
- **Amphotericin B** is also acceptable first-line treatment.[2–7] Dosing is typically 1–5 mg/kg/d depending on specific formulation.
  - Lipid formulations are better tolerated compared to amphotericin B deoxycholate, though nephrotoxicity and electrolyte derangements remain common side effects.
  - Amphotericin B is good empiric therapy when a fungal infection is suspected but the fungal pathogen has not yet been identified.
- Optimal duration of therapy is poorly characterized. Generally, patients should be maintained on an oral triazole (voriconazole, posaconazole, or isavuconazole) for at least 6–12 weeks only after immunosuppression has ended and there has been resolution of the lesions.
- **Caspofungin, micafungin, and anidulafungin** may also be used as salvage therapy in patients who do not respond to standard antifungal therapy.[3,5,7]
- Combination therapy has not been shown to be more effective than single-agent therapy.
- **Surgical resection** of infected tissue should be considered when there is massive hemoptysis or localized focus of infection, especially if further immunosuppression is planned.

Subacute and Chronic Necrotizing Aspergillosis

GENERAL PRINCIPLES

- Subacute aspergillosis is a more indolent form of invasive infection characterized by local invasion of lung tissue. Unlike IPA, CNA is **slowly progressive and vascular invasion or extrathoracic dissemination is unusual**.
- Subacute aspergillosis most commonly affects elderly patients with **underlying chronic lung disease**, particularly chronic obstructive pulmonary disease (COPD). Other risk factors include pulmonary TB, prior lung resection, prior radiation therapy, pneumoconiosis, and cystic fibrosis.[1,3,11–13]
- Patients with mild immunosuppression due to diabetes mellitus, chronic liver disease, corticosteroid therapy, alcohol abuse, and connective tissue disease are at increased risk.[1,3,11–13]

DIAGNOSIS

- Patients with CNA typically present with constitutional symptoms, including fever, malaise, fatigue, and weight loss of 1–6 months' duration.
- Patients may have chronic productive cough. If vascular invasion is present, hemoptysis of varying severity may also be present.
- Occasionally, patients are asymptomatic, and the diagnosis is made incidentally.
- Patients must meet all of the following criteria in order to make the diagnosis[1,2]:
  - Chronic pulmonary or systemic symptoms, including at least one of: weight loss, productive cough, or hemoptysis.
  - No overt immunocompromising conditions.
  - Cavitary pulmonary lesion with evidence of paracavitary infiltrates, new cavitary formation, or expansion of cavity size over time.
  - Elevated levels of inflammatory markers.
  - Isolation of *Aspergillus* from pulmonary or pleural cavity, or positive serum *Aspergillus* serology.
  - Exclusion of other pulmonary pathogens.

DIAGNOSTIC TESTING

- **Serum IgG antibodies** to *A. fumigatus* are variably positive during the course of the disease.
- As with IPA, diagnosis requires the **histologic demonstration of tissue invasion** by the fungus as well as the growth of *Aspergillus* on culture. However, transbronchial biopsy specimens and percutaneous aspirates have poor yield, and thoracoscopic or open lung biopsy is rarely performed, resulting in delayed diagnosis.[1,2,11–13]
- Radiographic findings are variable, though **CXR and chest CT** commonly show consolidation, pleural thickening, and cavitary lesions in the upper lobes. Aspergilloma may be seen in half of patients. The radiographic findings may progress over weeks to months.[2,3,11–13]

TREATMENT

- **Oral Voriconazole** 200 mg bid is the current primary therapy for CNA.
  - Alternative treatment regimens include:
    - Posaconazole
      - Delayed-release tables: 300 mg PO every 12 hours × 2 doses (loading dose), followed by 300 mg PO daily.
      - Suspension: 400 mg PO every 12 hours
    - Isavuconazole: 372 mg PO/IV every 8 hours × 6 doses, then 372 mg PO/IV daily
    - Itraconazole
      - Capsules: 200 mg PO every 12 hours
      - Oral solution: 2.5 mg/kg every 12 hours
  - Therapeutic drug monitoring should be utilized when serum concentration testing is available.
- The duration of therapy is usually prolonged but optimal duration and criteria for discontinuing therapy are currently unclear.[1-7]
- Markers for response to therapy include weight gain, improved energy levels, improved pulmonary symptoms, decreasing inflammatory markers, decreasing total serum IgE levels, and improvement or resolution of radiographic abnormalities.[3,4,7,12,13]
- **Surgical resection** may be considered in a very limited population, including young healthy patients with limited disease and good pulmonary reserve, patients not tolerating antifungal therapy, and patients with residual localized disease despite antifungal therapy.

Aspergilloma

GENERAL PRINCIPLES

- An aspergilloma is a fungal ball composed of hyphae, mucus, inflammatory cells, fibrin, and tissue debris. An aspergilloma is the **most common form of pulmonary aspergillosis**.[1,2]
- It usually occurs in patients with **pre-existing cavitary lung disease**. Rare cases of de novo aspergilloma in patients without pre-existing cavitary lung disease have been reported.[1-5]
- Risk factors include TB, sarcoidosis, neoplasm, cystic fibrosis, or severe emphysema.

DIAGNOSIS

- Most patients with aspergilloma have few clinical symptoms.
- When symptoms develop, **hemoptysis** is the most clinically important and is usually mild but may become severe. Bleeding usually occurs from bronchial vessels lining the lung cavity.[1-5]
- Patients may also experience chest pain, dyspnea, malaise, and fever.

DIAGNOSTIC TESTING

- Sputum cultures for *Aspergillus* are positive in only 50% of cases due to the limited communication between the cavity and the bronchial tree.[1,2]
- Serum IgG antibodies are very sensitive but may be negative in patients on corticosteroid therapy.[1-5]
- *Aspergillus* antigen has been found in the BAL fluid of patients with aspergilloma, but the diagnostic utility is variable.
- On CXR, aspergillomas classically appear as an upper lobe intracavitary mass surrounded by a radiolucent crescent, known as a crescent sign.
- However, these radiographic findings may also appear in other conditions, including neoplasm, abscess, cystic echinococcosis, and granulomatosis with polyangiitis.

TREATMENT

- Treatment of aspergilloma, most commonly a triazole antifungal, may be considered when there is progression of cavity size or when patients become symptomatic.[1-5]
- Inhaled, intracavitary and endobronchial instillations of antifungal agents have been attempted and have failed to demonstrate benefit in the clinical course, morbidity, or mortality.
- Medical therapy is frequently insufficient to resolve aspergillomas; in these cases, surgical resection is required for clinical resolution. Surgical intervention is most commonly considered when patients have recurrent and/or life-threatening hemoptysis.
- Tranexamic acid (TXA) and/or bronchial artery embolization should be considered in patients with life-threatening hemoptysis.

Allergic Bronchopulmonary Aspergillosis

GENERAL PRINCIPLES

- Unlike the previously discussed forms of pulmonary aspergillosis, ABPA is a **hypersensitivity reaction** rather than a true infection.
- The pathogenesis is not completely understood, but specific IgE-mediated type I hypersensitivity reactions, specific IgG-mediated type III hypersensitivity reactions, and abnormal T-lymphocyte cellular immune responses have all been implicated.[13-15]
- It most commonly occurs in patients with **asthma or cystic fibrosis**.[13-15]

DIAGNOSIS

- Patients with ABPA usually present with episodic wheezing, occasional productive cough, fever, and chest pain.
- Patients may also complain of expectoration of thick brown plugs, which are *Aspergillus*-laden mucoid bronchial casts.

Fungal Pulmonary Infections

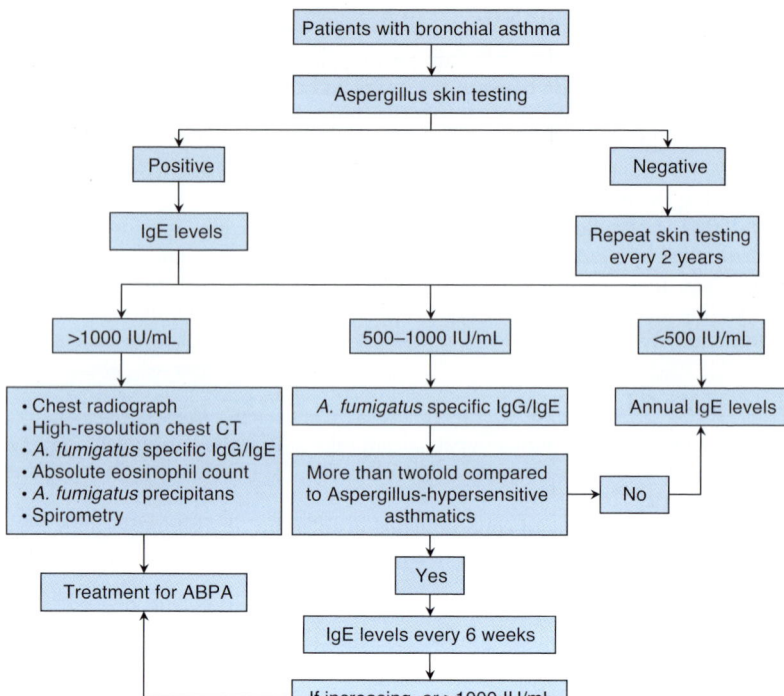

Figure 14-1 Diagnostic evaluation for allergic bronchopulmonary aspergillosis (ABPA). (With permission from Agarwal R. Allergic bronchopulmonary aspergillosis. *Chest.* 2009;135:805–826.)

- Patients in whom ABPA is suspected should undergo a specific diagnostic evaluation, outlined below in Figure 14-1.[1,13–15]
- Patients with ABPA can be classified as those with **central bronchiectasis** (ABPA-CB) and those without (ABPA-**seropositive**).
- The minimal diagnostic criteria for ABPA-CB include asthma, skin reactivity to *Aspergillus* antigens, serum IgE >1000 IU/mL, elevated serum *A. fumigatus*–specific IgG and IgE, and CB.[1,3,13–15]
- The minimal diagnostic criteria for ABPA-seropositive include asthma, skin reactivity to *Aspergillus* antigens, serum IgE >1000 IU/mL, history of transient pulmonary infiltrates, and elevated serum *A. fumigatus*–specific IgG and IgE.[13–15]

DIAGNOSTIC TESTING

- Early detection of ABPA prior to the development of irreversible bronchiectasis can help to minimize the severity of disease. A delay in diagnosis may result in irreversible pulmonary damage.

- **Serum IgE and IgG levels** are useful in diagnosing ABPA.
- CXRs may be clear or show **transient migratory infiltrates** that occur during acute exacerbations, frequently in the upper lobes. The ring sign and tram lines are radiographic findings that signify the thickened and inflamed bronchi.
- **Chest CT** scan may show mucoid impaction, bronchial thickening, or bronchiectasis. Findings typically occur in a central, upper lobe distribution.

TREATMENT

- ABPA treatment is intended to limit acute exacerbations and prevent progressive lung injury.
- **Glucocorticoids continue as the mainstay in treatment of ABPA.**[13–15]
- Although there is little data to guide the dosing or duration of therapy, lower doses of glucocorticoids have been associated with more frequent relapses.
- Current recommendations are to treat with prednisone 0.5 mg/kg/d PO daily for 2 weeks, followed by a slow taper over 3–6 months.
- Total serum IgE can be used as a marker of disease activity and should be checked 6–8 weeks after starting glucocorticoid therapy, then every 8 weeks for 1 year after that to determine a baseline serum IgE level.
- Itraconazole, 200 mg bid, for 16 weeks up to 6 months has been used as a steroid-sparing or adjunct therapy.[7]
  - Although oral itraconazole has been shown to reduce IgE levels, it has not been demonstrated to improve lung function.
  - Itraconazole is the most studied antifungal for ABPA treatment. However, other triazoles have shown better tolerability and better *Aspergillus* activity. Posaconazole, voriconazole, and isavuconazole can be considered alternative therapies.
  - Relapse after discontinuation of antifungal therapy is common.
  - Coadministration of a triazole and glucocorticoid can result in Cushing syndrome due to triazole inhibition of CYP450.
- Most patients with ABPA will have clinical presentations and lab testing that support the use of biologic asthma therapies. These agents include anti-interleukin (IL)-5, anti-IgE, and anti–IL-4 subunit antibodies. Long-term safety and efficacy studies are in progress; however, they can be considered for patients with frequent ABPA recurrences/exacerbations or in patients unable to wean off steroid therapy.

Blastomycosis

GENERAL PRINCIPLES

- Blastomycosis is a fungal infection caused by species from the genus *Blastomyces*.
- *Blastomyces dermatitidis* is the most commonly isolated species in North America, though other species including *Blastomyces gilchristii* and *Blastomyces helicus* may also be encountered clinically.
- *Blastomyces* spp. are dimorphic fungi, existing as mold in ambient environmental temperatures and convert to a broad-based budding yeast at mammalian body temperatures.

- *Blastomyces* spp. are commonly found in moist soil close to bodies of fresh water and/or decaying organic matter (i.e., detritus).
- Historically, *Blastomyces* was thought to be geographically restricted to hyperendemic regions along the Ohio and Mississippi river valleys. However, more recent data suggests the geographic distribution of *Blastomyces* spp. is expanding.[16-19]
- Like many of the other fungal pulmonary infections, infection most commonly occurs when the conidia are aerosolized and inhaled, although cases of transmission by direct inoculation have also been documented.[16-19]
- Hosts with impaired cell-mediated immunity are at greater risk of developing disseminated disease.
- Unlike histoplasmosis, most cases of clinically apparent blastomycosis are not self-limited and should be treated once diagnosis is made. Mortality rates in untreated disease approach 60%.

DIAGNOSIS

Clinical Presentation

- Clinical presentations of blastomycosis infection are **highly variable** and range from mild to fatal disseminated disease.[1,16-19]
- Most primary infections are asymptomatic or mild and resolve without treatment. Of those who are symptomatic, the infection most frequently manifests as a mild, self-limited pulmonary infection.[18]
- Patients seeking medical attention often present with cough, fever, night sweats, weight loss, chest pain, dyspnea, myalgias, and hemoptysis. Patients with widely disseminated or miliary disease may present with acute respiratory distress syndrome (ARDS).
- Common sites of disseminated disease include the bone, joints, genitourinary system, and central nervous system (CNS), but blastomycosis can involve virtually any organ.
- Approximately half of patients with disseminated disease have either ulcerative or verrucous skin lesions.[16-19]

Diagnostic Testing

- Diagnosing blastomycosis remains difficult due to the nonspecific symptoms and diagnostic delay is common. Blastomycosis is often not considered until the patient has failed to respond to one or more courses of antibiotics.
- Isolation of *Blastomyces* from sputum, BAL fluid, tracheal secretions, or skin lesions is diagnostic. However, growth on culture media may take 4–5 weeks, dramatically reducing its clinical utility.
- **Microscopic examination** of sputum, aspirate, or tissue shows the classic broad-based budding yeast, and can lead to more rapid, putative diagnosis.
- A urine antigen assay has a reported sensitivity of 93% and a specificity of 79% but histoplasmosis and other fungal pathogens are cross-reactive with the assay resulting in a false positive.[16-19]
- Serologic testing for blastomycosis has limited clinical utility. Serologic testing should be interpreted cautiously; consultation with infectious disease and pulmonary specialists is recommended.

- Chest radiography is highly variable frequently demonstrating alveolar or mass-like infiltrate, often with cavitation, and can sometimes be mistaken for malignancy.

Treatment
- In patients with non-CNS and non–life-threatening disease, **itraconazole** 200 mg TID for 3 days (loading dose) followed by maintenance dosing of 200 mg every 12–24 hours for 6–12 months.[7,16–19]
- In patients with severe, life-threatening diseases, a liposomal formulation **amphotericin B** is recommended for initial therapy. Typical dosing range is 3–5 mg/kg daily.[4] Once satisfactory clinical response has been documented, patients may be switched to itraconazole for a total of 1 year of therapy.
- Serum levels of itraconazole should be evaluated after therapy initiation.
- In immunosuppressed patients, lifelong suppressive therapy may be considered if the immunosuppression cannot be corrected.

Candidiasis

GENERAL PRINCIPLES
- *Candida* are commensal fungi of the skin and the upper respiratory, gastrointestinal, and genitourinary tracts. Due to their presence as commensal organisms, isolation of *Candida* spp. from cultures of these areas is common and often expected.
- *Candida albicans* is the major pathogenic species.
- The taxonomic nomenclature *Candida* spp. has changed to reflect more accurate phylogeny. Clinically relevant name changes include: *Pitchia kudriavzevii* (formerly *C. krusei*) and *Nakaseomyces glabrata* (formerly *C. glabrata*).
- **Isolated pulmonary candidiasis is rare and pulmonary involvement is usually secondary to disseminated candidiasis.**[1,20–26]
- Risk factors for developing disseminated candidiasis include intensive care unit hospitalization, hematologic and solid organ malignancy, hematopoietic stem cell and solid organ transplantation, use of central venous catheters, antibiotic therapy, total parenteral nutrition, and prior fungal colonization.[1,20–26]
- Definitive diagnosis of pulmonary candidiasis requires obtaining tissue via bronchoscopy or open lung biopsy and **histologic documentation of invasion of the bronchi or lungs**.
- If pulmonary candidiasis is suspected, consultation with infectious disease and pulmonary specialists is recommended to assist with diagnosis and treatment.

Coccidioidomycosis

GENERAL PRINCIPLES
- *Coccidioides immitis* is a dimorphic fungus that is historically geographically restricted to hyperendemic areas of the southwestern US.
- Infection occurs via inhalation of arthroconidia.

- Coccidioidomycosis has five primary manifestations: **acute pneumonia, chronic progressive pneumonia, pulmonary nodules and cavities, extrapulmonary nonmeningeal disease, and meningitis.**[27–30]
- Pregnancy and immunosuppression due to advanced HIV, stem cell transplant, solid organ transplantation, use of tumor necrosis factor-α (TNF-α) antagonists, prolonged glucocorticoid exposure, and malignancy are risk factors for acquiring coccidioidomycosis.[27–30]

DIAGNOSIS

- Approximately 60% of patients who become infected with *Coccidioides* are asymptomatic, and of those who are symptomatic, the vast majority develops acute **pneumonia**.[27–30]
- Symptoms develop 1–3 weeks after exposure, and are nonspecific, including fever, sore throat, cough, fatigue, and pleuritic chest pain; rarely, patients present with ARDS.
- It is sometimes associated with rashes, most classically erythema nodosum, and erythema multiforme in a necklace pattern around the neck.[27–30]
- Approximately 1–4% of patients fail to recover from acute pneumonia, and continue to have chronic progressive pneumonia, characterized by fever, weight loss, and productive cough.[27–30]
- Over the course of infection, the pneumonic process may consolidate to form a pulmonary **nodule or a cavity**. The majority of patients are asymptomatic, but hemoptysis, cough, fever, night sweats, weight loss, and localized chest wall pain may be presenting symptoms.
- In ≤5% of immunocompetent hosts, coccidioidomycosis progresses to **disseminated disease**.[27–30] The most common sites of dissemination include the skin, bones, joints, lymph nodes, and meninges. Diagnosis of disseminated disease is frequently delayed by weeks to months after the initial pulmonary symptoms. Patients with meningitis often present with headaches, mental status changes, and cranial nerve palsies.
- Prognosis, even in immunocompetent hosts, is grave if not diagnosed and treated promptly.

DIAGNOSTIC TESTING

- Diagnosis of coccidioidomycosis can be made in three ways: **identification of the spherules** in a cytology or biopsy specimen, **isolation of the organism from culture**, or positive **serologic testing**.[27–30]
- Identifying spherules in sputum, BAL fluid, or other body fluid is indicative of disease, as *Coccidioides* is not a commensal organism.[27–30]
- Active cultures of pathogenic *Coccidioides* pose an infection risk for laboratory personnel.
- Serologic testing with enzyme-linked immunoassay (EIA) of *Coccidioides* IgM and IgG antibodies is the most common diagnostic test. Positive EIA testing is sensitive, but positive results should be further evaluated by immunodiffusion. A titer ≥1:16 should prompt investigation for disseminated disease.[27–30]
- Negative serology does not rule out coccidiomycosis due to less-than-perfect sensitivity.

- CXRs in acute pneumonia most frequently reveal dense, upper lobe infiltrates; hilar, and mediastinal lymphadenopathies are not uncommon.
- In chronic pneumonia, CXRs may show persistent infiltrates, fibrosis, cavitation, hilar lymphadenopathy, and pleural changes.
- In cavitary disease, CXR classically shows a thin-walled lesion without an air–fluid level. In 90% of patients, the cavities are solitary and in 70% they are usually 2–4 cm in size.[1,28]
- In disseminated disease, CXR most commonly shows diffuse reticulonodular infiltrates, although miliary infiltrates, nodules, and cavities may be seen.

TREATMENT

- In immunocompetent patients with mild symptoms, antifungal therapy is not indicated.[4]
- In immunocompetent patients with moderate pulmonary disease, recommended treatment is oral **fluconazole** 400 mg daily.[7,27–30]
- In patients with disseminated disease or severe pulmonary disease, a lipid formulation of **amphotericin B** should be used as initial treatment. Once clinically stable, patients may be transitioned to maintenance therapy with oral fluconazole for at least 12–18 months.[7,27–30]
- Lifelong suppressive therapy with an oral azole can be considered for immunosuppressed patients.[7]
- In patients who are asymptomatic but have nodules or cavitary lesions, serial chest radiography is recommended to monitor the size of the lesions.

Cryptococcosis

GENERAL PRINCIPLES

- Cryptococcosis is an opportunistic infection caused by *Cryptococcus neoformans* or *Cryptococcus gatti*, an encapsulated, budding yeast.
- *C. neoformans* is found worldwide and is classically associated with soil contaminated with pigeon droppings.
- Cryptococcosis occurs via inhalation of fungal propagules. In the absence of a robust immune response, the fungus can then disseminate. Dissemination commonly results in meningitis or meningoencephalitis.
- Risk factors for developing cryptococcosis include HIV infection, diabetes mellitus, chronic liver disease, hematologic malignancies, solid organ or hematopoietic stem cell transplantation, corticosteroid therapy, use of TNF-α antagonists, sarcoidosis, and connective tissue diseases.[31–34]

DIAGNOSIS

- Immunocompetent hosts infected by *Cryptococcus* are usually asymptomatic. Those with symptoms frequently complain of nonproductive cough, fever, malaise, chest pain, dyspnea, night sweats, and hemoptysis.

- Immunocompetent patients may have a self-limited disease that resolves over weeks to months, even without antifungal therapy.
- Immunocompromised patients often have disseminated disease at the time of diagnosis. Patients commonly present with CNS findings concerning for meningoencephalitis, fever, and cough.
- A very small minority of immunosuppressed patients presented with isolated pulmonary symptoms, although severe cases may present with acute respiratory failure.[31–34]

DIAGNOSTIC TESTING

- Definitive diagnosis of pulmonary cryptococcosis requires **culture** and identification of the organism from a sterile specimen but sensitivity may be poor.
- **Cryptococcal antigen** testing for localized pulmonary disease performs much worse compared to serum testing for disseminated disease or cerebrospinal fluid testing for meningoencephalitis.[31–34]
- **Culture of BAL fluid** has good diagnostic yield, though microscopic examination of the BAL smear with India ink often allows for rapid diagnosis. Testing of BAL fluid or sputum samples for cryptococcal antigen has yielded inconsistent results.[31–34]
- Radiographic findings of pulmonary cryptococcosis are variable, and dependent on the degree of immunosuppression in the patient.[1,31–34]
  - In immunocompetent patients: solitary or multiple pulmonary nodules and airspace consolidation.
  - In immunosuppressed patients: diffuse, interstitial, and lobar infiltrates are the most common findings.

TREATMENT

Because the risk of dissemination and recurrence is related to host immunity, treatment is based upon the status of patient immune function as well as the severity of disease. Treatment recommendations are outlined in Table 14-2.[34]

Fusariosis

GENERAL PRINCIPLES

- *Fusarium* spp. are colorless septate molds that inhabit soil, water, and detritus worldwide.
- *Fusarium solani* and *Fusarium oxysporum* are the most commonly encountered pathogenic species, though there are several clinically relevant species.
- **Disseminated disease is nearly exclusive to immunocompromised patient populations.** Pulmonary involvement usually occurs in the context of disseminated disease.[35]
- Risk factors include hematologic malignancies (particularly acute myeloid or lymphocytic leukemia), hematopoietic stem cell or solid organ transplantation, and profound neutropenia.[35–37]

TABLE 14-2 TREATMENT RECOMMENDATIONS FOR PULMONARY CRYPTOCOCCOSIS

Disease Severity	Immune Status	Recommended Treatment
Mild to moderate		Fluconazole 400 mg daily for 6–12 mo[a]
Severe or progressive[b]	HIV positive	**Induction:** amphotericin B 0.7–1 mg/kg daily **PLUS** flucytosine (100 mg/kg daily in 4 divided doses) for 2 wk (4–6 wk if intolerant to flucytosine) **OR** Liposomal amphotericin B 3–4 mg/kg **PLUS** flucytosine (100 mg/kg daily in 4 divided doses) for 2 wk (4–6 wk if intolerant to flucytosine) **Consolidation:** fluconazole 400 mg daily for 8 wk **Maintenance:** fluconazole 200 mg daily for ≥1 y **OR** itraconazole 400 mg daily for ≥1 y
	Organ transplant recipient	**Induction:** liposomal amphotericin B 3–4 mg/kg daily **PLUS** flucytosine (100 mg/kg daily in 4 divided doses) for 2 wk **OR** Liposomal amphotericin B 6 mg/kg daily for 4–6 wk **OR** Amphotericin B 0.7 mg/kg daily for 4–6 wk **Consolidation:** fluconazole 400–800 mg daily for 8 wk **Maintenance:** fluconazole 200–400 mg daily for 6–12 mo

(*continued*)

TABLE 14-2	TREATMENT RECOMMENDATIONS FOR PULMONARY CRYPTOCOCCOSIS (Continued)		
Disease Severity	**Immune Status**	**Recommended Treatment**	
	Non–HIV-infected and nontransplant	**Induction:** amphotericin B 0.7–1 mg/kg daily **PLUS** flucytosine (100 mg/kg daily in 4 divided doses) for ≥4 wk (≥6 wk if intolerant to flucytosine) **OR** Liposomal amphotericin B 3–4 mg/kg with flucytosine if possible for ≥4 wk **Consolidation:** fluconazole 400–800 mg daily for 8 wk **Maintenance:** Fluconazole 200 mg daily for 6–12 mo	

[a]For immunocompetent patients, itraconazole 200 mg bid, voriconazole 200 mg bid, and posaconazole 400 mg bid acceptable if patient intolerant to or inappropriate for fluconazole.

[b]In immunocompromised patients must rule out meningitis.

[c]Possible alternative induction therapies include amphotericin B plus fluconazole, fluconazole plus flucytosine, fluconazole, and itraconazole.

Adapted from Perfect JR, Dismukes WE, Dromer F, et al. Clinical practice guidelines for the management of cryptococcal disease: 2010 update by the Infectious Diseases Society of America. *Clin Infect Dis.* 2010;50:291–322.

- Despite aggressive therapy, mortality remains as high as 100% in patients with disseminated disease and persistent neutropenia.[35]

DIAGNOSIS

- Pulmonary manifestations are like those seen with aspergillosis including allergic disease (i.e., allergic bronchopulmonary fusariosis), allergic pneumonitis, cavity colonization, and pneumonia.[37]
- Classically, disseminated infection presents refractory fevers in a patient with prolonged neutropenia and new skin lesions. Up to 75% of patients have cutaneous involvement. The characteristic cutaneous findings are bulls-eye lesions with central necrosis mimicking ecthyma gangrenosum.[35–37]

- Patients with pulmonary involvement may also have pleuritic chest pain, nonproductive cough, and shortness of breath.
- While isolation of the organism in culture is helpful in diagnosis, *Fusarium* spp. can also be a contaminant.
- **Blood cultures are positive in about 40% of cases with invasive disease.**[35]
- Diagnosis of fusariosis relies upon **histopathologic examination of the affected tissue,** which shows hyaline, acute-branching, septate hyphae, and sickle-shaped multiseptate macroconidia.
- Radiography findings are variable, and may show nonspecific alveolar or interstitial infiltrates, cavities, and nodules.

TREATMENT

- In disseminated disease, susceptibility testing is necessary to optimize antifungal therapy, as species-dependent resistance to amphotericin B and the triazoles may occur. Empiric combination therapy with liposomal formulation of amphotericin B and voriconazole is recommended. Step-down therapy should be tailored based on species-level identification and antifungal susceptibility testing.
- Local debridement may be necessary for progressive soft tissue infection.
- Immune reconstitution is often vital to patient's recovery from fusariosis. Mitigating iatrogenic immunosuppression is strongly recommended, when feasible.
- Glucocorticoids are associated with worse outcomes for patients with fusariosis and should be avoided.

Histoplasmosis

GENERAL PRINCIPLES

- *Histoplasmosis capsulatum* is a dimorphic fungus that grows as a mold in soil, bird roosts, bat caves, and other environmental foci. In human tissues at 37 °C, it grows as yeast that replicates via narrow-based budding.[1,38]
- Historically, *Histoplasma* was thought to be geographically restricted to hyperendemic regions of southeastern, mid-Atlantic, and central US. However, it is now well established that *Histoplasma* has a worldwide distribution.
- Severity of the illness depends upon both the host immunity and degree of exposure.
- HIV infection with a CD4 count <150/μL, use of immunosuppressive agents (particularly TNF-α antagonists), hematologic malignancies, and solid organ transplantation are risk factors for disseminated histoplasmosis.[38,39]

DIAGNOSIS

- **Most patients with acute histoplasmosis are asymptomatic or have mild pulmonary symptoms for which they never seek medical care.**
- Symptomatic patients seeking medical care are frequently misdiagnosed with community-acquired pneumonia resulting in delayed diagnoses. Histoplasmosis diagnosis is often made weeks to months after initial presentation and after several failed courses of antibiotics.[38]

- Patients who develop severe pneumonia present with fevers, chills, chest pain, cough, dyspnea, and hypoxia. The clinical course can rapidly progress to ARDS.
- A subset of elderly patients with emphysema is at increased risk of developing chronic cavitary pulmonary histoplasmosis.[38] Patients usually present with fever, fatigue, anorexia, weight loss, productive cough, hemoptysis, and other symptoms mimicking reactivation pulmonary TB.
- Progression to disseminated disease is typically limited to patients with significant immunosuppression.[39]

DIAGNOSTIC TESTING

- Isolation of *Histoplasma* from **culture** with use of a specific DNA probe for verification remains the diagnostic gold standard. However, fungal **growth in culture may take 4–6 weeks**.[38,39]
- Detection of *H. capsulatum* polysaccharide **antigen in urine** is the preferred rapid test, with a sensitivity of >90% in patients with disseminated disease.[1,38-41] Sensitivity decreases in those with only pulmonary disease to 75%.[39] While the specificity has been reported as 99%, false positives can occur in patients with other fungal infections.[38]
- Complement fixation and immunodiffusion assays of histoplasmosis antibodies in the serum may be useful in immunocompetent patients and in those with chronic infection. Serologic testing may be negative during early infection.[39]
- Microscopically, *Histoplasma* appears as 2–4-μm budding oval yeast on silver or periodic acid–Schiff staining of histopathology specimens.[38,39]
- Chest radiography frequently shows patchy infiltrates with hilar or mediastinal lymphadenopathy in mild histoplasmosis and diffuse reticulonodular infiltrates in severe pneumonia.
- Cavitary disease can appear as unilateral or bilateral upper lobe infiltrates or cavities and is associated with extensive fibrosis in the lower lung fields.

TREATMENT

- Treatment of immunocompetent patients with mild-to-moderate acute pulmonary histoplasmosis is often not necessary.
- For patients who have symptoms for >1 month, treatment with itraconazole for 6–12 weeks is recommended.[1,7,38-41]
- In patients with severe acute pulmonary histoplasmosis or progressive disseminated histoplasmosis:
  ○ Induction therapy with lipid formulation of amphotericin B 3–5 mg/kg daily for 1–2 weeks is recommended.
  ○ After induction therapy, step-down therapy is continued with itraconazole 200 mg PO every 8 hours for 3 days, then 200 mg every 12 hours for a total of 12 weeks.[7,38-41]
- A short course of **methylprednisolone** 0.5–1 mg/kg daily for 1–2 weeks may be useful in patients with ARDS.[7,38-41]
- Those with chronic cavitary pulmonary histoplasmosis should be treated with itraconazole 200 mg every 8 hours for 3 days, then 200 mg every 12 hours for 18–24 months with close monitoring for relapse.[38-41]

COMPLICATIONS

- In some cases, acute histoplasmosis infection may result in either granulomatous mediastinitis or fibrosing mediastinitis.
- **Granulomatous mediastinitis** is characterized by persistently enlarged lymph nodes that sometimes coalesce into a large, caseating lesion. Patients are frequently asymptomatic, and the disease does not progress to fibrosing mediastinitis. Itraconazole 200 mg PO every 12 hours for 6–12 months is often used but its benefit has not been proven.[40]
- **Fibrosing mediastinitis** is a rare complication of acute histoplasmosis infection and is thought to be caused by an exuberant fibrosing response to the infection. The progressive tissue fibrosis eventually results in entrapment of the great vessels and/or bronchi, resulting in heart failure, pulmonary emboli, superior vena cava syndrome, dyspnea, cough, wheezing, and hemoptysis. Fibrosing mediastinitis is notoriously resistant to treatment; antifungal administration, blood vessel or airway stenting, and surgical intervention have been shown to improve outcomes.

Mucormycosis

GENERAL PRINCIPLES

- Mucormycosis is an invasive fungal infection most commonly caused by fungi from the genera *Mucor*, *Rhizopus*, *Rhizomucor*, *Cunninghamella*, and *Saksenaea*.
- Mucormycosis occurs **primarily in immunocompromised patients**.
- Mucormycetes have a worldwide distribution and are commonly found in soil and on decaying organic material.
- Inhalation of sporangiospores is the typical route of entry.
- Risk factors include diabetes, chronic renal failure, hematologic malignancies, stem cell transplantation, solid organ transplantation, iron overload/deferoxamine, neutropenia, graft versus host disease, corticosteroids, IV drug use, advanced HIV, and trauma.[1,42–49]
- Despite aggressive measures, the prognosis of mucormycosis is grave, with mortality up to about 90%, depending on the site of infection and host characteristics.[43]

DIAGNOSIS

- Pulmonary mucormycosis is less common than rhinocerebral mucormycosis or cutaneous mucormycosis. However, all presentations can lead to disseminated disease. Pulmonary mucormycosis frequently presents with nonspecific symptoms, including cough, fever, and hemoptysis, which can be mistaken for IPA.
- Pulmonary mucormycosis often demonstrates multiple pulmonary nodules with pleural effusions. Massive hemoptysis may occur because of fungal invasion of the pulmonary artery.[48]

DIAGNOSTIC TESTING

- Blood, sputum, and nasal swabs are usually of little diagnostic utility because the organisms are extremely difficult to isolate and culture.

- The diagnosis usually **requires tissue biopsy with histopathologic examination**. Mucormycetes appear as thin-walled, ribbonlike nonseptated hyphae that branch at right angles.
- CXRs are rarely normal but the findings are variable. Infiltrates, consolidations, and cavitary lesions may all be seen.

TREATMENT

- Liposomal formulation of **amphotericin B** is the mainstay of therapy for mucormycosis. Typical dosing ranges from 3–5 mg/kg daily, and is continued until resolution of all visible lesions, and throughout immunosuppression.[7,42–49]
- **Posaconazole** and isavuconazole have also been shown to have activity against the agents of mucormycosis and have been used with success.[7,42–49]
- Voriconazole is not active against *Mucorales*.
- Aggressive **surgical debridement** of necrotic tissue is usually beneficial and sometimes vital for survival. However, clinical condition of the patients can sometimes make surgical intervention difficult.
- Iatrogenic immunosuppression should be minimized or discontinued, when possible.[43]

Pneumocystis Pneumonia

GENERAL PRINCIPLES

- *P. jirovecii*, previously known as *Pneumocystis carinii*, is an opportunistic, ascomycetous, nonfilamentous fungal pathogen of the lungs.
- The cell wall of this organism lacks ergosterol. This explains that *P. jirovecii* is resistant to amphotericin B and triazole antifungals as it lacks ergosterol in its cell wall.[50–52]
- *P. jirovecii* has a worldwide distribution, though the natural reservoir of the organism remains unknown. It can be found in the pulmonary system of many mammals, including humans.
- Risk factors include advanced HIV infection (CD4 count <200 cells/mL and/or CD4% <14%). Additional risk factors include hematologic and solid organ malignancy, use of immunosuppressive therapies, and history of recent transplant—within the past 6 months.[41]

DIAGNOSIS

- *Pneumocystis* pneumonia classically presents with fever, nonproductive cough, and dyspnea.
- Onset is often insidious, with patients having symptoms for weeks to months before coming to medical attention.
- Spontaneous pneumothorax can occur in patients with *Pneumocystis* pneumonia. In a small percentage of patients, their initial symptoms are pleuritic chest pain and severe dyspnea from the pneumothorax.

- On physical examination, lung auscultation is typically normal or with discrete crackles. Commonly, patients can be observed oxygenating well at rest but experience acute episodes of hypoxia with minimal exertion (e.g., conversation, standing).

DIAGNOSTIC TESTING

- Initial laboratory diagnostics are frequently nondiagnostic but may show an **elevated lactate dehydrogenase**.
- *Pneumocystis* remains difficult to reliably isolate in culture. Diagnosis continues to rely upon microscopic detection of the organism in a respiratory specimen, such as induced sputum or BAL fluid. The current gold standard technique uses **fluorescein-labeled monoclonal anti-*Pneumocystis* antibodies in histologic examination**. The sensitivity and specificity of BAL indirect fluorescence antibody staining are approximately 90–95%, but significantly less for induced sputum.[51,52]
- Assays testing for (1-3)-β-d-glucan, a cell wall component, are often very elevated in *Pneumocystis* pneumonia. However, these tests are not specific because (1-3)-β-d-glucan is highly conserved across both pathogenic and commensal fungi.
- **CXRs** classically show bilateral, diffuse reticular or granular opacities.
- **Chest CT** typically shows ground-glass opacities with patchy distribution that predominate the **perihilar** regions. Thin-walled cysts may be seen in 10–30% of patients, which predispose patients to developing pneumothoraces.[52]

TREATMENT

- Given its high mortality if untreated, **empiric treatment should be started once the diagnosis is considered**. Short courses of empiric treatment (<48 hours) should not impair diagnosis.
- The treatment of choice is **trimethoprim-sulfamethoxazole (TMP-SMX)**. Typical dosing range is 15–20 mg/kg daily of the TMP component divided into 3 or 4 doses.
- Treatment duration should be for 14 days for patients without HIV and 21 days for patients living with HIV.[1,7,50–52]
- Adjunctive glucocorticoid treatment is well studied and improves mortality among patients living with HIV with moderate to severe *Pneumocystis* pneumonia.
- Given the high likelihood of benefit, glucocorticoid treatment is typically recommended for most patients with moderate to severe *Pneumocystis* pneumonia regardless of HIV status.
- Moderate to severe disease is defined as patients having arterial oxygen partial pressure ≤70 mm Hg or A–a gradients ≥35 mm Hg while breathing room air.
- In those who are sulfa allergic or otherwise unable to tolerate TMP-SMX, alternative regimens include: TMP plus dapsone, primaquine plus clindamycin, atovaquone, and pentamidine.[7,50–52]
- TMP-SMX is highly effective as **primary prophylaxis** against *P. jirovecii* and should be considered in immunocompromised patients at risk of developing *Pneumocystis* pneumonia, including HIV-positive patients with CD4 counts

<200, organ transplant recipients, patients on chemotherapeutic regimens, and patients on prolonged steroid regimens. Oral prophylaxis consists of one double-strength tablet (160 mg TMP with 800 mg SMX) daily through additional dosing schedules and regimens are available depending on clinical situation.[50–52]

REFERENCES

1. Guarner J, Brandt ME. Histopathologic diagnosis of fungal infections in the 21st century. *Clin Microbiol Rev*. 2011;24:247–280.
2. Zmeili OS, Soubani AO. Pulmonary aspergillosis: a clinical update. *Q J Med*. 2007; 100:317–334.
3. Segal BH. Aspergillosis. *N Engl J Med*. 2009;360:1870–1884.
4. Patterson TF, Thompson III GR, Denning DW, et al. Practice guidelines for the diagnosis and management of aspergillosis: 2016 update by the Infectious Diseases Society of America. *Clin Infect Dis*. 2016;63:e1–e60.
5. Donnelly JP, Chen SC, Kauffman CA, et al. Revision and update of the consensus definitions of invasive fungal disease from the European Organization for Research and Treatment of Cancer and the Mycoses Study Group Education and Research Consortium. *Clin Infect Dis*. 2020;71:1367–1376.
6. Lamoth F, Calandra T. Pulmonary aspergillosis: diagnosis and treatment. *Eur Respir Rev*. 2022;31:220114.
7. Limper AH, Knox KS, Sarosi GA, et al. An official American Thoracic Society statement: treatment of fungal infections in adult pulmonary and critical care patients. *Am J Respir Crit Care Med*. 2011;183:96–128.
8. Pfeiffer CD, Fine JP, Safdar N. Diagnosis of invasive aspergillosis using a galactomannan assay: a meta-analysis. *Clin Infect Dis*. 2006;42:1417–1427.
9. Leeflang MM, Debets-Ossenkopp YJ, Visser CE, et al. Galactomannan detection for invasive aspergillosis in immunocompromized patients. *Cochrane Database Syst Rev*. 2008:CD007394.
10. D'Haese J, Theunissen K, Vermeulen E, et al. Detection of galactomannan in bronchoalveolar lavage fluid samples of patients at risk for invasive pulmonary aspergillosis: analytical and clinical validity. *J Clin Microbiol*. 2012;50:1258–1263.
11. White PL, Wingard JR, Bretagne S, et al. Aspergillus polymerase chain reaction: systematic review of evidence for clinical use in comparison with antigen testing. *Clin Infect Dis*. 2015;61(8):1293–1303.
12. Smith NL, Denning DW. Underlying conditions in chronic pulmonary aspergillosis including simple aspergilloma. *Eur Respir J*. 2011;37:865–872.
13. Denning DW. Chronic forms of pulmonary aspergillosis. *Clin Microbiol Infect*. 2001; 7:25–31.
14. Agarwal R. Allergic bronchopulmonary aspergillosis. *Chest*. 2009;135:805–826.
15. Schwartz HJ, Greenberger PA. The prevalence of allergic bronchopulmonary aspergillosis in patients with asthma, determined by serologic and radiologic criteria in patients at risk. *J Lab Clin Med*. 1991;117:138–142.
16. Saccente M, Woods GL. Clinical and laboratory update on blastomycosis. *Clin Microbiol Rev*. 2010;23:367–381.
17. Chapman SW, Dismukes WE, Proia LA, et al. Clinical practice guidelines for the management of blastomycosis: 2008 update by the Infectious Diseases Society of America. *Clin Infect Dis*. 2008;46:1801–1812.
18. McKinnell JA, Pappas PG. Blastomycosis: new insights into diagnosis, prevention, and treatment. *Clin Chest Med*. 2009;30:227–239.
19. Bradsher RW Jr. Pulmonary blastomycosis. *Semin Respir Crit Care Med*. 2008;29:174–181.
20. Darouiche RO. Candida in the ICU. *Clin Chest Med*. 2009;30:287–293.

21. Cruciani M, Serpelloni G. Management of Candida infections in the adult intensive care unit. *Expert Opin Pharmacother*. 2008;9:175–191.
22. Haron E, Vartivarian S, Anaissie E, Dekmezian R, Bodey GP. Primary Candida pneumonia. Experience at a large cancer center and review of the literature. *Medicine (Baltimore)*. 1993;72:137–142.
23. Azoulay E, Timsit JF, Tafflet M, et al. Candida colonization of the respiratory tract and subsequent pseudomonas ventilator-associated pneumonia. *Chest*. 2006;129: 110–117.
24. Kontoyiannis DP, Reddy BT, Torres HA, et al. Pulmonary candidiasis in patients with cancer: an autopsy study. *Clin Infect Dis*. 2002;34:400–403.
25. Wood GC, Mueller EW, Croce MA, Boucher BA, Fabian TC. Candida sp. isolated from bronchoalveolar lavage: clinical significance in critically ill trauma patients. *Intensive Care Med*. 2006;32:599–603.
26. Pappas PG, Kauffman CA, Andes D, et al. Clinical practice guidelines for the management of candidiasis: 2009 update by the Infectious Diseases Society of America. *Clin Infect Dis*. 2009;48:503–535.
27. Galgiani JN, Ampel NM, Blair JE, et al. Coccidioidomycosis. *Clin Infect Dis*. 2005; 41:1217–1223.
28. Parish JM, Blair JE. Coccidioidomycosis. *Mayo Clin Proc*. 2008;83:343–349.
29. Spinello IM, Munoz A, Johnson RH. Pulmonary coccidioidomycosis. *Semin Respir Crit Care Med*. 2008;29:166–173.
30. Ampel NM. Coccidioidomycosis: a review of recent advances. *Clin Chest Med*. 2009; 30:241–251.
31. Shirley RM, Baddley JW. Cryptococcal lung disease. *Curr Opin Pulm Med*. 2009; 15:254–260.
32. Huston SM, Mody CH. Cryptococcosis: an emerging respiratory mycosis. *Clin Chest Med*. 2009;30:253–264.
33. Brizendine KD, Baddley JW, Pappas PG. Pulmonary cryptococcosis. *Semin Respir Crit Care Med*. 2011;32:727–734.
34. Perfect JR, Dismukes WE, Dromer F, et al. Clinical practice guidelines for the management of cryptococcal disease: 2010 update by the Infectious Diseases Society of America. *Clin Infect Dis*. 2010;50:291–322.
35. Nucci M, Anaissie E. Fusarium infections in immunocompromised patients. *Clin Microbiol Rev*. 2007;20:695–704.
36. Ahearn DG, Zhang S, Stulting RD, et al. Fusarium keratitis and contact lens wear: facts and speculations. *Med Mycol*. 2008;46:397–410.
37. Nucci F, Nouér SA, Capone D, Anaissie E, Nucci M. Fusariosis. *Semin Respir Crit Care Med*. 2015;36:706–714.
38. McKinsay DS, McKinsey JP. Pulmonary histoplasmosis. *Semin Respir Crit Care Med*. 2011;32:735–744.
39. Kauffman CA. Histoplasmosis. *Clin Chest Med*. 2009;30:217–225.
40. Wheat LJ, Freifeld AG, Kleiman MB. Clinical practice guidelines for the management of patients with histoplasmosis: 2007 update by the Infectious Diseases Society of America. *Clin Infect Dis*. 2007;45:807–825.
41. Swartzentruber S, Rodes L, Kurkjian K, et al. Diagnosis of acute pulmonary histoplasmosis by antigen detection. *Clin Infect Dis*. 2009;49:1878–1882.
42. Lee FY, Mossad SB, Adal KA. Pulmonary mucormycosis: the last 30 years. *Arch Intern Med*. 1999;159:1301–1309.
43. Sun HY, Singh N. Mucormycosis: its contemporary face and management strategies. *Lancet Infect Dis*. 2011;11:301–311.
44. Aboutanos MB, Joshi M, Scalea TM. Isolated pulmonary mucormycosis in a patient with multiple injuries: a case presentation and review of the literature. *J Trauma*. 2003; 54:1016–1019.

45. Pagano L, Offidani M, Fianchi L, et al. Mucormycosis in hematologic patients. *Haematologica*. 2004;89:207–214.
46. Cornely OA, Alastruey-Izquerdo A, Arenz D, et al. Global guideline for the diagnosis and management of mucormycosis: an initiative of the European Confederation of Medical Mycology in cooperation with the Mycoses Study Group Education and Research Consortium. *Lancet Infect Dis*. 2019;19:e405–e421.
47. Pyrgos V, Shoham S, Walsh TJ. Pulmonary zygomycosis. *Semin Respir Crit Care Med*. 2008;29:111–120.
48. Quan C, Spellberg B. Mucormycosis, pseudallescheriasis, and other uncommon mold infections. *Proc Am Thorac Soc*. 2010;7:210–215.
49. D'Avignon LC, Schofield CM, Hospenthal DR. Pneumocystis pneumonia. *Semin Respir Crit Care Med*. 2008;29:132–140.
50. Krajicek BJ, Thomas CF Jr, Limper AH. Pneumocystis pneumonia: current concepts in pathogenesis, diagnosis, and treatment. *Clin Chest Med*. 2009;30:265–278.
51. Catherinot E, Lanternier F, Bougnoux ME, Lecuit M, Couderc LJ, Lortholary O. Pneumocystis jirovecii pneumonia. *Infect Dis Clin N Am*. 2010;24:107–138.
52. Ewald H, Raatz H, Boscacci R, Furrer H, Bucher HC, Briel M. Adjunctive corticosteroids for Pneumocystis jiroveci pneumonia in patients with HIV infection. *Cochrane Database Syst Rev*. 2015;2015(4):CD006150.

Viral Respiratory Infections

15

Alison M. Hixon and M. Cristina Vazquez-Guillamet

GENERAL PRINCIPLES

- Viral respiratory infections account for nearly 50% of all acute respiratory illnesses. Most infections are self-limited.
- Approximately 200 antigenically distinct viruses cause multiple clinical syndromes ranging from common cold, pharyngitis, croup (i.e., laryngotracheobronchitis), tracheitis, bronchitis, bronchiolitis, and pneumonia.
- This chapter will introduce the major respiratory viruses encountered in clinical practice, assist in differentiating viral and bacterial respiratory infections, and guide antiviral therapy where specific therapy exists.
- See Table 15-1 for common respiratory viruses.

Classification in the Normal Host
Upper Respiratory Tract Infections (URTIs)
- **Rhinosinusitis** is an upper respiratory tract infection defined as inflammation of the mucosa of the nasal passage and paranasal sinuses lasting up to 4 weeks.
  - **The most common etiology is viral.** Bacteria can secondarily infect an inflamed sinus cavity, but this only accounts for 0.5–2% of cases. Invasive fungi, may rarely cause fulminant disease in immunocompromised hosts characterized by tissue invasion and necrosis.[1]
  - Since management of **acute viral rhinosinusitis** (AVRS) is supportive, the focus for the clinician should be on identifying those cases with **acute bacterial rhinosinusitis** (ABRS). Viral etiologies include rhinovirus, adenovirus, parainfluenza virus (PIV), influenza virus, human coronavirus (HCoV), and enterovirus.
  - The most common bacteria associated with ABRS are *Streptococcus pneumoniae (S. pneumoniae)* and *Haemophilus influenzae (H. influenzae)*.[1]
  - Significant complications of ABRS are rare and include orbital cellulitis, cavernous sinus thrombosis, osteomyelitis, meningitis, and brain abscess. These complications represent medical emergencies that require hospitalization.
  - **The diagnosis is clinical.** Acute rhinosinusitis of any etiology presents with three major symptoms: nasal congestion or blockage, purulent rhinorrhea, and facial pain or pressure.
  - AVRS symptoms typically peak within 2–3 days of onset, decline gradually thereafter, and disappear within 10–14 days. Any pattern that deviates from the "classical" viral disease progression could suggest a bacterial infection.
  - Three criteria may help distinguish ABRS from AVRS[2]:
    - Persistent signs and symptoms lasting for ≥10 days.

TABLE 15-1 COMMON RESPIRATORY VIRUS INFECTIONS

Virus	Syndrome	Subtypes	Risk Factors	Incidence
Adenovirus	Keratoconjunctivitis, pharyngitis, croup, pharyngoconjunctival fever, tonsillitis, pneumonia	**Subgroup C** (AdV-1, 2, 5, 6), **subgroup B** (AdV-3, 7, 11, 16, 21), **subgroup E** (AdV-4)	Immunosuppressed, close quarters (barracks, daycares)	Year-round; peak in winter/spring
Coronavirus	URTI, pneumonia, ARDS	**SARS-CoV-2 (COVID-19), SARS-CoV-1,** MERS-CoV, HCoV-OC43, HCoV-229E, HCoV-NL63, NCoV-HKU1	Age, racial/ethnic minorities, immunosuppressed, asthma, cystic fibrosis, chronic lung disease, heart disease, chronic liver disease, obesity (BMI > 30), diabetes, smoking, pregnancy, dementia, physical inactivity, disabilities	Year-round for COVID-19; late fall to early spring for other HCoVs
CMV	Asymptomatic, mild URTI, pneumonia, systemic		Immunosuppressed, HIV	
Influenza virus	URTI, systemic symptoms, pneumonia, ARDS	A, B	Pregnant, elderly, young children	Late fall to early spring

hMPV	Common cold, bronchiolitis, pneumonia, otitis media (children)		Immunosuppressed, prematurity, cardiopulmonary disease, elderly
PIV	Rhinitis, pharyngitis, croup, bronchitis, pneumonia	PIV1, PIV2, PIV3, PIV4	COPD, asthma	PIV1 biannual in fall; PIV3 annual in spring/summer
RSV	Rhinitis, conjunctivitis, otitis media, apnea (infants), bronchiolitis, pneumonia	A, B	Infant (<6 mo), cardiopulmonary disease, COPD, asthma, elderly, immunosuppressed	Late fall to early spring
Rhinovirus/Enterovirus	Common cold, bronchitis, bronchiolitis, pneumonia	Many	COPD, asthma, cystic fibrosis	Year-round; peaks in fall and spring

URTI, upper respiratory tract infection; ARDS, acute respiratory distress syndrome; BMI, body mass index; CMV, cytomegalovirus; HIV, human immunodeficiency virus; hMPV, human metapneumovirus; PIV, parainfluenza virus; COPD, chronic obstructive pulmonary disease; RSV, respiratory syncytial virus.

- Severe symptoms for 3–4 consecutive days at the beginning of illness: high fever (≥39 °C), purulent rhinorrhea, or facial pain.
- Double-sickening: new onset of fever or increased nasal discharge following a typical viral URTI that lasted 5–6 days and was initially improving.
  ○ Imaging studies such as plain radiographs and CT scans are of little diagnostic value in uncomplicated acute rhinosinusitis and are not routinely recommended. An abnormal radiographic finding cannot distinguish between a viral or bacterial etiology.
  ○ Cultures obtained by sinus aspiration are not indicated for uncomplicated ABRS. They could be performed if the patient has failed to respond to initial empiric antimicrobial therapy.
  ○ Intranasal saline irrigation with either physiologic or hypertonic saline can be beneficial in symptomatic control, although the evidence supporting it is weak.[3]
  ○ Topical or systemic decongestants, antihistamines, and mucolytics are frequently used for symptom control. However, there are no significant data to support their use. Topical decongestants (i.e., phenylephrine, oxymetazoline) should not be used for more than 3 consecutive days to avoid rebound congestion and tachyphylaxis.
  ○ Intranasal corticosteroids have been shown to provide a modest relief in symptoms when compared to placebo and should be strongly considered in patients with allergic rhinitis.
  ○ Antibiotics may be beneficial for patients with a clinical diagnosis of AVRS and who have severe/persistent symptoms (>7 days), temperature ≥39 °C, or double-sickening.[2]
- **Pharyngitis/tonsillitis** is inflammation of the pharynx or tonsils, commonly referred to as a "sore throat."
  ○ **The most common etiology is viral.** Like rhinosinusitis, the focus for the clinician should be distinguishing viral versus bacterial pharyngitis.
    - Symptoms suggestive of a viral etiology include rhinorrhea, cough, oral ulcers, and hoarseness.
    - Common viral etiologies include rhinovirus, HCoV, adenovirus, herpes simplex virus (HSV), PIV, and influenza. Epstein–Barr virus (EBV), coxsackievirus, and acute HIV have also been identified.
    - Diagnostic testing of viral pharyngitis should be restricted to cases where symptoms fail to resolve within 1–2 weeks or for surveillance cultures during endemic virus outbreaks.
    - Treatment is mostly supportive with hydration, antipyretics, and analgesia. Topical anesthetics and lozenges alleviate throat pain.
  ○ Antibiotics should generally only be used for pharyngitis in cases of documented Group A β-hemolytic streptococcal (GAS) bacterial infection.[4]
    - The Infectious Diseases Society of America (IDSA) recommends rapid strep testing whenever there is consideration of GAS pharyngitis, except when only overt viral features are present.[4]
    - The **modified Centor criteria** can be used to estimate the probability of GAS pharyngitis. One point each is given for the following: temperature >38 °C, absence of cough, anterior cervical lymphadenopathy, and tonsillar swelling or exudate. The modification adds one point for ages 3–14 and subtracts one point for ages ≥45; ages 15–44 have no effect on the score. The

risk of streptococcal infection with ≤0 points is 1–2.5%; 1 point, 5–10%; 2 points, 11–17%; 3 points, 28–35%; and ≥4 points, 21–53%.[5]
- Negative rapid strep tests should be confirmed with throat culture in children >3 years old and adolescents due to a higher risk of developing acute rheumatic fever. In adults, a backup culture is unnecessary because both the rate of GAS pharyngitis and the risk of rheumatic fever are low.[4]
○ Less frequent in immunocompetent patients, physicians may encounter fungal oropharyngeal infection caused by *Candida* spp., commonly referred to as "thrush." Thrush can be recognized by adherent thick white patches on the palate and tongue. Risk factors include inhaled corticosteroid use without appropriate mouth rinsing, systemic steroids, antibiotics, severe xerostomia, and poor denture hygiene. Adults presenting with thrush should be screened for HIV.[6]

Lower Respiratory Tract Infections (LRTIs)
- **Bronchitis**
  ○ Bronchitis is inflammation of the large airways or bronchi.
  ○ It is classified as either acute or chronic:
    - **Chronic bronchitis** is a nonspecific clinical term with several meanings and is usually not due to infection.
      □ In the general context of chronic obstructive pulmonary disease (COPD), it is defined as cough with sputum production for 3 months in each of the 2 prior years without other explanation—it may or may not be associated with demonstrable airflow obstruction on pulmonary function testing.[7]
      □ In an even broader context, chronic bronchitis can imply a productive cough for >8–12 weeks. Chronic cough is discussed in detail in Chapter 7.
    - **Acute bronchitis** is a self-limited infection with cough as the predominant symptom usually lasting up to 3 weeks but can be as long as 6 weeks. Significant rhinorrhea, fever, dyspnea, tachypnea, or hypoxemia suggests an alternative diagnosis.[8]
      □ **Ninety percent of cases of acute bronchitis are viral,** most commonly PIV, influenza, adenovirus, HCoV including severe acute respiratory syndrome coronavirus 2 (SARS-CoV-2), human metapneumovirus (hMPV), PIV, respiratory syncytial virus (RSV), and rhinovirus. When caused by bacteria, mostly the organisms are *Mycoplasma pneumoniae, Chlamydia pneumoniae,* and *Bordatella pertussis (B. pertussis).* Superinfection with typical respiratory pathogens (i.e., *S. pneumoniae, H. influenzae,* and *M. catarrhalis*) is known to occur but is uncommon.
      □ Treatment is supportive with antitussives, expectorants, and possibly inhaled bronchodilators, despite a paucity of data to support their use.
      □ **Routine use of antibiotics is discouraged.** Likewise, there is limited value in treating smokers without COPD with antibiotics. An important exception is when *B. pertussis* is known or suspected to limit spread to unvaccinated infants and children. Unless started early, antibiotic treatment has little impact on the course of pertussis in immunocompetent, previously vaccinated adolescents and adults.
      □ Inhaled bronchodilators may be beneficial in patients who have airflow obstruction and wheezing.[9]

- **Bronchiolitis**[10]
  - Bronchiolitis, inflammation of the small airways or bronchioles, **is almost exclusively viral,** and typically occurs in <2-year-olds, though has been reported in adults.
  - **RSV is the most common etiology,** but other viruses include rhinovirus, hMPV, adenovirus, human bocavirus (HBoV), and influenza.
  - Treatment is primarily supportive with supplemental oxygen. Continuous positive airway pressure and high-flow nasal cannula therapy may provide effective ventilatory support and decrease the need for intubation.[10]
  - **RSV** vaccination is recommended in selected patient populations.[11]
  - Several studies have evaluated the effectiveness of inhaled bronchodilators, systemic corticosteroids, inhaled hypertonic saline, and heliox. None of these therapies demonstrated a consistent benefit on mortality or length of hospitalization. Lung transplant or hematopoetic stem cell transplant recipients with lower respiratory tract disease may benefit from oral ribavirin, although the data are limited.[12]
- **Pneumonia**[13–15]
  - Pneumonia, inflammation of the air sacs of the lungs, is a clinical diagnosis based on symptoms and radiographic findings.
  - 50–70% of childhood pneumonia and up to 30% of adult pneumonia cases have been attributed to a viral etiology. Likely organisms include SARS-CoV-2, influenza, RSV, rhinovirus, hMPV, PIV, and adenovirus.
  - Symptoms typically include fever, tachypnea, tachycardia, and clinical findings of lung involvement on examination such as rhonchi, or rales. Other symptoms may include cough, rhinorrhea, sinus congestion, chills, and myalgias.
  - CXR may demonstrate consolidation due to alveolar or interstitial infiltrates in a lobar or multilobar distribution.[16]
  - Viral pneumonia may be complicated by secondary bacterial pneumonia or concurrent viral and bacterial infection.
  - No specific clinical findings clearly differentiate viral from bacterial pneumonia. A high fever (>38.5 °C), high respiratory rate, lobar consolidation on chest radiography, and significantly elevated levels of C-reactive protein (CRP), white blood cell (WBC) count, and procalcitonin (PCT) suggest bacterial etiology.[16,17]
  - Mild cases improve with supportive management on an outpatient basis, while severe cases may necessitate admission to an intensive care unit (ICU), respiratory support with mechanical ventilation, or other aggressive measures.
  - Empiric antibiotics should be given in cases of severe pneumonia while awaiting confirmatory testing, narrowed as soon as possible to target the causal pathogen.
  - Patients presenting to the emergency department or hospitalized with pneumonia should receive intranasal swab polymerase chain reaction (PCR) testing for viral causes, especially treatable viral causes.
  - Specific antiviral therapies are discussed in more detail below.

Respiratory Virus Infections in Special Adult Populations
- **Pregnancy**
  - Pregnancy-related changes to the immune and endocrine systems can increase susceptibility to certain viral and bacterial infections. Pregnant women are at

risk for more severe infections and have higher morbidity and mortality from infection than their nonpregnant counterparts.[18,19]
- Treatment is supportive with hydration, oxygen, blood pressure, and, if necessary, mechanical ventilation. Specific antiviral therapy should be used if available.
- Antipyretics help to prevent fetal tachycardia and congenital abnormalities related to high maternal fevers.
- Because of the high risk of COVID-19–related complications in pregnancy, pregnant women should be offered the same COVID-19 treatments as nonpregnant adults. Most COVID-19 therapies have not demonstrated concerns in animal models or human trials, with the exception of the mutagenic antiviral molnupiravir, which should be avoided.[20]
- **Ribavirin is contraindicated in pregnancy, in those trying to conceive, and in male partners of pregnant women** due to animal models showing teratogenicity and deleterious effects on germ cells, although data in humans is limited.[21]
- Controlled data on the safety of many other antiviral compounds in pregnancy are lacking. Most (oseltamivir, zanamivir, ganciclovir, cidofovir) are classified as category C by the U.S. Food and Drug Administration (FDA) and should be used only when the benefits of therapy outweigh the risks. Acyclovir is classified as category B but is recommended only for cases of serious infection and not for routine use in pregnancy.
- Killed or inactivated vaccines have been shown to be safe in pregnancy, especially during seasonal outbreaks when benefits outweigh small risks. **Influenza and COVID-19 vaccinations should be offered during pregnancy. RSV vaccination in pregnancy (weeks 32–36 during the RSV season September–January) protects the infant from getting severe disease.**[22–24]

- **Chronic lung diseases**
  - Chronic lung diseases include asthma, COPD, and interstitial lung disease (ILD).
  - Viral respiratory infections can lead to exacerbations, as well as more severe respiratory infections and prolonged disease courses in these patients.
  - SARS-CoV-2, RSV, influenza, hMPV, rhinovirus, and parainfluenza are common culprits.
  - Influenza, COVID-19, and RSV vaccinations are recommended in appropriate patients.
- **Immunocompromised**[25]
  - There are many forms of acquired and innate immune deficiencies that can have varied susceptibility to and ability to mount an immune response against viral respiratory infections.
  - Classic symptoms, such as fever, may be absent in this population, and disease may progress faster and may be more severe.
  - All immunocompromised persons should be offered vaccination, although vaccines may have variable efficacy depending on the arm of the immune system affected.[26]
  - As circulating antibodies are a primary defense against viral infections, persons with a reduced ability to produce or maintain antibodies are particularly high risk. Populations with lower rates of seropositivity following vaccination are solid organ transplant recipients and those receiving B-cell–depleting therapy (rituximab).[27]

- Solid organ transplant recipients are at increased risk for developing respiratory infections from reactivated, latent viruses such as cytomegalovirus (CMV), HSV-1, EBV, and varicella zoster virus (VZV), and adenovirus.[15]
- Immunocompromised persons may shed viruses following infection for much longer (weeks to months) than immunocompetent persons (days to weeks) and may require longer periods of isolation both in and out of the hospital.

Prevention

- **Vaccination** remains the best means of preventing viral respiratory illness, but few vaccines are available.
- Vaccines stimulate both humoral and cellular immune responses, the primary result of which are circulating neutralizing antibodies against viral epitopes. Some vaccines also stimulate immunity through T-cells, memory B-cells, and nonneutralizing antibodies that contribute to the development and durability of the immune response.
- In absence of vaccines, hand hygiene, social distancing, and face masks have been shown to reduce the spread of viral infections to varying degrees that are likely dependent on population-level adherence and user technique.[28,29]
- **Influenza** vaccine
  - Vaccine strains change yearly; thus, influenza vaccines must be modified annually.
  - Annual flu vaccines are strongly recommended, especially in pregnant women, children <5 years old, adults >50 years old, people with chronic medical conditions (e.g., chronic respiratory disease, cardiovascular disease, diabetes, obesity, renal disease, immunosuppression), health care workers, residents of long-term care facilities, and people who live with or care for patients at high risk for severe influenza (including children under 6 months of age who cannot be vaccinated). Patients with egg allergy, regardless of severity are unlikely to require medical care when vaccinated.[30]
  - Options include injectable inactivated split-virus injected (recommended for all people >6 months old) and live attenuated virus inhaled (for healthy, nonpregnant people aged 2–49). Live vaccines should be avoided in patients who are immunosuppressed.
  - High-dose influenza vaccination is recommended in adults ≥65 years old due to higher risk of influenza-related complications.[30]
- **SARS-CoV-2** vaccine
  - There are two types of vaccines currently approved for COVID-19, mRNA and protein subunit. The initial vaccines to become available during the COVID-19 pandemic targeted the original COVID-19 variant. However, as the virus continues to mutate to evade the immune system, vaccine updates have been required to protect against subsequent variants.[31]
  - It is likely that booster vaccination to prevent severe disease will continue to be required periodically as the virus continues to evolve.
- **RSV** vaccine
  - Two monoclonal antibody vaccines (nirsevimab, palivizumab) against RSV are approved for infants <8 months old and children 8–19 months old at increased risk for severe RSV. Protection from this passive immunization lasts approximately 6 months.

- Two recombinant protein vaccines against RSV are approved for adults. Both vaccines are currently only recommended in adults ≥60 years old. One is also approved for high-risk pregnant women from 32–36 weeks gestation during RSV season. Neither vaccine is yet approved for immunocompromised or other high-risk adults <60 years old.[11,23]
- RSV vaccination should optimally be given just before or during the RSV season.
- **Varicella zoster virus** vaccine
  - Vaccination is available as primary prevention to prevent infection, that is, "chickenpox," as well as secondary prevention to protect those who had chickenpox from later developing reactivated varicella, that is, "shingles."
  - The chickenpox vaccine is a live, attenuated vaccine given in two doses. It is contraindicated in pregnant women, immunosuppressed patients, and patients who have other acute illness.
  - The shingles vaccine is a two-dose recombinant vaccine recommended for immunocompetent adults ≥50 years old and immunocompromised adults ≥19 years old. Given limited data, it is currently not recommended in pregnancy.
- **Adenovirus** vaccine: A live, oral vaccine against adenovirus strains 4 and 7 is available only to U.S. Military personnel aged 17–50 years.
- Additional information regarding specific vaccines is available on the Centers for Disease Control and Prevention (CDC) website (www.cdc.gov/vaccines/index.html).[32]

Diagnosis

- Diagnosis may be possible, based on clinical grounds alone and particularly during seasonal outbreaks. Various testing strategies are discussed in Table 15-2.

TABLE 15-2 DIAGNOSTIC STRATEGIES FOR VIRAL RESPIRATORY INFECTIONS

Diagnostic Test	Test Principle	Advantages	Disadvantages
PCR • Single • Multiplex	Amplification of a portion of the viral genome in a patient sample	High sensitivity High specificity Rapid Can detect multiple pathogens (multiplex) in single sample Can differentiate between viral strains/serotypes Can quantitate viral copies present in sample	Availability of equipment

(*continued*)

TABLE 15-2. DIAGNOSTIC STRATEGIES FOR VIRAL RESPIRATORY INFECTIONS (Continued)

Diagnostic Test	Test Principle	Advantages	Disadvantages
Antibody-mediated • Direct or indirect antibody • ELISA	Antibody detection of viral protein in a patient sample or cell culture inoculated with the patient sample	Relatively good sensitivity Relatively good specificity	
Viral culture	Inoculation of cells with a patient sample and detection of virus by antibody or pathogenic change such as plaque formation	Specificity Confirms presence of live virus in sample	Sensitivity Incubation periods long Not all viruses culturable
Serology	Detection and titer of patient antibodies to a specific virus	Useful for epidemiologic surveys	Requires acute and convalescent sera Difficult to differentiate serotype
Cytopathology	Pathologic appearance of virus infection in patient cell sample	Can detect virus-induced cellular changes in absence of positive culture (e.g., CMV, RSV)	Requires tissue biopsy

PCR, polymerase chain reaction; ELISA, enzyme-linked immunosorbent assay; CMV, cytomegalovirus; RSV, respiratory syncytial virus.

- **Radiographic** findings are not pathognomonic for specific viral etiologies.
- Diagnostic specimens can be collected from nasopharyngeal or oral swabs, nasal washings, induced sputum, nasopharyngeal or tracheal aspirates, bronchial washings, bronchoalveolar lavage (BAL), endobronchial brush biopsy, or lung biopsy.
    - In children, nasopharyngeal swabs and washings have similar sensitivities for detection of respiratory viruses by PCR.
    - In adults, nasopharyngeal swab is more sensitive than throat swab and lower respiratory samples are more sensitive than upper respiratory samples in cases of bronchitis or pneumonia.
- Viral culture remains the gold standard for diagnosing many viral infections. However, prolonged incubation times required to grow the virus in the laboratory preclude the utility of viral culture in many cases.
- Multiplex PCR testing is becoming more common, due to its high sensitivity, specificity, and rapidity.
- Direct and indirect fluorescence antibody-based assays and enzyme-linked immunosorbent assays (ELISA) are also useful for detection of certain viral pathogens.
- Cytopathology may also aid diagnosis by demonstrating cytopathologic effect (adenovirus), giant cells (CMV) or syncytial formation (RSV) in tissue specimens.

Treatment
Supportive Care
- Supportive care with adequate hydration and symptom control are mainstays of treatment.
    - Nasal steroids, antipyretics, antihistamines, decongestants, analgesics, and bronchodilators are sometimes helpful in appropriate patients.
    - Steroids may be useful for significant wheezing.
    - Nebulized epinephrine can be used in cases of stridor.
- In severe cases, transfer to an ICU and ventilatory support may be necessary.

Specific Antiviral Therapies
- Targeted antiviral therapies exist for some viral respiratory illnesses such as SARS-CoV-2 influenza, CMV, HSV, RSV, and adenovirus.
- These drugs target specific viral proteins including DNA polymerases, proteases, ion channels, and enzymes.
- Table 15-3 lists common viral respiratory pathogens, directed antiviral therapies, and vaccines, if available.

SPECIAL CONSIDERATIONS: SPECIFIC VIRAL PATHOGENS
Adenovirus
- **Virology:** Adenovirus is a nonenveloped, double-stranded DNA virus. There are 51 different serotypes with six subgroups, A–F. Adenoviruses of subgroup C primarily infect the upper respiratory tract while viruses in subgroups B and E cause disease of the lower respiratory tract. They can integrate into the host genome leading to latent infection.[33]

TABLE 15-3 TARGETED ANTIVIRAL THERAPIES FOR VIRAL RESPIRATORY PATHOGENS

Virus	Vaccine	Antiviral Compound	Viral Target	Comment
Adenovirus	N	Cidofovir	DNA polymerase	For solid organ and bone marrow transplant patients
CMV	N	Ganciclovir	DNA polymerase	First-line therapy
		Cidofovir	DNA polymerase	
		Foscarnet Letermovir Maribavir	DNA polymerase	For ganciclovir resistance; nephrotoxic
HSV	N	Ganciclovir, valganciclovir	DNA polymerase	First-line therapy
		Foscarnet	DNA polymerase	For ganciclovir resistance; nephrotoxic
Influenza	Y	Oseltamivir, zanamivir, peramivir, baloxavir	Neuraminidase	Effective against influenza A and B; can be used for prophylaxis
		Amantadine, rimantadine	Ion channel	No longer recommended due to high levels of resistance
PIV	N	Ribavirin	Purine RNA nucleotide	Infants, high-risk patients

TABLE 15-3 TARGETED ANTIVIRAL THERAPIES FOR VIRAL RESPIRATORY PATHOGENS (Continued)

Virus	Vaccine	Antiviral Compound	Viral Target	Comment
RSV	Y	Palivizumab, nirsevimab	Fusion protein	Can be used for prophylaxis
		Ribavirin	Purine RNA nucleotide	Infants, high-risk patients
SARS-CoV-2	Y	Nirmatrelvir-ritonavir	Proteases	Multiple drug interactions
		Molnupiravir	Viral RNA mutagen	Contraindicated in pregnancy
		Remdesivir	RNA polymerase	Intravenous infusion
VZV	Y	Acyclovir	DNA polymerase	First-line therapy; nephrotoxic
		Foscarnet	DNA polymerase	For ganciclovir resistance; nephrotoxic

CMV, cytomegalovirus; HSV, herpes simplex virus; PIV, parainfluenza virus; RSV, respiratory syncytial virus; SARS, severe acute respiratory syndrome; VZV, varicella zoster virus.

- **Epidemiology**
  - Adenoviruses have a worldwide distribution, and infections are more frequent in winter and spring.
  - At least 5–10% of acute respiratory infections in children, and 1–7% in adults, are attributed to adenoviruses so that by age 10 most individuals have serologic evidence of adenoviral infection.
  - Epidemics of adenovirus acute respiratory disease (ARD) have been reported among military recruits, immunocompromised patients, and in daycare settings.
  - Transmission occurs via fomites, aerosolized particles, and the fecal–oral route. Adenoviruses can cause persistent infections, and the virus may be shed in the feces for months.
  - Adenoviral infections have been transmitted to kidney and liver transplant recipients, suggesting that reactivation of latent virus (most likely in the gastrointestinal [GI] tract) may be another important mode of transmission.

- Vertical transmission has been reported in infants who were exposed to infected cervical secretions.
- **Clinical presentation**
  - The presentation depends on the age and immune status of the infected host.
  - Adenovirus can cause upper respiratory tract illnesses such as coryza, pharyngitis, and croup but can also cause lower respiratory tract disease.
  - **Pharyngoconjunctival fever** is an adenovirus syndrome presenting with pharyngitis, conjunctival injection, fever, and cervical lymphadenopathy.
  - **Keratoconjunctivitis** presenting as pink eye without purulent discharge is caused by adenovirus serotypes 8, 19, and 37.
  - GI symptoms are caused by other adenovirus serotypes.
  - Adenovirus is **the most common cause of tonsillitis in infants**. Exudative tonsillitis and palpable cervical adenopathy may be seen, making differentiation from strep throat in older children difficult.
  - Pneumonia is most common in infants but rare in immunocompetent adults.
  - Complications include bronchiectasis in children and **ARD** in young adults. ARD is especially common in close-quarter dwellings. Patients with ARD develop fever, pharyngitis, cough, hoarseness, and conjunctivitis.
  - Bone marrow transplant patients may develop a wide range of respiratory clinical syndromes. Solid organ transplant recipients may develop asymptomatic shedding, all manner of respiratory syndromes, and even fatal disseminated disease. Adenoviral pneumonia is a well-known early complication of lung transplantation.
- **Diagnosis**
  - The diagnosis is difficult to make on clinical grounds alone. PCR-based assays on blood are the test of choice.
  - Viral culture is the historical gold standard. All adenoviruses except serotypes 40 and 41 cause a characteristic cytopathic effect in culture. Samples for culture can be obtained from nasopharyngeal swabs or aspirates, throat washings or swabs, rectal swabs, urine, cerebrospinal fluid (CSF), or tissue biopsies. Cultures may take up to a week for completion and may not detect adenovirus in cases where there may be a low viral load (e.g., immunocompromised hosts). Because prolonged shedding may be seen in immunocompromised patients without overt disease, culture positivity should be interpreted with respect to the clinical situation.
  - Histopathology may provide definitive diagnosis of adenovirus in tissue biopsies and can be supplemented by other detection techniques (PCR, immunohistochemistry).
- **Treatment**
  - There are no approved antiviral treatments for adenovirus. Brincidofovir, a lipid conjugate of cidofovir showed promising results in phase II and open-label phase III trials.[34]
  - Cell-mediated immunity is critical in controlling adenovirus infection. Immune reconstitution, reducing immunosuppression, and donor leukocyte infusions may improve survival in life-threatening adenovirus infections.
  - In case reports and small series of solid organ transplant and bone marrow transplant patients, cidofovir may be an option to treat adenoviral infections, especially when therapy is initiated early.[35]

Coronaviruses
- **Virology**
  - Coronaviruses are positive-sense, single-stranded ribonucleic acid (RNA) viruses encased in a crown-like envelope with a diameter of 80–160 nm.
  - Coronaviruses have high rates of recombination and mutation compared to other RNA viruses, which likely contributes to the ability of these viruses to jump between and adapt to new species.
  - Primary sites of replication include the lungs and intestinal tract.
- **Epidemiology**[35,36]
  - Endemic HCoV
    - There are four endemic coronaviruses that likely entered the population within the last 1000 years and are now well-adapted to humans.
    - In temperate climates, they cause disease in late fall, winter, and early spring and are associated with outbreaks every 2–4 years.
  - **Severe acute respiratory syndrome virus-1 (SARS-CoV-1)**
    - SARS-CoV-1 is a zoonotic infection thought to be spread from bats (natural reservoir) and palm civets (incidental host) to humans (accidental host).
    - In late 2002 and into 2003, an outbreak of SARS-CoV emerged in China and Hong Kong and spread globally, causing more than 8000 cases with a case fatality rate of 9.6%.[29]
  - **Middle East respiratory syndrome virus (MERS-CoV)**
    - MERS-CoV is a zoonotic infection thought to be spread from bats (natural reservoir) and dromedary camels (incidental host) to humans (accidental host).
    - Since emerging from the Saudi Arabian Peninsula in 2012, it has caused disease in 27 countries with a 35% case fatality rate.
  - **Severe acute respiratory syndrome virus-2 (SARS-CoV-2)**
    - SARS-CoV-2 emerged from Wuhan, China in late 2019 to cause the global COVID-19 pandemic, resulting in the death of over 6.9 million people at the time of this publication.
    - The virus has continued to mutate and evolve, with new variants of concern continuing to rise at a rapid pace as the virus adapts to living in humans.
- **Clinical presentation**
  - Endemic HCoVs
    - The four older endemic strains are responsible for 10–20% of cases of the common cold and are spread in a manner like that of rhinoviruses (RV), via direct contact with infected secretions or via large aerosol droplets.
    - Infection is often asymptomatic and self-limited, although more severe infections can occur in infants, the elderly, or the immunocompromised.
  - **SARS-CoV-1 and MERS:** These viruses primarily cause LRTI, including severe pneumonia. Much of the pathogenesis is believed to derive from a significant host response to infection rather than from direct damage by the virus itself. Potential complications include secondary bacterial infection and acute respiratory distress syndrome (ARDS).
  - **COVID-19 (SARS-CoV-2)**
    - Infection spans a spectrum from asymptomatic to cold-like symptoms to severe pneumonia resulting in ARDS. A prominent feature of COVID-19 compared to other CoVs is loss of taste and smell.

- COVID-19 illness can be classified by severity.
  - **Asymptomatic**—Positive test but no symptoms.
  - **Mild**—Symptoms include sore throat, rhinorrhea, fatigue, but no signs of lower respiratory tract disease such as shortness of breath or infiltrates on chest imaging.
  - **Moderate**—Symptoms of lower respiratory tract infection on clinical exam and chest imaging but does not require oxygen.
  - **Severe**—Requires oxygen to maintain normal oxygen saturation, respiratory rate >30, or infiltrates >50% of lungs on imaging.
  - **Critical**—Respiratory failure, shock, and multiorgan failure requiring intensive care. This includes patient requiring high-flow oxygen, noninvasive positive-pressure ventilation, mechanical ventilation, extracorporeal membrane oxygenation (ECMO).
- **Diagnosis**
  - RT-PCR or nucleic acid amplification testing (NAAT) is the gold standard diagnostic test for all HCoVs.
  - Other diagnostic tests include serologic detection and antigen detection, but these are less useful clinically.
  - Rapid antigen tests can be used for screening or detecting continued viral shedding. These tests are more accurate for symptomatic infections, are approximately 65% sensitive and 99% specific, and have been shown to reliably detect new COVID-19 variants.[37]
- **Treatment**
  - Patients with suspected HCoV, should be placed on contact, droplet, and airborne precautions.
  - Treatment for the endemic HCoVs is primarily supportive with symptom management, hydration, and ventilatory support.
  - There are no FDA-approved antivirals against endemic HCoVs, SARS-CoV-1, or MERS-CoV.
  - The COVID-19 pandemic resulted in rapid testing of antiviral and immunomodulatory therapies against SARS-CoV-2. Antiviral medications below are discussed by the CDC for treatment of COVID-19. The most current guidelines can be found at https://www.cdc.gov/covid/treatment/index.html.[38]
  - Antivirals should be given within 5–7 days of symptom onset in patients who are at high risk of progressing to severe disease.
    - **Nirmatrelvir-ritonavir** is a viral protease inhibitor approved for use in children and adults ≥12 years and ≥40 kg at high risk for severe symptoms within 5 days of symptoms onset.
    - **Molnupiravir** is a viral RNA mutagen approved for use only in adults ≥18 years and should be avoided in pregnant women.
    - **Remdesivir** is an inhibitor of viral RNA polymerase approved for use in both adults and children.
  - Immunomodulators are given in severe COVID-19, where disease is thought to be driven by an excessive host inflammatory response.
    - **Dexamethasone** is a potent glucocorticoid approved for use in adults and children. It is unclear which second-line agent is superior.
    - **Baricitinib** is a janus kinase (JAK) tyrosine kinase inhibitor, which is a major activator of inflammatory pathways. It is approved for use in adults with severe COVID-19 and sometimes used off-label in children.

- **Tocilizumab** binds interleukin (IL)-6 receptors, preventing IL-6 signaling, which is a major driver of fever and inflammation. It is approved for use in adults and children.
- Selection of therapies for COVID-19 is stratified by treatment setting: outpatient or inpatient.
  - The goal of **outpatient treatment** is to prevent progression to severe disease requiring hospitalization.
    - Persons at high risk of developing severe COVID-19 include those >65 years old, racial/ethnic minorities, immunocompromised hosts, and underlying respiratory disease or cardiovascular disease.
    - Those at high risk should be offered treatment with either nirmatrelvir-ritonavir, molnupiravir, or remdesivir.
    - Both nirmatrelvir-ritonavir and molnupiravir have been shown to significantly reduce the likelihood of hospitalization and death from COVID-19 by approximately 25–75%.[39]
    - Remdesivir has been found to reduce the risk of hospitalization and mortality by up to 87%, although coordinating outpatient infusions may present a challenge.[40]
    - All persons who test positive for COVID-19 or suspect they are infected should isolate to prevent the spread of disease.
  - **Inpatient treatment** is stratified by illness severity with the goal of reducing symptom progression and mortality.
    - Hospitalized patients found to incidentally have **asymptomatic COVID-19** should not receive COVID-19–specific therapies.
    - Patients with **mild-to-moderate COVID-19 hospitalized for reasons other than COVID-19** and with risk factors for progression to severe COVID-19 should be offered the same antiviral treatments as nonhospitalized patients.
    - Patients hospitalized **due to moderate COVID-19**, but do not require oxygen, should receive remdesivir.[41]
    - Patients with **severe COVID-19** and a new or increased oxygen requirement by standard nasal cannula should receive remdesivir plus dexamethasone.[42,43]
    - Patients **with severe or critical COVID-19** with a rapidly increasing oxygen requirement or those requiring high-flow nasal cannula or non-invasive positive-pressure ventilation should receive dexamethasone along with either baricitinib (preferred) or tocilizumab. Remdesivir should be considered in immunocompromised patients within 10 days of symptom onset or if there is concern for continued viral shedding by antigen testing. **Baricitinib** has been shown to decrease mortality in severe COVID-19 by up to 30–40%.[44,45] **Tocilizumab** was shown to slow disease progression in several trials, although benefit on mortality has been more mixed. Tocilizumab may be more beneficial in critically ill COVID-19 patients requiring ICU-level care.[46] The ACTIV-1 IM trial suggested a survival benefit for using **Abatacept** and **infliximab** in addition to a **corticosteroid** in critically ill COVID-19 patients, however, the trial was not designed to examine this endpoint, so additional studies to confirm these data are required.[47]

- Critically ill patients with COVID requiring, mechanical ventilation, or ECMO, should receive dexamethasone and either baricitinib or tocilizumab.
- COVID-19 has been shown to significantly increase the risk of thrombosis, including venous thromboembolism (VTE), stroke, and myocardial infarction.
  - Noncritically ill patients with COVID-19 who require oxygen have improved survival with therapeutic anticoagulation.[48]
  - However, critically ill patients with COVID-19 have not been shown to have a survival benefit from therapeutic anticoagulation. Decisions should be catered to the specific patient regarding prophylactic or therapeutic dosing.[49]
  - Routine measurement of D-dimer is not recommended to risk-stratify patients for anticoagulation.

Cytomegalovirus

- **Virology:** CMV, a member of the *Herpesviridae* family, is a large, enveloped double-stranded DNA virus with a diameter of 120–200 nm.
- **Epidemiology**[50]
  - CMV infects over 50% of adults in the US and Canada by the age of 50 years. Seroprevalence rates of CMV reach 100% in countries with lower socioeconomic status.
  - After acute infection, it remains dormant in human immune progenitor cells. Alterations to the immune system that occur with stress, illness, and aging can result in reactivation.
  - Congenital CMV is the most common intrauterine infection in the US and is the number one cause of congenital hearing loss.
- **Clinical presentation**
  - Primary CMV infection usually is asymptomatic or mild URTI in immunocompetent hosts.
  - In immunocompromised persons, CMV manifests in many organ systems and can cause severe pneumonitis, hepatitis, colitis, esophagitis, and encephalitis.
  - As CMV can reactivate at low levels in times of physical stress, it is important to distinguish between CMV reactivation and active CMV disease. It is unclear if treatment for CMV reactivation provides significant benefits.
  - CMV pneumonitis may occur in up to 15% of transplant populations. The disease is usually severe with hypoxemia, a high incidence of respiratory failure, and a mortality rate exceeding 80%. Patients may present with focal infiltrates, bilateral patchy infiltrates, or diffuse interstitial infiltrates.[51]
  - Pulmonary manifestations are also seen in HIV patients but have become less prevalent with the advent of highly active antiretroviral therapy. CMV is often identified in patients presenting with *Pneumocystis jirovecii* pneumonia, although the virus may not contribute to the severity of disease or symptoms.
  - Clinical laboratory features of CMV include elevation of serum transaminases, relative lymphopenia, atypical lymphocytes, and thrombocytopenia and suggest CMV over other viral infections.
- **Diagnosis**
  - Quantitative PCR is the most widely available method of detecting and monitoring CMV in blood and other tissues. Both the initial viral load and rate

of increase are important features to distinguish reactive versus active CMV, although there are no formal guidelines specifying diagnostic cut-offs.[52]
- Although PCR is now more commonly used for detection of CMV, the gold standard for confirming CMV pneumonitis is histopathology as giant CMV-infected pneumocyte inclusions. Immunohistochemical stains for CMV have also been developed.
- **Treatment**[51]
  - First-line treatment for CMV is IV **ganciclovir** and is the preferred agent for the induction phase in hospitalized patients. Oral **valganciclovir** can also be used as initial therapy in those able to take medications by mouth, or as an extension following induction therapy with IV ganciclovir. Therapy typically lasts 2–4 weeks.
  - Other agents effective against CMV include foscarnet, cidofovir, letermovir, maribavir, and CMV immune globulin (Cytogam).
    - Foscarnet is nephrotoxic and usually reserved for cases of ganciclovir-resistant CMV.
    - Cidofovir is considered a second-line therapy. It is nephrotoxic and should be given along with IV fluids and probenecid.
    - Letermovir and maribavir have been developed due to highly resistant CMV. Letermovir inhibits the viral terminase complex making it less toxic. It has been approved for CMV prophylaxis in hematopoietic stem cell transplant patients. Maribavir targets the viral kinase UL 97 and is currently approved for the treatment of posttransplant CMV infections.
    - Cytogam is reserved for cases of life-threatening CMV infection (e.g., transplant patients with severe disease).

Herpesviruses: HSV-1, EBV, VZV

- The *Herpesviridae* family includes HSV-1, HSV-2, VZV, EBV, and human herpesvirus-8 (HHV-8, the causative agent of Kaposi sarcoma).
- In certain ICU populations (immunocompromised, ARDS, chronically ventilated, postsurgical, or burn), HSV-1 is an important cause of respiratory tract infection.
- EBV infection has been implicated in the development of posttransplant lymphoproliferative disease.
- VZV manifests with chickenpox on primary exposure and as zoster with reactivation. Primary pneumonias are rare but have a high mortality rate. Immunocompromised patients are at greatest risk of VZV pulmonary infection.

Influenza Virus

- **Virology**
  - Influenza is an acute respiratory illness caused by type A or type B influenza virus infection.
  - They are negative-strand, segmented RNA virus in the *Orthomyxoviridae* family, subdivided into antigenic subgroups based on the properties of the hemagglutinin (HA) and neuraminidase (NA) glycoproteins.
  - Influenza viruses circulate in humans, birds, and swine. New influenza strains can arise from reassortment of viral gene products in coinfected organisms (e.g., a pig coinfected with an avian strain and a swine strain).

- **Epidemiology**
  - Influenza traditionally occurs in a seasonal, epidemic form in the winter months.
  - Pandemic influenza arises periodically with strains more highly pathogenic than the seasonal variants (e.g., 1918 H1N1 Spanish influenza, 1957 H2N2 Asian influenza, 1968 H3N2 Hong Kong influenza, and 2009 H1N1 influenza).
- **Clinical presentation**
  - Most cases of influenza are mild, self-limited upper respiratory infections. The incubation period ranges from 1–3 days.
  - Typical symptoms include fever, myalgias, fatigue, and headache, with respiratory symptoms such as rhinorrhea, sore throat, and cough. GI symptoms, including vomiting, and diarrhea, may also occur, especially in children.
  - Severe cases may present with dyspnea, hemoptysis, purulent sputum, rapidly progressive hypoxemia, primary and secondary pneumonia, respiratory failure, and ARDS.
  - Pneumonia may be primary (viral pneumonitis) or secondary to bacterial coinfection, notably *S. aureus, S. pneumoniae, Streptococcus pyogenes,* and *H. influenzae.* Patients with primary influenza pneumonia usually have persistent or worsening symptoms, high fevers, and dyspnea. Patients with secondary bacterial pneumonias may show initial improvement in their symptoms before developing worsening fever and respiratory complaints.
- **Diagnosis**[53]
  - Clinical symptoms during seasonal epidemics provide a high degree of clinical suspicion.
  - Common radiographic findings include bilateral patchy, interstitial, and alveolar infiltrates. Ground-glass opacities may also be present.
  - Rapid detection of influenza can be made by RT-PCR. Multiple testing of samples from various sites (nasopharyngeal swab, tracheal aspirate, and bronchial lavage) can improve diagnostic yield.
- **Treatment**[53]
  - Acetaminophen is recommended over salicylates (to avoid Reye syndrome in patients <18 years old). Antitussives may also be used, and adequate hydration is essential.
  - Antibiotics are reserved for bacterial superinfections.
  - NA inhibitors have activity against types A and B and are most effective if prescribed within 48 hours of symptom onset. They reduce viral shedding and time to symptom relief.
    - **Oseltamivir** is an oral therapy approved for both inpatient and outpatient use. Higher doses and longer durations can be considered in more severe diseases.[39–41]
    - **Zanamivir** is an inhaled therapy that is not recommended for severe or progressive disease or hospitalized patients. It can cause bronchospasm and should be avoided in patients with underlying respiratory conditions.[41]
    - **Peramivir** is an IV medication that can be considered for off-label use for hospitalized patients with severe influenza who cannot tolerate or absorb oseltamivir.
    - **Baloxavir** can be considered for postexposure prophylaxis if given within 48 hours of exposure or for treatment if given within 48 hours of symptom onset.

- Due to high levels of resistance, amantadine or rimantadine against influenza A is no longer recommended.

Metapneumovirus[54]
- hMPV is a member of the *Paramyxoviridae* (like RSV and PIV).
- Discovered in 2001, it is now recognized as a cause of UTRI and LRTI, primarily in children of whom 90–100% have evidence of infection by age 10. hMPV has been implicated in 10% of all hospitalized cases of respiratory viral infections.
- **Clinical presentation** ranges from the cold-like symptoms to bronchiolitis and severe pneumonia.
- **Diagnosis** is by RT-PCR, direct immunofluorescence, and/or viral culture.
- There are no approved targeted therapies. Ribavirin has been studied though there is no strong evidence that treatment modifies disease outcomes.

Parainfluenza Virus[54]
- **Virology:** PIV is another member of *Paramyxoviridae* with four major serotypes: PIV1, PIV2, PIV3, and PIV4. PIV3 is the most prevalent serotype, with 90–100% of children being seropositive by age 5.
- **Epidemiology**
  - PIV causes ~20% of acute respiratory tract infections in hospitalized children, ranking as the second most common etiology for LRTI in this patient population. Up to 10% of acute LRTI in hospitalized adults can be attributed to PIV.
  - Spread occurs easily through large droplet inhalation.
  - PIV1 generally causes epidemics biennially during the fall, while PIV3 occurs in annual spring and summer epidemics. PIV2 and PIV4 occur in less predictable patterns. However, studies in adults suggest year-round circulation of all four serotypes.[47]
- **Clinical presentation**
  - PIV causes URTI and LRTI in adults and children. It primarily infects nasal and oropharyngeal epithelial cells, with subsequent distal spread to the large and small airways. The incubation period is typically 2–8 days.
  - **PIV1 and PIV2 are the primary causes of childhood croup**. Symptoms last up to 4 days. Stridor, dyspnea, and respiratory distress can develop in severe cases.
  - PIV3 is associated with bronchiolitis and pneumonia and is often mistaken for RSV.
  - In adults, PIV usually causes a mild URTI but LRTI is possible, especially in the setting of chronic lung disease.
  - Immunocompromised hosts are susceptible to serious PIV infections, including pneumonia and disseminated infections.[55]
  - Complications may include secondary bacterial pneumonia, sinusitis, otitis media, meningitis, pericarditis, myocarditis, and Guillain–Barré syndrome.
- **Diagnosis:** PIV is often diagnosed clinically, although RT-PCR has become more common. As with other respiratory viruses, viral culture is the gold standard but clinically not necessary.
- **Treatment**[56]
  - There are no antiviral agents with specific activity against PIV. Ribavirin has been trialed in bone marrow transplant recipients, but few data exist on

efficacy. Combination therapy with ribavirin and immunoglobulin has not altered the duration of illness or mortality.
- **Steroids** are recommended in children with severe croup and can decrease length of hospitalization, need for additional therapies, and need for intubation. Nebulized epinephrine can be added if stridor or respiratory distress is present.

Respiratory Syncytial Virus
- **Virology**
  - RSV is an enveloped, single-stranded, negative-sense RNA virus of the *Paramyxoviridae* family.
  - RSV can be divided into two distinct antigenic groups (RSV-A and RSV-B), both of which are present during outbreaks.
  - RSV primarily infects airway epithelial cells. Following cellular entry and replication, it is transmitted through fusion of neighboring cells into large multinucleated syncytia.
- **Epidemiology**[11,57]
  - RSV is the most common cause of LRTIs in infants and young children. The highest rates of illness are seen in infants aged 1–6 months, with peak rates occurring at 3 months. Risk factors include preterm birth, male sex, immunodeficiency, lack of breastfeeding, and overcrowding.
  - In adults, >5% of adult LRTIs are attributable to RSV, especially in elderly and immunocompromised patients.
  - Outbreaks occur in late fall through early spring.
  - Transmission occurs by contact with respiratory secretions or large droplets and fomites.
  - Previous infection with RSV does not confer complete protection against reinfection. Humoral immunity may reduce the severity of subsequent RSV infections. Elderly patients who have lower antibody titers are more likely to develop symptomatic disease.
- **Clinical presentation**
  - RSV URTIs present with cough, coryza, rhinorrhea, conjunctivitis, and otitis media.
  - Apneic episodes may be seen in infants admitted with RSV infections, though the exact mechanism remains unclear and may precipitate sudden infant death syndrome.
  - **LRTIs present with bronchospasm, bronchiolitis,** pneumonia, and, in severe cases, respiratory failure. Patients at risk for LRTI include infants, children with underlying structural lung and heart disease, pre-existing asthma or COPD, institutionalized elderly patients, and immunocompromised patients.
- **Diagnosis**
  - RT-PCR is the diagnostic test of choice because of its rapidity, sensitivity, and specificity.
  - Viral culture from nasal or throat swabs, tracheal aspirates, bronchial washings, or BAL specimens remains the gold standard for diagnosis. Culture may take days to weeks before identification of virus by immunofluorescence staining.
- **Treatment**[58]
  - Bronchodilators may be used in adults with underlying asthma/COPD.

- Mechanical ventilation may be required in some patients with severe disease.
- The evidence for steroids is not compelling but may still be considered in severe disease.
- **Palivizumab and nirsevimab** are monoclonal antibodies against RSV that are approved for prevention of RSV in infants less than 2 years of age. There is limited data to support the use of monoclonal antibodies in adults with RSV, although they may be considered off-label for prophylaxis in high-risk, immunocompromised adults.
- **Ribavirin** is available in oral and inhaled aerosolized formulations.
  - Aerosolized ribavirin is FDA s for use in infants and children with RSV. However, given the lack of positive outcome data and high drug cost, the American Academy of Pediatrics currently recommends against ribavirin for pediatric RSV.
  - Oral ribavirin may be considered in patients with hematologic malignancies, hematopoietic stem cell and lung transplant recipients as off-label option.[59]

Rhinoviruses and Enteroviruses
- **Virology**[60]
  - RV and enteroviruses (EV) are nonenveloped, single-stranded RNA viruses in the *Picornaviridae* family.
  - RVs and some EVs preferentially grow at nasal passage and upper airway temperatures.
  - Other EVs, preferential grow and replicate in the oropharynx and intestinal tract.
  - RVs are classified into species A, B, and C. There are 100 different serotypes in RV-A and RV-B. A third lineage, RV-C, discovered in 2006 includes over 50 strains.
  - EVs are classified into species A-L, that are further divided into dozens of serotypes that cause a wide array of human disease. Of note, Enterovirus A–C contain the coxsackie viruses, which cause hand, foot, and mouth disease (HFMD). Enterovirus C contains all poliovirus serotypes. Enterovirus B contains the echoviruses.
  - Both RVs and EVs can be transmitted via direct contact with infected secretions. Subsequent self-inoculation of the nasal or conjunctival mucosa leads to infection. Transmission by fomites and aerosolized virus may also occur.
  - EVs can also be spread by fecal–oral transmission.
- **Epidemiology**
  - **RV/EV are responsible for about half of common colds.**
  - Infection rates are highest among young children and infants, with an average of six infections per year. Infection rates decrease with advancing age except in the 20s, when another peak is seen. Risks for infections include contact with small children.
  - RV infections peak in autumn and spring in North America and Europe. They are more active during the rainy season in tropical regions of the world. No one strain predominantly circulates at any one time.
  - Some EVs demonstrate seasonality, circulating predominantly in the summer and fall.
  - Despite any anecdotal evidence and popular beliefs, cold temperature exposure, fatigue, and sleep deprivation have not been associated with increased rates of transmission.

- **Clinical presentation**
  - Incubation period is 1–2 days.
  - Symptoms may include rhinorrhea and sneezing (50–70%), sore throat (50%), malaise, headaches, diarrhea, rash, and otitis media. Symptoms generally last 7–10 days but minor symptomatology can linger and viral shedding may occur for up to 3 weeks.
  - Hoarseness and cough are less common but can occur due to upper airway irritation or concurrently with sinusitis and bronchitis. Fever, chills, and myalgias are unusual and should prompt a search for other potential causes.
  - The nasal mucosa becomes edematous and hyperemic and produces a mucoid discharge. The nasal turbinates often become engorged, which can lead to sinus cavity obstruction and occasionally bacterial superinfection.
  - RV/EV may also cause LRTI. Causation is hard to discern, as coinfection with other viruses is common.
  - EV-D68 and EV-A71 infection is associated with the development of polio-like paralysis known as acute flaccid myelitis (AFM) in a small number of cases (<0.1%).[61]
- **Diagnosis**
  - Infection is usually diagnosed clinically as a common cold, although with poor specificity. Viral diagnosis can be confirmed by RT-PCR from nasal swab or nasal washing but generally unnecessary.
  - Most PCR testing does not distinguish between RVs and EVs.
  - Identification of specific RVs and EVs is not routinely performed.
- **Treatment:** There are no antivirals approved. Treatment is supportive and symptom based.

Complications

- **Postviral cough**
  - Cough is a common symptom during acute viral URTI and LRTI.
  - **Many cases of subacute cough (persisting for 3–8 weeks) are due to postviral cough,** which may not respond well to common antitussive therapy.
  - Although postviral cough is a common etiology for subacute cough, other potential causes can be considered (see Chapter 7).
  - In patients with asthma or COPD, cough may be a manifestation of a prolonged exacerbation.
- **Postviral wheeze/asthma**
  - Postviral wheezing/asthma is more common in children and may continue up to 1 year after resolution of the infection.
  - For most patients, wheezing will spontaneously resolve over time.
  - Multiple studies have implicated infantile rhinovirus and RSV infections in the subsequent development of asthma in children and teens.[62]
- **Post-COVID conditions**
  - Post-COVID conditions (PCC), also called "long COVID syndrome," is broadly defined as the development or continuation of symptoms after resolution of a COVID-19 infection. Symptoms can include fatigue, memory concerns, muscle pains, shortness of breath, postural tachycardia, and headaches.
  - Up to ~20% of adults may develop some spectrum of PCC, though most improve over the course of 2 weeks, but some can last for months to years.[63]

- Risk of developing PCC is highest in those hospitalized for COVID-19. Vaccination protects against the development of PCC.
- The pathophysiology is currently unclear but may be due to virus-induced endothelial dysfunction, microvascular clotting, immune dysregulation, development of autoimmunity, or a combination of mechanisms.[64]
- There are no specific medical tests for this condition. Evaluation should be directed toward the symptoms described.
- There are no current treatments beyond supportive care and patients should be carefully examined to exclude other causes.

REFERENCES

1. Sande MA, Gwaltney JM. Acute community-acquired bacterial sinusitis: continuing challenges and current management. *Clin Infect Dis.* 2004;39:S151–S158.
2. Chow AW, Benninger MS, Brook I, et al. IDSA clinical practice guideline for acute bacterial rhinosinusitis in children and adults. *Clin Infect Dis.* 2012;54:e72–e112.
3. King D, Mitchell B, Williams CP, Spurling GKP. Saline nasal irrigation for acute upper respiratory tract infections. *Cochrane Database Syst Rev.* 2015;2015:CD006821.
4. Shulman ST, Bisno AL, Clegg HW, et al. Clinical practice guideline for the diagnosis and management of group A streptococcal pharyngitis: 2012 update by the Infectious Diseases Society of America. *Clin Infect Dis.* 2012;55:e86–e102.
5. Centor RM, Witherspoon JM, Dalton HP, Brody CE, Link K. The diagnosis of strep throat in adults in the emergency room. *Med Decis Making.* 1981;1:239–246.
6. Pappas PG, Kauffman CA, Andes DR, et al. Clinical Practice Guideline for the Management of Candidiasis: 2016 Update by the Infectious Diseases Society of America. *Clin Infect Dis.* 2016;62:e1–e50.
7. Kim V, Criner GJ. Chronic bronchitis and chronic obstructive pulmonary disease. *Am J Respir Crit Care Med.* 2013;187:228–237.
8. Kinkade S, Long NA. Acute bronchitis. *Am Fam Physician.* 2016;94:560–565.
9. Becker LA, Hom J, Villasis-Keever M, van der Wouden JC. Beta2-agonists for acute cough or a clinical diagnosis of acute bronchitis. *Cochrane Database Syst Rev.* 2015;2015(9):CD001726.
10. Dalziel SR, Haskell L, O'Brien S, et al. Bronchiolitis. *Lancet.* 2022;400:392–406.
11. Melgar M, Britton A, Roper LE, et al. Use of respiratory syncytial virus vaccines in older adults: recommendations of the Advisory Committee on Immunization Practices–United States, 2023. *Morb Mortal Wkly Rep.* 2023;72:793–801.
12. Manothummetha K, Mongkolkaew T, Tovichayathamrong P, et al. Ribavirin treatment for respiratory syncytial virus infection in patients with haematologic malignancy and haematopoietic stem cell transplant recipients: a systematic review and meta-analysis. *Clin Microbiol Infect.* 2023;29:1272–1279.
13. Pagliano P, Sellitto C, Conti V, Ascione T, Esposito S. Characteristics of viral pneumonia in the COVID-19 era: an update. *Infection.* 2021;49:607–616.
14. Metlay JP, Waterer GW, Long AC, et al. Diagnosis and treatment of adults with community-acquired pneumonia. An Official Clinical Practice Guideline of the American Thoracic Society and Infectious Diseases Society of America. *Am J Respir Crit Care Med.* 2019;200:e45–e67.
15. File TM Jr, Ramirez JA. Community-acquired pneumonia. *N Engl J Med.* 2023;389:632–641.
16. Febbo J, Revels J, Ketai L. Viral pneumonias. *Radiol Clin North Am.* 2022;60(3):383–397.
17. Rhee C. Using procalcitonin to guide antibiotic therapy. *Open Forum Infect Dis.* 2017;4:ofw249.

18. Racicot K, Mor G. Risks associated with viral infections during pregnancy. *J Clin Invest.* 2017;127:1591–1599.
19. Yu W, Hu X, Cao B. Viral infections during pregnancy: the big challenge threatening maternal and fetal health. *Matern Fetal Med.* 2021;4:72–86.
20. Jamieson DJ, Rasmussen SA. An update on COVID-19 and pregnancy. *Am J Obstet Gynecol.* 2022;226:177–186.
21. Sinclair SM, Jones JK, Miller RK, Greene MF, Kwo PY, Maddrey WC. Final results from the ribavirin pregnancy registry, 2004–2020. *Birth Defects Res.* 2022;114:1376–1391.
22. Kalafat E, Heath P, Prasad S, Brien PO, Khalil A. COVID-19 vaccination in pregnancy. *Am J Obstet Gynecol.* 2022;227:136–147.
23. Kampmann B, Madhi SA, Munjal I, et al. Bivalent prefusion F vaccine in pregnancy to prevent RSV illness in infants. *N Engl J Med.* 2023;388:1451–1464.
24. Schrag SJ, Verani JR, Dixon BE, et al. Estimation of COVID-19 mRNA vaccine effectiveness against medically attended COVID-19 in pregnancy during periods of delta and omicron variant predominance in the United States. *JAMA Netw Open.* 2022; 5:e2233273.
25. Ison MG. Respiratory viral infections in the immunocompromised. *Curr Opin Pulm Med.* 2022;28:205–210.
26. Johnson AG, Amin AB, Ali AR, et al. COVID-19 incidence and death rates among unvaccinated and fully vaccinated adults with and without booster doses during periods of delta and omicron variant emergence—25 U.S. Jurisdictions, April 4–December 25, 2021. *Morb Mortal Wkly Rep.* 2022;71:132–138.
27. Fung M, Babik JM. COVID-19 in immunocompromised hosts: what we know so far. *Clin Infect Dis.* 2021;72:340–350.
28. Leung NHL, Chu DKW, Shiu EYC, et al. Respiratory virus shedding in exhaled breath and efficacy of face masks. *Nat Med.* 2020;26:676–680.
29. Tabatabaeizadeh SA. Airborne transmission of COVID-19 and the role of face mask to prevent it: a systematic review and meta-analysis. *Eur J Med Res.* 2021;26:1.
30. Grohskopf LA, Blanton LH, Ferdinands JM, Chung JR, Broder KR, Talbot HK. Prevention and control of seasonal influenza with vaccines: recommendations of the Advisory Committee on Immunization Practices—United States, 2023–24 Influenza Season. *MMWR Recomm Rep.* 2023;72:1–25.
31. Regan JJ, Moulia DL, Link-Gelles R, et al. Use of updated COVID-19 vaccines 2023–2024 formula for persons aged ≥6 months: recommendations of the Advisory Committee on Immunization Practices–United States, September 2023. *Morb Mortal Wkly Rep.* 2023;72(42):1140–1146.
32. Centers for Disease Control and Prevention. *Vaccines and Immunizations.* Accessed August 23, 2024. www.cdc.gov/vaccines/index.html
33. Lynch JP 3rd, Fishbein M, Echavarria M. Adenovirus. *Semin Respir Crit Care Med.* 2011;32:494–511.
34. Dodge MJ, MacNeil KM, Tessier TM, Weinberg JB, Mymryk JS. Emerging antiviral therapeutics for human adenovirus infection: recent developments and novel strategies. *Antiviral Res.* 2021;188:105034.
35. Forni D, Cagliani R, Clerici M, Sironi M. Molecular evolution of human coronavirus genomes. *Trends Microbiol.* 2017;25:35–48.
36. Tang G, Liu Z, Chen D. Human coronaviruses: origin, host and receptor. *J Clin Virol.* 2022;155:105246.
37. Jegerlehner S, Suter-Riniker F, Jent P, Bittel P, Nagler M. Diagnostic accuracy of a SARS-CoV-2 rapid antigen test in real-life clinical settings. *Int J Infect Dis.* 2021;109:118–122.
38. Centers for Disease Control and Prevention (CDC). *Types of COVID-19 Treatment.* Accessed August 23, 2024. https://www.cdc.gov/covid/treatment/index.html
39. Torti C, Olimpieri PP, Bonfanti P, et al. Real-life comparison of mortality in patients with SARS-CoV-2 infection at risk for clinical progression treated with molnupiravir or

nirmatrelvir plus ritonavir during the Omicron era in Italy: a nationwide, cohort study. *Lancet Reg Health Eur.* 2023;31:100684.
40. Gottlieb RL, Vaca CE, Paredes R, et al. Early remdesivir to prevent progression to severe Covid-19 in outpatients. *N Engl J Med.* 2022;386:305–315.
41. Chokkalingam AP, Hayden J, Goldman JD, et al. Association of remdesivir treatment with mortality among hospitalized adults with COVID-19 in the United States. *JAMA Netw Open.* 2022;5:e2244505.
42. Group RC, Horby P, Lim WS, et al. Dexamethasone in hospitalized patients with Covid-19. *N Engl J Med.* 2021;384:693–704.
43. Mourad A, Thibault D, Holland TL, et al. Dexamethasone for inpatients with COVID-19 in a national cohort. *JAMA Netw Open.* 2023;6:e238516.
44. Kalil AC, Patterson TF, Mehta AK, et al. Baricitinib plus remdesivir for hospitalized adults with Covid-19. *N Engl J Med.* 2021;384:795–807.
45. Marconi VC, Ramanan AV, de Bono S, et al. Efficacy and safety of baricitinib for the treatment of hospitalised adults with COVID-19 (COV-BARRIER): a randomised, double-blind, parallel-group, placebo-controlled phase 3 trial. *Lancet Respir Med.* 2021; 9:1407–1418.
46. Salama C, Han J, Yau L, et al. Tocilizumab in patients hospitalized with Covid-19 pneumonia. *N Engl J Med.* 2021;384:20–30.
47. O'Halloran JA, Ko ER, Anstrom KJ, et al. Abatacept, cenicriviroc, or infliximab for treatment of adults hospitalized with COVID-19 pneumonia: a randomized clinical trial. *JAMA.* 2023;330:328–339.
48. Investigators ATTACC, Investigators AC-4a, Investigators R-C, et al. Therapeutic anticoagulation with heparin in noncritically ill patients with Covid-19. *N Engl J Med.* 2021;385:790–802.
49. Investigators R-C, Investigators AC-4a, Investigators A, et al. Therapeutic anticoagulation with heparin in critically ill patients with Covid-19. *N Engl J Med.* 2021;385:777–789.
50. Fowler K, Mucha J, Neumann M, et al. A systematic literature review of the global seroprevalence of cytomegalovirus: possible implications for treatment, screening, and vaccine development. *BMC Public Health.* 2022;22:1659.
51. Kotton CN, Kumar D, Caliendo AM, et al. The Third International Consensus Guidelines on the management of cytomegalovirus in solid-organ transplantation. *Transplantation.* 2018;102:900–931.
52. Azevedo LS, Pierrotti LC, Abdala E, et al. Cytomegalovirus infection in transplant recipients. *Clinics (Sao Paulo).* 2015;70:515–523.
53. Uyeki TM, Bernstein HH, Bradley JS, et al. Clinical Practice Guidelines by the Infectious Diseases Society of America: 2018 Update on diagnosis, treatment, chemoprophylaxis, and institutional outbreak management of seasonal influenza. *Clin Infect Dis.* 2019;68: e1–e47.
54. de Zwart A, Riezebos-Brilman A, Lunter G, et al. Respiratory syncytial virus, human metapneumovirus, and parainfluenza virus infections in lung transplant recipients: a systematic review of outcomes and treatment strategies. *Clin Infect Dis.* 2022;74:2252–2260.
55. Shah DP, Shah PK, Azzi JM, Chemaly RF. Parainfluenza virus infections in hematopoietic cell transplant recipients and hematologic malignancy patients: a systematic review. *Cancer Lett.* 2016;370:358–364.
56. Branche AR, Falsey AR. Parainfluenza virus infection. *Semin Respir Crit Care Med.* 2016;37:538–554.
57. Griffiths C, Drews SJ, Marchant DJ. Respiratory syncytial virus: infection, detection, and new options for prevention and treatment. *Clin Microbiol Rev.* 2017;30:277–319.
58. Gatt D, Martin I, AlFouzan R, Moraes TJ. Prevention and treatment strategies for respiratory syncytial virus (RSV). *Pathogens.* 2023;12:154.
59. Trang TP, Whalen M, Hilts-Horeczko A, Doernberg SB, Liu C. Comparative effectiveness of aerosolized versus oral ribavirin for the treatment of respiratory syncytial virus

infections: a single-center retrospective cohort study and review of the literature. *Transpl Infect Dis*. 2018;20:e12844.
60. Baggen J, Thibaut HJ, Strating JRPM, van Kuppeveld FJM. The life cycle of non-polio enteroviruses and how to target it. *Nat Rev Microbiol*. 2018;16:368–381.
61. Messacar K, Abzug MJ, Dominguez SR. The emergence of enterovirus-D68. *Microbiol Spectr*. 2016;4.
62. Jartti T, Bønnelykke K, Elenius V, Feleszko W. Role of viruses in asthma. *Semin Immunopathol*. 2020;42:61–74.
63. Ford ND, Slaughter D, Edwards D, et al. Long COVID and significant activity limitation among adults, by age–United States, June 1–13, 2022, to June 7–19, 2023. *Morb Mortal Wkly Rep*. 2023;72:866–870.
64. Davis HE, McCorkell L, Vogel JM, Topol EJ. Long COVID: major findings, mechanisms and recommendations. *Nat Rev Microbiol*. 2023;21:133–146.

Cystic Fibrosis

16

James McMenimen and Jeffrey J. Atkinson

GENERAL PRINCIPLES

Definition
Cystic fibrosis (CF) is an **autosomal recessive** disorder caused by mutations in the **cystic fibrosis transmembrane conductance regulator gene** (CFTR), resulting in dysfunction in numerous exocrine organs.

Epidemiology
- CF is the most common lethal inherited disease affecting the white population.
- The incidence is ~1 in 3500 to 1 in 5000 live births in the US and Canada. Approximately 1000 new cases are diagnosed annually in the US and the overall prevalence is just under 30,000 patients.[1-3]
- Newborn screening has been widely adopted and accounted for ~60% of new diagnoses in 2022 and 91.6% of diagnoses in children less than 6 months old. Interestingly, this rate has remained relatively stable over the past decade.[1] Early asymptomatic diagnosis may have better pulmonary function during early childhood.[3]
- Aside from newborn screening, most cases are identified in babies born with meconium ileus or young children who present with respiratory symptoms, most commonly recurrent pulmonary infections.
- Despite broad utilization of newborn screening, up to 10% of patients are diagnosed at age 10 or older.[1,4] These patients are more likely to present with nonclassic CF symptoms including bronchiectasis without pancreatic insufficiency, recurrent or chronic pancreatitis, or infertility (azoospermia with congenital absence of the vas deferens).
- There have been substantial improvements in survival of people with CF in the past decades with innovation in therapeutics. The median predicted survival age has been increasing and is predicted to be 68.2 years (95% confidence interval 63.0–76.2 years) for individuals born between 2018 and 2022 in the US.[1]

Pathophysiology
- **CF is a multisystem disease, with highly variable disease presentation.**
- Progressive lung disease and chronic respiratory tract infection, however, are the major cause of morbidity and mortality.[2]
  - Pulmonary disease is related to abnormal electrolyte transport in airways, resulting in decreased airway surface liquid and impaired mucociliary clearance.

Infection, inflammation, and chronic airway obstruction ultimately result in bronchiectasis, chronic infection, and premature death.[5]
- Thickened secretions in the pancreatic and biliary ducts result in malabsorption, maldigestion, diabetes, and occasionally liver disease.
* A genetic mutation in the CFTR gene leading to an abnormal protein is the basic molecular defect responsible for CF.
  - The CFTR gene is located on chromosome 7.
  - CFTR is a cyclic AMP-regulated chloride ion channel on the apical surface of epithelial cells that primarily plays a role in chloride transport.
  - In CF, this protein is missing or malfunctioning, leading to abnormal chloride transport.
  - Abnormal function leads to **decreased chloride secretion** and increased sodium absorption on the apical surface of epithelial cells. This results in **thickened secretions** in airways, sinuses, pancreatic ducts, biliary ducts, intestines, sweat ducts, and reproductive tract.[5]
  - CFTR also plays a role in the regulation of other ion channels that may be important in the pathogenesis of CF.
  - Many of the specific mechanisms by which the molecular defect of CF leads to clinical disease remain unclear and are the subject of current investigations.
  - CFTR mutations can be divided into five classes, based on the effect of the mutation on CFTR protein production and function.[1]
    - Class I mutations lead to defective protein production. These are often nonsense, frameshift, or splicing mutations leading to complete absence of CFTR protein. G542X, W1282X, and R533X are examples of nonsense mutations.
    - Class II mutations lead to defective protein processing. The CFTR protein is produced but is prevented from trafficking properly.
      - F508del, N1303K are examples.
      - **The most common CFTR mutation is F508del,** which is a deletion of three nucleotides that encode phenylalanine (F) at amino acid 508. This mutation is **found in over 80% of patients with CF in the US** (44.0% homozygotes and 41.4% heterozygotes).[1]
    - Class III mutations lead to defective regulation of the CFTR protein. CFTR is present on the membrane; however, channel activity is diminished. G551D is the most common example.
    - Class IV mutations lead to defective conduction of the CFTR protein. CFTR is produced, localized, and regulated normally; however, ion conductance and channel opening are reduced. R117H is the most common example.
    - Class V mutations cause decreased numbers of normally functioning CFTR protein. A455E is an example.
    - Information about specific mutations and reported phenotypes can be found on the CFTR2 website.[6]
* Classifying mutations based on **theratype**, or the pattern of response to a CFTR modulator is becoming more common. This is evaluated by administration of drug to genetically modified cells in culture. Theratype classes include mutations responsive to potentiators (ivacaftor), correctors (lumacaftor, tezacaftor, elexacaftor), or nonresponders.

DIAGNOSIS
Clinical Presentation
Pulmonary
- Nearly all patients have **chronic sinusitis** in radiographic studies. Nasal polyposis is common.
- **Chronic lower airway infections** are characteristics of this disease.
  - Chronic infection causes inflammation, increased mucus secretion and obstruction, and direct destruction of pulmonary parenchyma.
  - Pulmonary infections with *Haemophilus influenzae* and *Staphylococcus aureus* are common early in the disease process.
  - Later, ***Pseudomonas aeruginosa* becomes the dominant lung pathogen in a majority of CF patients.** Progressive inflammation, lung damage, decline in lung function, and progressive dyspnea are most closely correlated with this organism.
  - Infection with other gram-negative organisms such as *Burkholderia cenocepacia* can lead to a fulminant course with a high mortality rate.
  - Colonization with *Aspergillus fumigatus* is common but invasive disease from this organism is relatively rare.
  - CF patients are at higher risk for infection with nontuberculous mycobacteria, with prevalence of 12.7%. The most common strains identified are *Mycobacterium avium* complex and *Mycobacterium abscessus*.[7]
- **Acute exacerbation of CF** is a common presentation of pulmonary disease.
  - The typical exacerbation presents with some combination of symptoms, including increased cough, changing sputum, increased shortness of breath, decreased exercise tolerance, and weight loss. Low-grade fever is common but not universal.
  - The specific factors causing exacerbations are unclear but viral infections have been implicated in some studies.[8]
  - Occasionally, a reduction in pulmonary function on spirometry may be the only abnormality noted.
  - CXRs are often unchanged during exacerbations but are useful to exclude other pulmonary complications of CF.
- **Pneumothorax** is a relatively common pulmonary complication that presents in CF.
  - The incidence of pneumothorax rises with increasing age secondary to worsening lung disease. Approximately 3.4% of CF patients will experience pneumothorax (1 in 167 patients per year).[9]
  - Patients typically present with chest pain and dyspnea (but may present atypically) because of decreased compliance in the CF lung.
- A second pulmonary complication is minor **hemoptysis** (<240 mL), which is common (9.1% of patients) and often occurs with acute exacerbations of this disease.[10]
  - Approximately 4% of CF patients will experience massive, life-threatening hemoptysis (>500 mL/24 h) during their lifetime (1 in 115 patients per year).[11]
  - Hypertrophic bronchial arteries from chronic inflammation are the typical source of bleeding.
  - Patients presenting with hemoptysis should be treated with antibiotics.
  - Intractable, life-threatening or frequent recurrent hemoptysis may require an evaluation for palliative bronchial artery embolization.

- **Respiratory failure** is the most concerning pulmonary presentation of CF. Unless reversible etiologies are responsible, this complication often indicates end-stage lung disease and carries a poor prognosis for recovery.

Gastrointestinal
- Approximately 90% of CF patients exhibit **exocrine pancreatic insufficiency**.
  - Patients with pancreatic insufficiency have **significantly lower life expectancies** than those with pancreatic sufficiency.
  - Pancreatic sufficiency is more common in patients who present later in life.[4]
  - Pancreatic exocrine insufficiency can lead to steatorrhea, chronic malnutrition, and various vitamin deficiencies.
  - Fat-soluble vitamins A, D, E, and K are most commonly affected. Vitamin A deficiency can lead to visual deficiencies such as night blindness, and in severe cases xerophthalmia, keratomalacia, and complete blindness. Vitamin D deficiency can lead to poor bone mineralization. Vitamin E deficiency can lead to ataxia and absent deep tendon reflexes.
- **Gastroesophageal reflux disease** is more common in CF patients than healthy control subjects and is possibly linked to worsening lung disease.[12]
- Another presentation of GI disease is the **distal intestinal obstruction syndrome** (DIOS), which can be considered an adult equivalent of meconium ileus.
  - Colicky abdominal pain with a palpable mass is a typical presentation.
  - Radiographic patterns consistent with partial or complete obstruction can be seen on obstructive series.
  - Caution must be exercised, however, because these signs and symptoms are present in other abdominal conditions that present in CF patients. Empiric treatment of DIOS while evaluation is underway for other conditions is recommended.
- Volvulus, intussusception, and rectal prolapse can occur.
- Cholelithiasis and cholecystitis are seen.
- CF can be associated with an asymptomatic increase in alkaline phosphatase and a mild transaminitis in up to one-third of patients, whereas biliary cirrhosis is much less common.
- A small percentage of patients do have significant **liver disease**, ~6%.[1]

Endocrine and Reproductive
- **Men are usually infertile** secondary to obstructive azoospermia. Patients who are diagnosed at older ages may present with only **congenital absence of the vas deferens**.
- **Women have reduced fertility** because of thick cervical mucus as well as other, less understood factors.
- Puberty can be late in onset in the setting of malnutrition.
- **Osteoporosis** occurs in approximately one-third of adult CF patients.
- **Diabetes mellitus** is common in CF, affecting 29.7% of adults.[2]
  - Diabetes in CF is primarily due to deficient insulin production, although insulin resistance may play a role as well.
  - CF patients may be dependent on insulin for glucose control but diabetic ketoacidosis is rare.

Diagnostic Criteria
- The diagnosis of CF is based on **clinical presentation** coupled with confirmatory testing.
- At least one criterion from each set of features is required to diagnose CF[13]:
  - Compatible clinical feature of CF (persistent colonization/infection with typical organisms, chronic cough and sputum production, persistent CXR abnormalities, airway obstruction, sinus abnormalities/polyps, clubbing, meconium ileus, DIOS, rectal prolapse, pancreatic insufficiency/pancreatitis, jaundice/biliary cirrhosis, malnutrition, acute salt depletion, chronic metabolic alkalosis, obstructive azoospermia) **OR**
  - Positive family history **OR**
  - Positive newborn screening test

  AND
  - Elevated sweat chloride >60 mmol/L on two occasions **OR**
  - Presence of two disease-causing mutations in CFTR **OR**
  - Abnormal nasal transepithelial potential difference test

Differential Diagnosis
- Primary ciliary dyskinesia: bronchiectasis, sinusitis, and infertility are common. Gastrointestinal (GI) symptoms are limited and sweat chloride levels are normal. Dextrocardia or situs inversus totalis can be seen.
- Shwachman–Diamond syndrome: pancreatic insufficiency, cyclic neutropenia, and short stature are seen. Sweat chloride levels are normal.
- Young syndrome: bronchiectasis, sinusitis, and azoospermia. Respiratory symptoms are mild, and there is a lack of GI symptoms. Sweat chloride testing is normal.
- Immunoglobulin deficiency leads to recurrent sinus and pulmonary infections and can cause bronchiectasis. GI symptoms are absent and sweat chloride testing is normal.
- Idiopathic bronchiectasis.
- Chronic rhinosinusitis.
- Chronic idiopathic pancreatitis.

Diagnostic Testing
- Diagnosis of CF is usually made during childhood. Approximately 10% of patients are diagnosed after age 10.[4] In 2022, ~60% of new diagnoses were made from newborn screening.[1]
- **Pilocarpine iontophoresis,** or **sweat testing,** is the most common confirmatory test and is **the gold standard** for CF diagnosis.[13]
  - A quantitative test with a **chloride value of >60 mmol/L** on two occasions is consistent with CF.
  - Other conditions produce abnormal sweat tests but can usually be differentiated from CF based on their clinical presentation.
  - Borderline or nondiagnostic results should prompt repeat or additional testing depending on clinical suspicion.
- Genetic testing for CF is available but usually is not used as the initial diagnostic test. There are >1800 known mutations and a number of unknown mutations that can lead to CF disease.

- **Two mutations on different alleles must be present to diagnose CF.**
  - Commercially available probes, while identifying >90% of abnormal genes in the White Northern European population, test for a minority of known CF mutations.
  - Full gene sequencing is available, but interpretation may be complex.
- Other diagnostic evaluation can support the presence of CF but is generally neither specific nor sensitive for the diagnosis.
- **Pulmonary function tests** show an obstructive pattern early in the disease and tend to change to a mixed obstructive and restrictive pattern in more advanced diseases.
- Early in the disease, radiographic testing tends to show hyperinflated lungs. Bronchiectasis and mucus plugging is a later finding.
- **Sputum cultures** are typically positive for multiple organisms, including *P. aeruginosa, S. aureus,* nontypeable *H. influenzae, Stenotrophomonas maltophilia, Burkholderia species,* and mucoid variants of *P. aeruginosa*. Use of special culture media to identify fastidious organisms is recommended. Nontuberculous mycobacteria are frequently isolated and may be pathogenic.[7]
- Testing for pancreatic insufficiency and malabsorption is not commonly done, as the diagnosis based on history, vitamin deficiency, and response to pancreatic enzyme supplementation is often sufficient for diagnosis. Seventy-two-hour stool collections for fecal fat or measurement of fecal elastase levels can be helpful in situations where the diagnosis is not clear.

TREATMENT

- The overall goals of CF therapy are to improve quality of life, decrease number and frequency of exacerbations and hospitalizations, reduce the rate of decline in lung function, and prolong life expectancy.
- **Comprehensive care at an accredited CF care center is recommended.**

Pulmonary

- **CFTR modulators** treat the underlying cause of disease by improving production, intracellular processing, or function of defective CFTR protein. These medications have significantly improved clinical outcomes in patients with specific CFTR mutations.[14–18]
  - **Elexacaftor-Tezacaftor-Ivacaftor (ETI)** is a triple-drug combination that is part of highly effective modulator therapy for patients with at least one F508del mutation and any other CFTR mutation that is responsive. This is ~92% of people with CF in the US.[1]
  - Approved for use in patients greater than 2 years of age with eligible CFTR genotype.
  - A phase III randomized, double-blind, placebo-controlled trial demonstrated an increase in percentage of predicted FEV_1 by 13.8 points at 4 weeks of treatment and 14.3 points at 24 weeks of treatment. There was also a 63% decrease in pulmonary exacerbations with ETI compared to placebo.[14]
  - For adults, ETI is administered as two tablets of 100 mg elexacaftor/50 mg tezacaftor/75 mg ivacaftor in morning and one tablet of ivacaftor 150 mg in evening ideally 12 hours apart. Absorption is significantly improved when the medication is administered with a fat-containing meal or snack.

- Adverse effects of ETI include hepatotoxicity (rise in transaminases and bilirubin) and mild increases in blood pressure. Hepatotoxicity should be suspected with rise in alanine aminotransferase (ALT)/aspartate aminotransferase (AST) greater than five times the upper limit of normal or rise in ALT/AST greater than three times the upper limit of normal with concomitant rise in bilirubin greater than two times the upper limit of normal. Therapy should be discontinued until resolved and risks and benefits should be considered prior to resumption.
- The US list prices for CFTR modulators such as ETI are over $250,000 per year, but financial assistance programs through pharmaceutical companies currently exist to offset portions of the cost.
- **Ivacaftor** was the first CFTR modulator approved by the U.S. Food and Drug Administration (FDA) for use in CF in January 2012.[16] It is now approved for use in patients with the G551D mutation who are >6 months old, which is present in ~5% of patients with CF and causes a class III mutation. It is a highly effective modulator therapy for individuals with a G551D mutation.
  - Developed using large-scale chemical screen for agents that increase chloride ion efflux in cells expressing a G551D CFTR mutant.
  - A phase III randomized, placebo-controlled trial demonstrated an increase in FEV_1 by 10.4% with ivacaftor compared to an FEV_1 decline of 0.2% in placebo controls after 24 weeks of treatment. Sweat chloride levels, frequency of CF exacerbations, and adverse events were all significantly lower in patients treated with ivacaftor. Weight gain was common in subjects receiving ivacaftor.
  - In adults, dosing is 150 mg every 12 hours.
  - Ivacaftor is best absorbed when combined with fat- and enzyme-containing meals, and the channel-modulating effects may decrease rapidly with missed doses. Reinforcement of proper use is crucial for optimal outcomes.
- **Tezacaftor-Ivacaftor** is a combination medication of potentiator (**ivacaftor**) and corrector (**tezacaftor**) that is approved by the FDA for individuals 6 years of age or older who have homozygous F508del mutations or ≥1 other mutation sensitive to tezacaftor-ivacaftor. ETI has been shown to have superior improvement in lung function to tezacaftor-ivacaftor,[18] but there are five mutations that are sensitive to tezacaftor-ivacaftor but do not benefit from the addition of elexacaftor: 711+3A>G, 2789+5G>A, 3272-26A>G, 3849+10kbC>T, E831X.
- **Lumacaftor-Ivacaftor** is a combination medication of potentiator (ivacaftor) and corrector (lumacaftor) that is approved for use in individuals who are homozygous for the F508del mutation who are greater than 1 year of age. A phase III randomized, double-blind, placebo-controlled clinical trial demonstrated an increase in percent predicted FEV_1 by 2.6–4.0% compared to those treated with placebo, and decrease in pulmonary exacerbations by 39%.[15]
- Significant drug interactions exist with CFTR modulator therapy. CYP3A4 inducers may decrease the serum concentration of modulators. CYP3A4 inhibitors may increase the serum concentration of modulators. Careful examination of drug interactions should be performed.
- Management of the acute pulmonary exacerbation is probably the most common reason for the hospital admission of CF patients.
- **Immunizations** should be kept up to date in an attempt to prevent exacerbations. **Yearly influenza vaccination** decreases the frequency of infection.[1]

- **Pulmonary rehabilitation,** when performed with exercise rehabilitation, may improve functional status and assist with airway clearance.
- **Inhaled bronchodilators** (e.g., albuterol, salmeterol, formoterol) are recommended for all CF patients, particularly in association with chest physiotherapy or other nebulized agents. Bronchodilators facilitate clearance of airway secretions and limit bronchial constriction seen in response to certain inhaled agents, such as hypertonic saline and dornase ALFA.
- **Respiratory therapy,** including chest percussion and postural drainage, has long been known to be efficacious in exacerbations.[19,20] Other techniques including percussors, pneumatic compression vests, and oscillating positive expiratory pressure devices such as the Flutter and Acapella are available to assist in airway clearance.
- **Hypertonic saline** (7%) is administered as an inhalation, and functions to improve mucociliary clearance of airway secretions.[21]
   - Hypertonic saline increases water content of secretions by creating a high osmotic gradient.
   - Mucus clearance is improved, with mild improvements in lung function and decreased incidence of respiratory exacerbations.
   - Albuterol should be administered prior to hypertonic saline to reduce bronchospasm. Patients with FEV_1 <40% should be given a test dose under observation before initiating therapy at home.
- **Inhaled recombinant DNase** (dornase alfa) digests extracellular DNA and reduces the viscosity of CF sputum.[22]
   - Shown to be effective in reducing sputum viscosity and improving pulmonary function.
   - In patients with normal pulmonary function, dornase ALFA has been shown to slow the rate of decline in lung function.
   - Dornase alfa decreases the incidence of respiratory tract infections requiring parenteral antibiotics.
   - Side effects include pharyngitis, laryngitis, rash, chest pain, and conjunctivitis.
- If lung function remains stable on CFTR modulator therapy, de-escalation of additional airway clearance therapies could be considered to limit the effect of treatment burden on individuals with CF.
- **Antibiotics** are the main treatment for acute exacerbations.[23]
   - Antibiotic use in CF patients differs from that in other patients. Higher doses of antibiotics are needed because of increased clearance and volumes of distribution. Longer courses of antibiotics of 14–21 days have been classically used. A randomized clinical trial suggested noninferiority of treatment with 10–14-day courses of antibiotics based on response to therapy in the form of percent predicted of FEV_1.[24]
   - Sputum culture results should guide antibiotic choice.
   - In general, antibiotics are selected based on respiratory tract cultures and susceptibilities, however:
     - The utility of in vitro susceptibility testing has been questioned, since there appears to be discordance between susceptibility testing and clinical response to antibiotics.
     - In a study published in 2003, treatment outcomes of patients experiencing a CF exacerbation with IV tobramycin or IV ceftazidime did not correlate with minimum inhibitory concentration (MIC) values of *P. aeruginosa* obtained from sputum cultures.[25]

- Oral antibiotics are appropriate for mild exacerbations. The main barrier in using oral antibiotics is the limited number of agents active against *Pseudomonas*. **Ciprofloxacin** (750 mg PO bid) is the oral antibiotic of choice against *Pseudomonas*. Use of this drug should be limited to 3-week courses given the rapid rise of resistant organisms when longer courses are used.
- For moderate to severe exacerbations or failed oral treatment courses, IV regimens are the standard of care.[23]
    - A typical two-drug regimen consists of an **aminoglycoside** (gentamicin/tobramycin, 3 mg/kg IV q8h or 10 mg/kg q24h following peak and trough levels) plus an **extended-spectrum penicillin** (piperacillin/tazobactam, 4.5 g IV q6h) or **cephalosporin** (cefepime, 2 g IV q8h).
    - Measurement of aminoglycoside peaks and troughs or other evaluations of aminoglycoside pharmacokinetics should be employed to optimize aminoglycoside dosing and prevent toxicity. **Once-daily dosing is preferred.**
    - Occasionally, **methicillin-resistant *S. aureus*** is isolated from the sputum. **IV vancomycin** (15 mg/kg adjusted to maintain a trough of ~0–15 mcg/mL) or **linezolid** (600 mg q12h, IV or PO) should be used for adequate coverage.
- Inhaled **tobramycin** in patients with chronic airways infection with *P. aeruginosa* used in 28-day cycles was shown to improve pulmonary function and decrease the rate of hospitalization.[26]
- **Inhaled aztreonam** in patients with chronic airways infection with *P. aeruginosa* has been shown to improve pulmonary function and increase the time until subsequent antibiotic treatment.[27]
- There is some evidence that home IV treatment can be as effective as hospital treatment.[23] However, the decision of inpatient versus outpatient treatment must be made on an individual basis. Resources available in the hospital such as intensive monitoring and chest physical therapy are generally unavailable at home.

- Inflammation in CF is an additional target for CF therapeutics.
    - Chronic treatment with **azithromycin** (500 mg three times a week) in patients chronically infected with *P. aeruginosa* has been shown to improve lung function and reduce days in the hospital for treatment of acute exacerbations.[28] Its use should be limited to patients with multiple cultures negative for nontuberculous mycobacteria.
    - One trial compared prednisone therapy 1 mg/kg versus 2 mg/kg versus placebo on alternate days. The prednisone group had a higher percentage of predicted forced vital capacity.[29] However, complications of steroid therapy, such as growth retardation and glycemic control, have limited the use of this therapy, and long-term use should be avoided.
    - High-dose ibuprofen has been used with some success in young patients with mild disease but is again limited by side effects including renal failure and peptic ulcer disease.[30]

- Treatment for chronic respiratory failure is usually supportive.
    - Oxygen therapy should be provided based on standard rest and exercise oxygen assessments.
    - Noninvasive ventilation or even intubation has been used as a bridge to lung transplantation.
    - **Bilateral lung transplantation** is the treatment of choice.[31] Success rates compare favorably to other indications for lung transplantation.

- Chronic sinusitis is common, and many patients benefit from nasal steroids. Nasal saline washes are helpful. Some patients may require functional endoscopic sinus surgery and nasal polypectomy.

Gastrointestinal

- Achieving **adequate nutrition** in CF patients affects both pulmonary status and overall mortality.
  - **Replacement of pancreatic** enzymes as supplements is important for this goal.[32]
  - The usual starting dose is 500 lipase units/kg/meal PO, which can be increased to maximum dose of 2500 units/kg/meal. Dosing is adjusted to achieve one to two semisolid stools per day and maintain adequate nutrition.
  - Acid suppression may be necessary in some patients as enzymes may be inactivated in an acidic environment, though supporting data are limited.[33]
  - Adequate proportions of fat and protein calories need to be ingested, which usually require increased caloric intake.
  - Dietary goals should aim for a body mass index of ≥50th percentile or in adult males ≥22 and females ≥23. Better lung function is associated with a higher body mass index (BMI). More severe disease and worse pancreatic function result in greater caloric deficits and intake recommendations should be tailored to the individual patient. Nutritional supplementation should be provided when appropriate.[1,32]
  - Fat-soluble vitamins should be provided in supplements.
- The preferred treatments for other GI complications are less clear.
  - Ursodeoxycholic acid probably has a role in the management of CF-induced cholestasis.
  - Management of end-stage liver disease and the resulting complications of portal hypertension are the same as in other etiologies of end-stage liver disease.
  - **DIOS** may be managed by oral administration of laxative electrolyte solutions such as magnesium citrate or polyethylene glycol. With the presence of complete obstruction, diatrizoate meglumine and diatrizoate sodium (hypaque) enemas can be used as both a diagnostic and a therapeutic maneuver.[34] Surgery is rarely required. Chronic daily polyethylene glycol laxative may be necessary to prevent recurrence.

Endocrine and Reproductive

- Glucose intolerance as well as **diabetes mellitus** is more common in CF patients. Screening with a 2-hour 75-g glucose tolerance test should be done yearly.[35] Management of CF-related diabetes mellitus generally relies on insulin therapy.
- **Osteopenia** should be managed with calcium and vitamin D supplementation. Bisphosphonate therapy is effective for **osteoporosis** in adult CF patients.[36]
- Most males are **infertile** secondary to obstructive azoospermia. Surgical sperm aspiration with intracytoplasmic sperm injection into the ova may be used to overcome male infertility.

Lung Transplantation

- In general, transplantation improves life expectancy in patients who have an estimated 5-year survival of 30% or less.[31]

- Criteria for referral to a lung transplantation center include[37]:
  - FEV_1 <40% predicted or FEV_1 <50% predicted with a rapid decline in FEV_1 or markers of shortened survival (6-minute walk <400 m, hypoxemia, hypercarbia, or pulmonary hypertension).
  - FEV_1 <40% predicted with >two exacerbations per year requiring IV antibiotics or one exacerbation requiring positive pressure ventilation.
  - FEV_1 <40% predicted with pneumothorax
  - FEV_1 <40% predicted with massive hemoptysis requiring intensive care unit (ICU) admission or bronchial artery embolization.
- Many transplant centers consider respiratory tract infection with *B. cepacia* complex to be a contraindication for lung transplantation in CF patients.

SPECIAL CONSIDERATIONS

- Corresponding with the increasing life expectancy and impacts of CFTR modulators, the incidence of pregnancy in CF patients is increasing.
- Women with good lung function and good nutritional status generally do well during pregnancy.[38]
  - FEV_1 <60% predicted and/or low BMI (<21 kg/m^2) is associated with more CF-related complications during and after pregnancy and more frequently delivered preterm newborns.[39] It remains unclear if women on CFTR modulator therapy will have similar outcomes.
  - Women should be encouraged to reach 90% of their ideal weight before their pregnancy.
  - Exacerbations should be treated aggressively. Cephalosporins and synthetic penicillins are generally safe. Aminoglycosides potentially cause fetal ototoxicity but may be necessary.
  - There is no data to suggest CFTR modulators should be held during pregnancy or breastfeeding. Shared decision-making discussions regarding risk and benefit should occur during pregnancy until adequate outcomes are available.[36]
- Families should be counseled on the genetic risk of CF. All children of a parent with CF carry a single CF mutation; their chances of having CF disease depend on the genetics of the affected parent's partner. Early data on CFTR modulators suggest methods utilized in some states (immunoreactive trypsinogen) for newborn screening may give false-negative results to children born to CFTR modulator-treated mothers.

COMPLICATIONS

- **Pneumothorax** is an indication for hospital admission.[40]
  - If small (<20% of the hemithorax volume), pneumothoraces can be managed conservatively with serial CXRs.
  - BiPAP treatment should be withheld until the pneumothorax has resolved. Airplane travel, weight lifting, and spirometry should be avoided for 2 weeks after the pneumothorax has resolved.
  - In general, airway clearance measures utilizing positive expiratory pressure (flutter valve), intrapulmonary percussive ventilation, and exercise should be avoided in most instances of large pneumothorax.

- If the pneumothorax enlarges or is symptomatic, a chest tube should be placed.
- Obliterative procedures such as pleurodesis should be considered for persistent and recurrent pneumothoraces.
- Surgical pleurodesis is preferred over chemical pleurodesis.
- **Hemoptysis** is usually minor and responds to conservative treatment with IV antibiotics.[40]
  - Moderate to massive hemoptysis may require a more interventional approach.
  - Basic treatment involves correction of coagulation parameters, withholding chest physiotherapy, and stopping inhaled antibiotics.
  - Bronchial artery embolization plays an important role in massive hemoptysis or palliation of recurrent hemoptysis. A small study showed decreased bleeding and pulmonary exacerbations as well as increased quality of life when early bronchial artery embolization was used.[41] Bronchoscopy is not recommended prior to bronchial artery embolization.
  - Repeated embolization in the setting of recurrent hemoptysis is frequently successful, and atypical sources of neovascularization should be considered in patients with prior embolization and persistent bleeding. CT angiograms may not always be able to localize a bleeding lesion, but may assist with defining quantity of collaterals.
  - Surgery is the last option if bronchial artery embolization fails to control the bleeding.

REFERENCES

1. Cystic Fibrosis Foundation. *Patient Registry Annual Data Report to the Center Directors, 2022.* 2023. Accessed August 23, 2024. https://www.cff.org/medical-professionals/patient-registry
2. Strausbaugh SD, Davis PB. Cystic fibrosis: a review of epidemiology and pathobiology. *Clin Chest Med.* 2007;28:279–288.
3. Stephenson AL, Swaleh S, Sykes J, et al. Contemporary cystic fibrosis incidence rates in Canada and the United States. *J Cyst Fibros.* 2023;22:443–449.
4. Gilljam M, Ellis L, Corey M, Zielenski J, Durie P, Tullis DE. Clinical manifestations of cystic fibrosis among patients with diagnosis in adulthood. *Chest.* 2004;126:1215–1224.
5. Grasemann H, Ratjen F. Cystic fibrosis. *N Engl J Med.* 2023;389(18):1693–1707.
6. *Clinical and Functional Translation of CFTR.* 2023. Accessed August 24, 2024. http://www.cftr2.org
7. Floto RA, Olivier KN, Saiman L, et al. US Cystic Fibrosis Foundation and European Cystic Fibrosis Society consensus recommendations for the management of non-tuberculous mycobacteria in individuals with cystic fibrosis: executive summary. *Thorax.* 2016;71:88–90.
8. Collinson J, Nicholson KG, Cancio E, et al. Effects of upper respiratory tract infections in patients with cystic fibrosis. *Thorax.* 1996;51:1115–1122.
9. Flume PA, Strange C, Ye X, Ebeling M, Hulsey T, Clark LL. Pneumothorax in cystic fibrosis. *Chest.* 2005;128:720–728.
10. Efrati O, Harash O, Rivlin J, et al. Hemoptysis in Israeli CF patients—prevalence, treatment, and clinical characteristics. *J Cyst Fibros.* 2008;7:301–306.
11. Flume PA, Yankaskas JR, Ebeling M, Hulsey T, Clark LL. Massive hemoptysis in cystic fibrosis. *Chest.* 2005;128:729–738.
12. Robinson NB, DiMango E. Prevalence of gastroesophageal reflux in cystic fibrosis and implications for lung disease. *Ann Am Thorac Soc.* 2014;11:964–968.
13. Farrell PM, White TB, Ren CL, et al. Diagnosis of cystic fibrosis: consensus guidelines from the Cystic Fibrosis Foundation. *J Pediatr.* 2017;181.

14. Middleton PG, Mall MA, Dřevínek P, et al. Elexacaftor–tezacaftor–ivacaftor for cystic fibrosis with a single Phe508del allele. *N Engl J Med*. 2019;381:1809–1819.
15. Wainwright CE, Elborn JS, Ramsey BW, et al. Lumacaftor–Ivacaftor in patients with cystic fibrosis homozygous for phe508delCFTR. *N Engl J Med*. 2015;373:220–231.
16. Ramsey BW, Davies J, McElvaney NG, et al. A CFTR potentiator in patients with cystic fibrosis and the G551D mutation. *N Engl J Med*. 2011;365:1663–1672.
17. Taylor-Cousar JL, Munck A, McKone EF, et al. Tezacaftor–Ivacaftor in patients with cystic fibrosis homozygous for phe508del. *N Engl J Med*. 2017;377:2013–2023.
18. Sutharsan S, McKone EF, Downey DG, et al. Efficacy and safety of elexacaftor plus tezacaftor plus ivacaftor versus Tezacaftor plus ivacaftor in people with cystic fibrosis homozygous for F508del-CFTR: a 24-week, multicentre, randomised, double-blind, active-controlled, phase 3B trial. *Lancet Respir Med*. 2022;10:267–277.
19. Flume PA, Robinson KA, O'Sullivan BP, et al. Clinical practice guidelines for Pulmonary Therapies Committee. Cystic fibrosis pulmonary guidelines: airway clearance therapies. *Respir Care*. 2009;54:522–537.
20. Main E, Rand S. Conventional chest physiotherapy compared to other airway clearance techniques for cystic fibrosis. *Cochrane Database Syst Rev*. 2023;5:CD002011.
21. Elkins MR, Robinson M, Rose BR, et al. A controlled trial of long-term inhaled hypertonic saline in patients with cystic fibrosis. *N Engl J Med*. 2006;354:229–240.
22. Fuchs HJ, Borowitz DS, Christiansen DH, et al. Effect of aerosolized recombinant human DNase on exacerbations of respiratory symptoms and on pulmonary function in patients with cystic fibrosis. The Pulmozyme Study Group. *N Engl J Med*. 1994;331:637–642.
23. Flume PA, Mogayzel PJ Jr, Robinson KA, et al. Cystic fibrosis pulmonary guidelines: treatment of pulmonary exacerbations. *Am J Respir Crit Care Med*. 2009;180:802–808.
24. Goss CH, Heltshe SL, West NE, et al. A randomized clinical trial of antimicrobial duration for cystic fibrosis pulmonary exacerbation treatment. *Am J Respir Crit Care Med*. 2021;204:1295–1305.
25. Smith AL, Fiel SB, Mayer-Hamblett N, Ramsey B, Burns JL. Susceptibility testing of Pseudomonas aeruginosa isolates and clinical response to parenteral antibiotic administration: lack of association in cystic fibrosis. *Chest*. 2003;123:1495–1502.
26. Ramsey B, Pepe MS, Quan JM, et al. Intermittent administration of inhaled tobramycin in patients with cystic fibrosis. Cystic Fibrosis Inhaled Tobramycin Study Group. *N Engl J Med*. 1999;340:23–30.
27. Retsch-Bogart GZ, Quittner AL, Gibson RL, et al. Efficacy and safety of inhaled aztreonam lysine for airway pseudomonas in cystic fibrosis. *Chest*. 2009;135:1223–1232.
28. Southern KW, Barker PM, Solis-Moya A, Patel L. Macrolide antibiotics for cystic fibrosis. *Cochrane Database Syst Rev*. 2012;11:CD002203.
29. Eigen H, Rosenstein BJ, FitzSimmons S, Schidlow DV. A multicenter study of alternate-day prednisone therapy in patients with cystic fibrosis. Cystic Fibrosis Foundation Prednisone Trial Group. *J Pediatr*. 1995;126:515–523.
30. Konstan MW, Byard PJ, Hoppel CL, Davis PB. Effect of high-dose ibuprofen in patients with cystic fibrosis. *N Engl J Med*. 1995;332:848–854.
31. Pilewski JM. Update on lung transplantation for cystic fibrosis. *Clin Chest Med*. 2022;43:821–840.
32. Stallings VA, Stark LJ, Robinson KA, et al. Evidence-based practice recommendations for nutrition-related management of children and adults with cystic fibrosis and pancreatic insufficiency: results of a systematic review. *J Am Diet Assoc*. 2008;108:832–839.
33. Ng SM, Franchini AJ. Drug therapies for reducing gastric acidity in people with cystic fibrosis. *Cochrane Database Syst Rev*. 2014;7:CD003424.
34. Colombo C, Ellemunter H, Houwen R, Munck A, Taylor C, Wilschanski M; ECFS. Guidelines for the diagnosis and management of distal intestinal obstruction syndrome in cystic fibrosis patients. *J Cyst Fibros*. 2011;10:S24–S28.

35. Moran A, Brunzell C, Cohen RC, et al. CFRD Guidelines Committee. Clinical care guidelines for cystic fibrosis-related diabetes: a position statement of the American Diabetes Association and a clinical practice guideline of the Cystic Fibrosis Foundation, endorsed by the Pediatric Endocrine Society. *Diabetes Care*. 2010;33:2697–2708.
36. Conwell LS, Chang AB. Bisphosphonates for osteoporosis in people with cystic fibrosis. *Cochrane Database Syst Rev*. 2012;4:CD002010.
37. Ramos KJ, Smith PJ, McKone EF, et al. CF Lung Transplant Referral Guidelines Committee. Lung transplant referral for individuals with cystic fibrosis: Cystic Fibrosis Foundation consensus guidelines. *J Cyst Fibros*. 2019;18:321–333.
38. Jain R, Kazmerski TM, Zuckerwise LC, et al. Pregnancy in cystic fibrosis: review of the literature and expert recommendations. *J Cyst Fibros*. 2022;21:387–395.
39. Cohen-Cymberknoh M, Gindi Reiss B, Reiter J, et al. Baseline cystic fibrosis disease severity has an adverse impact on pregnancy and infant outcomes, but does not impact disease progression. *J Cyst Fibros*. 2021;20:388–394.
40. Flume PA, Mogayzel PJ, Robinson KA, et al. Cystic fibrosis pulmonary guidelines: pulmonary complications: hemoptysis and pneumothorax. *Am J Respir Crit Care Med*. 2010;182:298–306.
41. Antonelli M, Midulla F, Tancredi G, et al. Bronchial artery embolization for the management of nonmassive hemoptysis in cystic fibrosis. *Chest*. 2002;121:796–801.

Hemoptysis   17

Rachel McDonald

GENERAL PRINCIPLES

Definition
- **Hemoptysis** refers to the expectoration of blood originating from the lower airway or lung.
- **Massive hemoptysis** is defined as the expectoration of large amounts of blood.
  - There is no consensus on the volume of blood needed to be classified as massive; prior definitions range from 100 mL to >600 mL over a 24-hour period.
  - Rather than a definition based on volume, massive hemoptysis now focuses on the clinical significance of hemoptysis. A clinical definition of massive hemoptysis is any amount of bleeding that causes difficulty with oxygenation or ventilation or causes hemodynamic instability.[1]
  - Massive hemoptysis can be life threatening and should be considered a medical emergency. Death is more commonly from asphyxiation with flooding of the alveoli resulting in refractory hypoxemia; however, death from exsanguination can also occur.
  - Massive hemoptysis accounts for about 1–5% of all patients presenting with hemoptysis.
- **The most common causes of hemoptysis in the US are bronchitis, bronchiectasis, bronchogenic carcinoma, tuberculosis (TB), and pneumonia. In the developing world, TB is the most common cause of hemoptysis.**
- The pulmonary circulation consists of dual blood supplies: the pulmonary and bronchial artery systems.
  - The pulmonary artery system is a low-pressure system with normal pressures of 15–20/5–10 mm Hg. It delivers blood from the right ventricle to the pulmonary capillary beds for oxygenation and returns it to the left atrium via the pulmonary veins.
  - Bronchial arteries arise from the aorta and thus exhibit systemic pressures. These are the main source of nutrients and oxygenation of lung tissue and hilar lymph nodes.
  - While distinct blood supplies, the bronchial and pulmonary arteries communicate with each other through small anastomoses.
- In patients with normal pulmonary artery pressures, bleeding from the pulmonary arterial system only accounts for about 5% of massive hemoptysis cases.
- **Risk factors** identified for in-hospital mortality include mechanical ventilation, pulmonary artery bleeding, cancer, aspergillosis, chronic alcoholism, and an admission CXR with infiltrates in more than two quadrants.[2]

DIAGNOSIS

- A thorough history, physical examination, and laboratory evaluation may help determine the correct etiology of the hemoptysis and guide optimal diagnostics.
- Processes that could be confused with hemoptysis, such as hematemesis or bleeding from the upper airway, must first be eliminated.

Clinical Presentation

- Important historical points to review include preexisting lung, cardiac, or renal disease, history of smoking cigarettes, prior hemoptysis, pulmonary symptoms, infectious symptoms, family history of hemoptysis or brain aneurysms (hereditary hemorrhagic telangiectasia), chemical exposures, travel history, TB exposures, bleeding disorders, use of anticoagulants or antiplatelets, and gastrointestinal or upper airway complaints.
- Signs that may aid in diagnosis include telangiectasias (hereditary hemorrhagic telangiectasia), skin rashes (vasculitis, rheumatologic diseases, infective endocarditis), splinter hemorrhages (endocarditis, vasculitis), clubbing (chronic lung disease, carcinoma), cardiac murmurs (endocarditis, mitral stenosis, congenital heart disease), and lower extremity edema (deep vein thrombosis).

Differential Diagnosis

The differential diagnosis of hemoptysis is presented in Table 17-1 (also see Chapter 18).

Diagnostic Testing

Laboratories

- Complete blood count: to assess the magnitude and acuity of bleeding and for thrombocytopenia.
- Renal function and urinalysis: to evaluate for evidence of pulmonary–renal syndromes.
- Coagulation profile: to assess for the presence of a coagulopathy.
- Pulse oximetry and an arterial blood gas: to assess oxygenation.

Imaging

- Common methods to evaluate hemoptysis include CXR, CT scan, and bronchoscopy.
- Performing a **CXR** first is reasonable for most patients.
  - A negative CXR may or may not be very helpful, depending on the clinical picture. For example, a nonsmoking young patient with a small amount of transient hemoptysis in the setting of acute bronchitis likely does not require further evaluation. In other patients, a normal CXR does not eliminate the possibility of a serious cause, including malignancy.[3]
  - Further imaging is appropriate in patients with significant or recurrent hemoptysis, risk factors for malignancy, or massive hemoptysis.[3–7]
- **CT chest with contrast**
  - The sensitivity of contrast-enhanced CT is better than CXR, particularly for certain diagnoses, such as bronchiectasis.[8–10]
  - A contrast-enhanced CT may reveal active extravasation and guide treatment decisions.

TABLE 17-1 CAUSES OF HEMOPTYSIS

Infection
Bronchitis
Endocarditis/septic emboli
Lung abscess
Mycetoma
Pneumonia (viral, tuberculous, fungal, necrotizing)
Parasitic infections

Malignancy
Primary bronchogenic carcinoma
Kaposi sarcoma
Lung metastases

Pulmonary
Bronchiectasis
Cystic fibrosis
Sarcoidosis

Trauma/foreign body
Broncholithiasis
Direct lung trauma
Foreign body
Vascular fistula

Cardiac/pulmonary vascular
Arteriovenous malformation
Pulmonary hypertension
Endocarditis
Mitral stenosis
Pulmonary artery rupture
Pulmonary embolism/infarction
Bronchial or pulmonary artery aneurysm

Miscellaneous
Amyloidosis
Cryptogenic
Endometriosis

Alveolar hemorrhage
Vasculitis
Behçet syndrome
Goodpasture syndrome
Granulomatosis with polyangiitis
Eosinophilic granulomatosis with polyangiitis
Henoch–Schönlein purpura
Microscopic polyangiitis

Rheumatologic
Rheumatoid arthritis
Systemic sclerosis
Systemic lupus erythematosus

Hematologic
Antiphospholipid antibody syndrome
Platelet disorders
Hematopoietic stem cell transplant
Primary and acquired coagulopathies

Medication/drugs/toxin exposure (penicillamine, cytotoxics, nitrofurantoin, amiodarone, retinoic acid, crack cocaine, solvents, anticoagulants, antiplatelets)
Idiopathic pulmonary hemosiderosis

- CT has better diagnostic yield when compared to bronchoscopy in some studies.[3,10–12]

Diagnostic Procedures
- **Bronchoscopy**
  - The diagnostic yield of bronchoscopy for hemoptysis is debated and likely depends on patient population. Flexible bronchoscopy in the acute setting versus delayed bronchoscopy has been shown to be more likely to visualize active bleeding (41% vs. 8%) and the site of bleeding (34% vs. 11%).[13]

- In patients with abnormal, but nonlocalizing CXRs, the diagnostic yield of bronchoscopy has been reported between 34–55%. In patients with moderate to severe hemoptysis, bronchoscopy was able to localize the site of bleeding in ~65% of patients. Bronchoscopy combined with CT scanning had a diagnostic yield of 93%.[8]
- In patients with a localizing CXR, the utility of bronchoscopy has been as high as 82%.[14]
- **Flexible bronchoscopy** has the advantage of better visualization of airways, ability to navigate into subsegments, and can be performed at the bedside. However, suctioning blood is inferior with flexible bronchoscopy compared to that with rigid bronchoscopy.
- **Rigid bronchoscopy** usually requires operating room resources, only allows direct visualization of larger airway but more therapeutic interventions may be possible.

TREATMENT

- **Nonmassive hemoptysis:** Treat the underlying cause (i.e., antibiotics for an infection, radiation therapy or laser therapy for an endobronchial tumor).
  - **Tranexamic acid** (TXA), either delivered intravenously or via nebulization, may decrease hemoptysis without an increase in adverse events. The administration of TXA can be considered while other treatment strategies are being considered.[15]
  - **Consideration of additional imaging including angiography should be considered in cases of recurrent hemoptysis, even in cases of nonmassive hemoptysis.**
    - Bronchial artery embolization has been shown to have similar success rates in cases of nonmassive hemoptysis as it does in cases of massive hemoptysis.[16]
    - Recurrent episodes of nonmassive hemoptysis may be a potential harbinger of the later development of massive hemoptysis. Interventions before life-threatening bleeding occurs should be considered.
- **Massive hemoptysis:** Management of massive hemoptysis should focus on **airway protection and stabilization, localization of bleeding, and bleeding control.** A patient with massive hemoptysis should be treated in an intensive care unit, even if not intubated.
- **Airway protection and stabilization**
  - Hemodynamic monitoring and continuous pulse-oximetry are essential. Oxygen supplementation should be used as necessary to maintain saturation.
  - Establishment of adequate IV access as well as blood typing and crossmatching of blood products should occur early in preparation for possible transfusion and hemodynamic support.
  - If the location is known, the patient should be placed in the **lateral decubitus position** with the affected side down.
  - If the patient is unable to maintain adequate oxygenation or ventilation, or is unable to protect the airway, endotracheal (ET) intubation should be considered.
  - A patient with massive hemoptysis often requires intubation, ideally with a large-diameter ET tube.

- ET tube positioning and selective mainstem intubation can be used to prevent aspiration of blood into the nonbleeding lung.
  - If bleeding occurs in the left lung, caution must be taken when placing a standard ET tube into the right mainstem bronchus due to the proximal position of the right upper lobe bronchus takeoff and risk of right upper lobe collapse.
  - Endobronchial blockers can be placed under bronchoscopic guidance in a mainstem bronchus or in the affected lobe to tamponade bleeding and protect the nonbleeding airways.
  - If available, a double-lumen ET tube may be preferable.
- Blood clots in the large bronchi can be life threatening even without decreases in hematocrit. Bronchoscopy with therapeutic aspiration may be required.
- The use of strong cough suppressants (e.g., opiates) may also be helpful.

- **Localization of the bleeding**
  - Localization is critical in the management of massive hemoptysis.
  - The presence of focal rhonchi or wheezes might suggest the site of bleeding.
  - Imaging and diagnostic procedures listed in the previous section are recommended.

- **Control of bleeding**
  - The patient's medication list should be reviewed for anticoagulants and antiplatelet agents. These medications should be held or reversed, if medically reasonable.
  - If a coagulopathy is present, correction with the use of appropriate factor replacement and platelet transfusions is appropriate.
  - In patients with a history of renal failure, desmopressin for possible platelet dysfunction should be considered.
  - Endoscopic interventions may be attempted include aspiration of blood and clots, iced saline lavage, endobronchial tamponade, and laser photocoagulation.

- **Pulmonary angiography and bronchial artery embolization** by interventional radiology may also be attempted.
  - This strategy is frequently used in massive hemoptysis or recurrent hemoptysis. The short-term success rate of bronchial artery embolization is estimated between 65% and 95%, but rebleeding can recur.[17–20] Risk of rebleeding differs according to underlying etiology of hemoptysis, with recurrent bleeding being most common in patients with chronic pulmonary aspergillosis, malignancy, and sarcoidosis.
  - Bronchial artery embolization is contraindicated if the anterior spinal artery arises from the bronchial artery, as this could lead to spinal cord ischemia. The overall risk of spinal cord ischemic injury is <1%. Bronchoscopy prior to angiography may be helpful in directing the radiologist to the affected area of lung if CT scan is equivocal.

- **Surgery**
  - Surgery is an option for a patient who can sustain a lobectomy or pneumonectomy.
  - Which patients should undergo surgical treatment is unclear; however, surgery can be considered in patients with recurrent hemoptysis or continued hemoptysis despite alternative therapies.
  - Mortality rates have been reported between 4% and 35%.[21]
  - Thoracic surgery consultation and evaluation should be obtained early in an unstable hemoptysis patient.

○ Operative complications include recurrence of hemoptysis, spinal cord injury/ischemia due to disruption of the anterior spinal arteries, bronchopleural fistula, infection, and prolonged mechanical ventilation.

REFERENCES

1. Charya AV, Holden VK, Pickering EM. Management of life-threatening hemoptysis in the ICU. *J Thorac Dis.* 2021;13:5139–5158.
2. Fartoukh M, Khoshnood B, Parrot A, et al. Early prediction of in-hospital mortality of patients with hemoptysis: An approach to defining severe hemoptysis. *Respiration.* 2012; 83:106–114.
3. Thirumaran M, Sundar R, Sutcliffe IM, Currie DC. Is investigation of patients with haemoptysis and normal chest radiograph justified? *Thorax.* 2009;64:854–856.
4. Poe RH, Israel RH, Marin MG, et al. Utility of fiberoptic bronchoscopy in patients with hemoptysis and a nonlocalizing chest roentgenogram. *Chest.* 1988;93:70–75.
5. O'Neil KM, Lazarus AA. Hemoptysis. Indications for bronchoscopy. *Arch Intern Med.* 1991;151:171–174.
6. Herth F, Ernst A, Becker HD. Long-term outcome and lung cancer incidence in patients with hemoptysis of unknown origin. *Chest.* 2001;120:1592–1594.
7. Ketai LH, Mohammed TL, Kirsch J, et al. ACR appropriateness criteria hemoptysis. *J Thorac Imaging.* 2014;29:W19–22.
8. Hirshberg B, Biran I, Glazer M, Kramer MR. Hemoptysis: etiology, evaluation, and outcomes in a tertiary referral hospital. *Chest.* 1997;112:440–444.
9. Tasker AD, Flower CD. Imaging the airways. Hemoptysis, bronchiectasis, and small airways disease. *Clin Chest Med.* 1999;20:761–773.
10. Revel MP, Fournier LS, Hennebicque AS, et al. Can CT replace bronchoscopy in the detection of the site and cause of bleeding in patients with large or massive hemoptysis. *Am J Roentgenol.* 2002;179:1217–1224.
11. Set PA, Flower CD, Smith IE, Chan AP, Twentyman OP, Shneerson JM. Hemoptysis: comparative study of the role of CT and fiberoptic bronchoscopy. *Radiology.* 1993;189:677–680.
12. Laroche C, Fairbairn I, Moss H, et al. Role of computed tomographic scanning of the thorax prior to bronchoscopy in the investigation of suspected lung cancer. *Thorax.* 2000;55:359–363.
13. Gong H Jr, Salvatierra C. Clinical efficacy of early and delayed fiberoptic bronchoscopy in patients with hemoptysis. *Am Rev Respir Dis.* 1981;124:221–225.
14. Hsiao EI, Kirsch CM, Kagawa FT, Wehner JH, Jensen WA, Baxter RB. Utility of fiberoptic bronchoscopy before bronchial artery embolization for massive hemoptysis. *Am J Roentgenol.* 2001;177:861–867.
15. Wand O, Guber E, Guber A, Shochet GE, Israeli-Shani L, Shitrit D. Inhaled Tranexamic acid for hemoptysis treatment: a randomized control trial. *Chest.* 2018;154(6):1379–1384.
16. Expert Panel on Thoracic Imaging; Olsen KM, Manouchehr-Pour M, Donnelly EF, et al. ACR appropriateness criteria hemoptysis. *J Am Coll Radiol.* 2020;17:S148–S159.
17. Cremaschi P, Nascimbene C, Vitulo P, et al. Therapeutic embolization of bronchial artery: a successful treatment in 209 cases of relapse hemoptysis. *Angiology.* 1993;44:295–299.
18. Jean-Baptiste E. Clinical assessment and management of massive hemoptysis. *Crit Care Med.* 2000;28:1642–1647.
19. Woo S, Yoon CJ, Chung JW, et al. Bronchial artery embolization to control hemoptysis: comparison of N-butyl-2-cyanoacrylate and polyvinyl alcohol particles. *Radiology.* 2013; 269:594–602.
20. Larici AR, Franchi P, Occhipinti M, et al. Diagnosis and management of hemoptysis. *Diagn Interv Radiol.* 2014;20:299–309.
21. Andréjak C, Parrot A, Bazelly B, et al. Surgical lung resection for severe hemoptysis. *Ann Thorac Surg.* 2009;88:1556–1565.

Diffuse Alveolar Hemorrhage

18

John Grotberg and Bryan D. Kraft

GENERAL PRINCIPLES

- Diffuse alveolar hemorrhage (DAH) encompasses a heterogeneous group of pulmonary and nonpulmonary disorders characterized by widespread intraalveolar bleeding.
- DAH is a medical emergency that can result in acute respiratory failure and death.
- The exact incidence and prevalence of DAH are unknown owing to the variety of underlying etiologies. The most common cause of DAH appears to be systemic vasculitis, in particular granulomatosis with polyangiitis (GPA); see Figure 18-1.[1,2]
- The pathogenesis of DAH varies depending on the underlying cause. Major categories include immune-mediated, which may include inflammation of the alveolar capillary endothelium (capillaritis), capillary stress failure in the setting of increased hydrostatic pressures (bland hemorrhage), and diffuse alveolar damage.
- Determining DAH etiology is important to identify the appropriate therapy.
- Differentiation from localized etiologies (Table 18-1) of pulmonary hemorrhage is difficult to ascertain on history and physical examination alone; diagnostic procedures such as chest imaging and fiberoptic bronchoscopy are often needed.

DIAGNOSIS

- Appropriate diagnosis of DAH requires high clinical suspicion and a thorough history and physical examination.
- **Rapid diagnosis of DAH is mandatory** given the potential for excessive morbidity (renal failure, restrictive and obstructive lung disease) and mortality rates approaching 70–80% in untreated subsets of patients.

Clinical Presentation

- DAH should be suspected when a patient presents with **hemoptysis, dyspnea, consistent imaging findings, and a predisposing condition,** such as an underlying connective tissue disorder, systemic vasculitis, or certain drug or occupational exposures.
- Hemoptysis, a presumed cardinal symptom of DAH, may be absent in up to one-third of cases despite pronounced and life-threatening alveolar hemorrhage.
- A **detailed past medical and surgical history, past and present medications** (prescribed and over the counter), **recreational drug use, occupational exposures,** and **complete review of systems** should be obtained. Amiodarone, retinoic acid, sirolimus, penicillamine, and crack cocaine have all been implicated as causative agents of DAH.[3]
- **Physical examination findings are nonspecific** and may include fever, hypoxemia, tachypnea, and diffuse crackles.

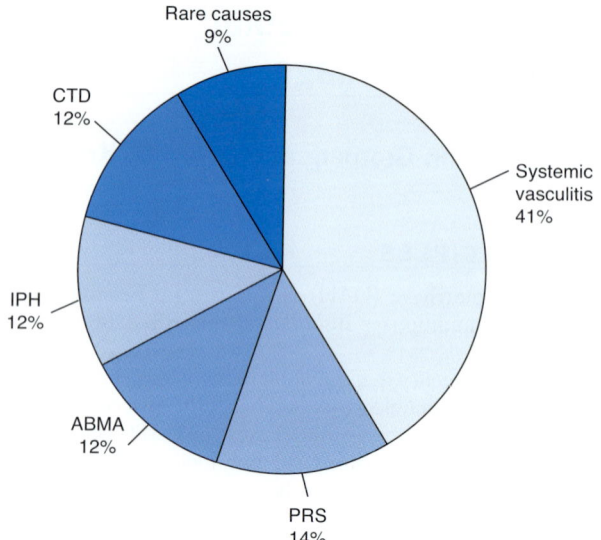

Figure 18-1 Causes of diffuse alveolar hemorrhage. ABMA, antibasement membrane antibody–mediated disease; CTD, connective tissue disease; IPH, idiopathic pulmonary hemorrhage; PRS, pulmonary–renal syndromes. (Data from Travis WD, Colby TV, Lombard C, Carpenter HA. A clinicopathologic study of 34 cases of diffuse pulmonary hemorrhage with lung biopsy confirmation. *Am J Surg Pathol*. 1990;14:1112–1125.)

TABLE 18-1	CAUSES OF LOCALIZED PULMONARY HEMORRHAGE

Aspiration of blood from the upper airway (e.g., epistaxis) or gastrointestinal tract (e.g., hematemesis) (may be difficult to distinguish from diffuse alveolar hemorrhage)
Neoplasm (e.g., primary bronchogenic, metastatic disease)
Cavitary lung disease (e.g., secondary to TB, aspergillosis)
Pulmonary infarction
Bronchitis
Bronchiectasis
Broncholithiasis
Necrotizing bronchopneumonia
Arteriovenous malformations

- Signs suggesting an underlying systemic disorder should be sought. These signs may include sinusitis, iritis, oral ulcers, arthritis, synovitis, palpable purpura or other skin changes, neuropathy, and cardiac murmurs.

Differential Diagnosis

DAH is infrequently the initial presentation of an underlying systemic disorder (Table 18-2 and Fig. 18-1).[1–14] Twenty percent of patients with systemic lupus

TABLE 18-2 CAUSES OF DIFFUSE ALVEOLAR HEMORRHAGE

Rheumatologic
Systemic lupus erythematosus[5]
Rheumatoid arthritis[6]
Mixed connective tissue disorder[6]
Systemic sclerosis
Juvenile rheumatoid arthritis
Polymyositis
Behçet disease
Cryoglobulinemia
Goodpasture syndrome
Granulomatosis with polyangiitis (Wegener granulomatosis)
Henoch–Schönlein purpura
Microscopic polyangiitis

Isolated Pulmonary Disease
Isolated pauci-immune pulmonary capillaritis
Idiopathic pulmonary fibrosis
Idiopathic pulmonary hemosiderosis
Acute lung transplant rejection
Pulmonary veno-occlusive disease
Pulmonary capillary hemangiomatosis
Acute respiratory distress syndrome
Pneumonia due to viral, bacterial, or fungal pathogens
Pulmonary infarcts

Renal
IgA nephropathy
Idiopathic glomerulonephritis
Poststreptococcal glomerulonephritis

Cardiac
Mitral valve disease
Aortic valve disease
Bacterial endocarditis
Congestive heart failure

Hematologic
Hematopoietic stem cell transplant[7]
Thrombotic thrombocytopenic purpura[8]
Idiopathic thrombocytopenic purpura
Disseminated intravascular coagulation
Cryoglobulinemia
Antiphospholipid antibody syndrome[9]
Multiple myeloma
Leukemia

Gastrointestinal
Ulcerative colitis

Medication/Drugs
Amiodarone[11]
Crack cocaine[3]
Nitrofurantoin
Penicillamine
Propylthiouracil
Phenytoin
Retinoic acid[12]
Sirolimus[13]
Anticoagulants
Antiplatelet agents

Occupational Exposures
Trimellitic anhydride
Radiation exposure
Asbestos
Welder pneumoconiosis

erythematosus (SLE) and 5–10% of patients with Goodpasture syndrome present with DAH as the initial or sole manifestation. Therefore, emphasis should be placed on the rheumatologic, renal, pulmonary, and cardiac review of systems.

Diagnostic Testing

Laboratories

- Laboratory evaluation is crucial for the diagnosis of DAH.
- Complete blood count
  - Anemia is commonly found, and repeated episodes of DAH may lead to an iron-deficiency anemia.
  - Thrombocytopenia.
- Coagulation parameters. Elevated coagulation parameters (e.g., prothrombin time, partial thromboplastin time) should raise the possibility of hemorrhage secondary to an acquired coagulopathy. An isolated elevation in partial thromboplastin time may indicate an antiphospholipid antibody syndrome (APLS).
- Basic metabolic profile to screen for renal dysfunction.
- Urinalysis with urine sediment assessment for dysmorphic red blood cells or casts.
- Drug screen should be obtained on all patients to rule out cocaine use.[3]
- **Serologic markers** should also be obtained and their selection guided by the differential diagnosis.
  - **Antineutrophil cytoplasmic antibodies** (ANCAas) (see Chapter 19)
    - Commonly found in GPA, microscopic polyangiitis (MPA), Churg–Strauss syndrome (CSS), and isolated pauci-immune capillaritis. ANCAs are occasionally seen in other disease states.[15]
    - Cytoplasmic ANCA (c-ANCA) screens for the definitive antibody test, antiproteinase 3 (PR3), and likewise for perinuclear ANCA (p-ANCA) and antimyeloperoxidase (MPO). The level of c-ANCA may sometimes be useful in following disease activity but this is not consistently the case. In a prior review, the sensitivity of c-ANCA in active GPA was 91% versus 63% in inactive disease. The specificity was equivalent in both situations and approached 99%.[16]
    - p-ANCA, antibodies directed against MPO, is less specific and may be associated with many clinical syndromes. p-ANCA is found in 80% of patients with MPA. p-ANCA has also been identified in 15–20% of patients with GPA and up to 20–30% of patients with Goodpasture syndrome.
  - **Antiglomerular basement membrane (Anti-GBM) antibodies**
    - Diagnostic for Goodpasture syndrome, characterized by antibodies (predominantly IgG) directed against the noncollagenous domain of type IV collagen, alpha 3.[17]
    - The sensitivity and specificity of anti-GBM approaches 98%. Two percent to 3% of patients with renal biopsy-proven Goodpasture syndrome may have negative serum anti-GBM, making renal (and not lung) biopsy the gold standard for diagnosis.[17,18]
  - **Serologic markers help to assess for SLE**
    - Antinuclear antibody (ANA)
    - Anti–double-stranded DNA (anti-dsDNA)
    - Complement levels (C3 and C4)

- **Serologic markers to help assess for APLS**
  - Lupus anticoagulant
  - Anti-cardiolipin antibodies
  - Anti–β-2-glycoprotein 1 antibodies

Imaging
- CXRs
  - Standard two-view CXRs in DAH are nonspecific for any of the underlying etiologies and often reveal bilateral alveolar infiltrates during the acute episode.
  - Pulmonary fibrosis or severe obstructive lung disease may develop in chronic, recurrent episodes of DAH. Accordingly, persistent interstitial infiltrates or hyperinflation may be evident on successive CXRs.
- Chest CT typically shows bilateral consolidative and/or ground glass opacities with sparing of the periphery. Pleural effusions are less common in contrast to heart failure.

Diagnostic Procedures
- **Pulmonary function testing** (PFTs)
  - PFTs are unnecessary in the diagnostic assessment but may demonstrate restriction and gas exchange abnormalities in chronic cases.
  - In active DAH, an increase in the diffusing capacity for carbon monoxide (DLCO) may be present attributed to the increased binding of carbon monoxide to intra-alveolar hemoglobin.
  - Varying degrees of hypoxemia result from the ventilation–perfusion abnormalities produced by the alveolar hemorrhage.
- **Fiberoptic bronchoscopy**
  - Bronchoscopy with **bronchoalveolar lavage** (BAL) is the diagnostic gold standard for DAH and helps to evaluate for infectious causes.
    - Criteria for DAH include progressively bloodier returns from three aliquots on sequential BAL or >20% hemosiderin-laden macrophages.[19]
    - False-positive results can occur in smokers (so-called "smokers' macrophages," the most common cause of hemosiderin-laden macrophages) and with distal bronchiolar sources of hemorrhage.[20]
    - Hemosiderin-laden macrophages may not be seen immediately if bronchoscopy is performed too early or too late. On average, 48–72 hours are necessary for hemosiderin-laden macrophages to be seen in alveoli and interstitial spaces. After 2–4 weeks, hemosiderin-laden macrophages generally clear.
  - The role of **bronchoscopic biopsies** is less significant for the differential diagnosis of DAH.
    - Only 17.6% of directed endobronchial biopsies were diagnostic of GPA in the setting of observed ulcerating tracheobronchitis.[21]
    - Transbronchial biopsies may be of low yield given small sample size.
- **Surgical lung biopsy** is reserved for rare occasions where the diagnosis is not clear from history, physical examination, and serologic markers, and in otherwise stable patients that are appropriate candidates for surgery.

- **Microscopic findings**[1,4,20]
    - The most common histologic finding in DAH is pulmonary capillaritis: fibrin thrombi occluding capillaries, fibrinoid necrosis of capillary walls, neutrophils and nuclear dust in the interstitium and surrounding alveoli, and interstitial red blood cells and hemosiderin. In one series of 34 patients with biopsy-proven DAH, 88% of patients displayed pulmonary capillaritis.[2]
    - Diffuse alveolar damage is a stereotypic response to lung injury, characterized by interstitial edema, intra-alveolar hyaline membranes, and type 2 alveolar cell hyperplasia in the acute phase.
    - Bland pulmonary hemorrhage is characterized by blood cells in the alveolar spaces without inflammation, necrosis, or destruction of the alveolar walls. Causes can include bleeding disorders, anticoagulation, and decompensated heart failure.
    - None of these patterns are pathognomonic for any specific disease and multiple histologic findings can be associated with the same disease process.

TREATMENT

- Treatment of DAH depends primarily on the underlying disorder.
- Therapies ranging from observation (in idiopathic pulmonary hemosiderosis) to high-dose corticosteroids and cytotoxic therapy (in ANCA-associated vasculitides).[1,22,23]
- Supportive care should be provided to all patients including reversal of coagulopathies if present.
- Patients requiring invasive mechanical ventilation may benefit from a higher PEEP strategy to mitigate alveolar hemorrhage.
- There may be some benefit to hemostatic agents in local or diffuse hemorrhage that is refractory to conventional therapy[24]:
    - Intravenous or nebulized tranexamic acid (TXA) or aminocaproic acid
    - Recombinant factor VIIa (FVIIa)
- Typical regimens for life-threatening alveolar hemorrhage due to pulmonary capillaritis include:
    - Methylprednisolone, 1 g daily for 3 days, followed by a slow prednisone taper over several months.
    - Rituximab 375 mg/m^2 once weekly for 4 weeks.[25]
    - Plasmapheresis is indicated in certain cases such as Goodpasture syndrome or APLS.[26–29]
    - Cyclophosphamide, 1–2 mg/kg daily initially, and subsequent prolonged maintenance therapy.
    - Also see Chapter 19.

REFERENCES

1. Lara AR, Schwarz MI. Diffuse alveolar hemorrhage. *Chest.* 2010;137:1164–1171.
2. Travis WD, Colby TV, Lombard C, Carpenter HA. A clinicopathologic study of 34 cases of diffuse pulmonary hemorrhage with lung biopsy confirmation. *Am J Surg Pathol.* 1990;14:1112–1125.
3. Haim DY, Lippmann ML, Goldberg SK, Walkenstein MD. The pulmonary complications of crack cocaine. A comprehensive review. *Chest.* 1995;107:233–240.
4. Green RJ, Ruoss SJ, Kraft SA, Duncan SR, Berry GJ, Raffin TA. Pulmonary capillaritis and alveolar hemorrhage. Update on diagnosis and management. *Chest.* 1996;110:1305–1316.

References | 211

5. Zamora MR, Warner ML, Tuder R, Schwarz MI. Diffuse alveolar hemorrhage and systemic lupus erythematosus: clinical presentation, histology, survival, and outcome. *Medicine.* 1997;76:192–202.
6. Schwarz MI, Zamora MR, Hodges TN, Chan ED, Bowler RP, Tuder RM. Isolated pulmonary capillaritis and diffuse alveolar hemorrhage in rheumatoid arthritis and mixed connective tissue disease. *Chest.* 1998;113:1609–1615.
7. Afessa B, Tefferi A, Litzow MR, et al. Diffuse alveolar hemorrhage in hematopoietic stem cell transplant recipients. *Am J Respir Crit Care Med.* 2002;166:641–645.
8. Martinez AJ, Maltby JD, Hurst DJ. Thrombotic thrombocytopenic purpura seen as pulmonary hemorrhage. *Arch Intern Med.* 1983;143:1818–1820.
9. Crausman RS, Achenbach GA, Pluss WT, O'Brien RF, Jennings CA. Pulmonary capillaritis and alveolar hemorrhage associated with the antiphospholipid antibody syndrome. *J Rheumatol.* 1995;22:554–556.
10. Ali A, Patil S, Grady KJ, Schreiber TL. Diffuse alveolar hemorrhage following administration of tirofiban or abciximab: a nemesis of platelet glycoprotein IIb/IIIa inhibitors. *Cathet Cardiovasc Interv.* 2000;49:181–184.
11. Vizioli LD, Cho S. Amiodarone-associated hemoptysis. *Chest.* 1994;105:305–306.
12. Nicolls MR, Terada LS, Tuder RM, Prindiville SA, Schwarz MI. Diffuse alveolar hemorrhage with underlying pulmonary capillaritis in the retinoic acid syndrome. *Am J Respir Crit Care Med.* 1998;158:1302–1305.
13. Vlahakis NE, Rickman OB, Morgenthaler T. Sirolimus-associated DAH. *Mayo Clin Proc.* 2004;79:541–545.
14. Barnett VT, Bergmann F, Humphrey H, Chediak J. Diffuse alveolar hemorrhage secondary to superwarfarin ingestion. *Chest.* 1992;102:1301–1302.
15. Gal AA, Velasquez A. Antineutrophil cytoplasmic autoantibody in the absence of Wegener's granulomatosis or microscopic polyangiitis: implications for the surgical pathologist. *Mod Pathol.* 2002;15:197–204.
16. Rao JK, Weinberger M, Oddone EZ, Allen NB, Landsman P, Feussner JR. The role of antineutrophil cytoplasmic antibody testing in the diagnosis of Wegener's granulomatosis. A literature review and meta-analysis. *Ann Intern Med.* 1995;123:925–932.
17. Hudson BG, Tryggvason K, Sundaramoorthy M, Neilson EG. Alport's syndrome, Goodpasture's syndrome, and type IV collagen. *N Engl J Med.* 2003;348:2543–2556.
18. Salama AD, Dougan T, Levy JB, et al. Goodpasture's disease in the absence of circulating anti-glomerular basement membrane antibodies as detected by standard techniques. *Am J Kidney Dis.* 2002;39:1162–1167.
19. De Lassence A, Fleury-Feith J, Escudier E, Beaune J, Bernaudin JF, Cordonnier C. Alveolar hemorrhage. Diagnostic criteria and results in 194 immunocompromised hosts. *Am J Respir Crit Care Med.* 1995;151:157–163.
20. Colby TV, Fukuoka J, Ewaskow SP, Helmers R, Leslie KO. Pathologic approach to pulmonary hemorrhage. *Ann Diagn Pathol.* 2001;5:309–319.
21. Daum TEA, Specks U, Colby TV, et al. Tracheobronchial involvement in Wegener's granulomatosis. *Am J Respir Crit Care Med.* 1995;151:522–526.
22. Jantz MA, Sahn SA. Corticosteroids in acute respiratory failure. *Am J Respir Crit Care Med.* 1999;160:1079–1100.
23. Metcalf JP, Rennard SI, Reed EC, et al. Corticosteroids as adjunctive therapy for diffuse alveolar hemorrhage associated with bone marrow transplantation. *Am J Med.* 1994;96:327–334.
24. Park JA. Treatment of diffuse alveolar hemorrhage: controlling inflammation and obtaining rapid and effective hemostasis. *Int J Mol Sci.* 2021;22:793.
25. Stone JH, Merkel PA, Spiera R, et al. Rituximab versus cyclophosphamide for ANCA-associated vasculitis. *N Engl J Med.* 2010;363:221–232.
26. Gallagher H, Kwan JT, Jayne DR. Pulmonary renal syndrome: a 4-year, single-center experience. *Am J Kidney Dis.* 2002;39:42–47.

27. Klemmer PJ, Chalermskulrat W, Reif MS, Hogan SL, Henke DC, Falk RJ. Plasmapheresis therapy for diffuse alveolar hemorrhage in patients with small-vessel vasculitis. *Am J Kidney Dis.* 2003;42:1149–1153.
28. Jayne DR, Gaskin G, Rasmussen N, et al. Randomized trial of plasma exchange or high-dosage methylprednisolone as adjunctive therapy for severe renal vasculitis. *J Am Soc Nephrol.* 2007;18:2180–2188.
29. Walsh M, Catapano F, Szpirt W, et al. Plasma exchange for renal vasculitis and idiopathic rapidly progressive glomerulonephritis: a meta-analysis. *Am J Kidney Dis.* 2011;57:566–574.

Pulmonary Vasculitis   19

Vladimir Despotovic

Vasculitis Overview

GENERAL PRINCIPLES

- This chapter discusses the pulmonary features of systemic vasculitides, primarily focusing on the antineutrophil cytoplasmic antibody (ANCA)-associated small-vessel vasculitides (**AAV**) **granulomatosis with polyangiitis (GPA), microscopic polyangiitis (MPA),** and **eosinophilic granulomatosis with polyangiitis (EGPA).**
- Other vasculitides with pulmonary manifestations will be described under special considerations.

Definition

- Systemic vasculitides feature inflammatory leukocytes damaging the walls of blood vessels. This damage can lead to **vessel wall inflammation and downstream tissue ischemia.**
- **Vasculitis is a pathologic finding, not a diagnosis.** Clinicians must determine the cause of the vasculitic condition.

Classification

- Vasculitides may be classified as **primary versus secondary processes**. Primary vasculitides are further classified by the size and type of involved blood vessels.
- **Primary vasculitis** occurs in the absence of an underlying illness and without identifiable etiology.
  - Several classification schemes have been described; the most common is derived from the 2012 revised **Chapel Hill Consensus Conference,** so-called "CHC criteria."[1]
  - While vasculitis may often affect vessels of more than one size, the CHC criteria organized the vasculitides based on the **size of the vessels primarily affected** (Table 19-1).[1] The small-vessel vasculitides are further subdivided into ANCA positive or ANCA negative.
- **Secondary vasculitis** occurs in the presence of an underlying condition, such as the capillaritis seen in systemic lupus erythematosus (SLE) or virus-induced vasculitis.

Epidemiology

- Although the primary systemic vasculitides are rare and epidemiologic studies have been difficult with evolving classification systems, the **frequency of vasculitic diagnoses has been increasing,** possibly because vasculitic syndromes are more readily recognized.

TABLE 19-1 CLASSIFICATION OF VASCULITIS

Large Vessel
Takayasu arteritis (TAK)
Giant-cell arteritis (GCA)

Medium Vessel
Polyarteritis nodosa (PAN)
Kawasaki disease (KD)

Small Vessel
Immune complex related
Hypersensitivity vasculitis[a]
IgA vasculitis (Henoch–Schönlein purpura) (IgAV)
Cryoglobulinemic vasculitis (CV)[b]
Hypocomplementemic urticarial vasculitis
Connective tissue disease–associated vasculitis

Antineutrophil cytoplasmic antibody (ANCA)-associated vasculitis (AAV)
Granulomatosis with polyangiitis (GPA)
Eosinophilic granulomatosis with polyangiitis (EGPA)
Microscopic polyangiitis (MPA)

Vasculitis associated with systemic disease
Lupus vasculitis
Rheumatoid vasculitis
Sarcoid vasculitis

Single-organ vasculitis (SOV)
Cutaneous leukocytoclastic angiitis (Hypersensitivity vasculitis)[a]
Primary central nervous system vasculitis
Isolated Aortitis

---
[a]Most often caused by medications, infections, and malignancies.
[b]Most often associated with hepatitis B and C, Epstein–Barr virus, plasma cell dyscrasias, chronic inflammatory/autoimmune disorders, and lymphoproliferative malignancies.

With permission from Jennette JC, Falk RJ, Bacon PA, et al. 2012 Revised International Chapel Hill Consensus Conference Nomenclature of Vasculitides. *Arthritis Rheum.* 2013;65:1–11.

- At a pooled incidence of 10 cases/100,000 adults, **giant-cell arteritis (GCA) represents the most common vasculitis**. GCA is followed in annual incidence by **AAV** with the combined incidence rate for GPA, MPA, and EGPA around 3.3 cases/100,000 in the US.[2]

DIAGNOSIS

- Clinicians should consider a diagnosis of vasculitis in patients whose clinical presentation includes **systemic symptoms** (e.g., fatigue, weakness, fever) as well as **evidence of organ dysfunction** (e.g., renal, neurologic, pulmonary). As the

clinical manifestations of the vasculitides are quite variable and overlap with many other disorders, a thorough history and physical examination is essential to aid in the diagnosis of vasculitis.
- **Pulmonary manifestations** of the systemic vasculitides may range from shortness of breath due to mild upper respiratory tract symptoms to respiratory failure from alveolar hemorrhage. While the lungs may not represent the only involved organ system in many cases, respiratory symptoms often motivate these patients to seek medical attention.[3]
- Basic **laboratory** tests for the vasculitides should include serum creatinine, liver function tests, complete blood count (CBC), muscle enzymes, erythrocyte sedimentation rate (ESR), C-reactive protein (CRP), viral hepatitis and HIV serologies, urinalysis, and urine toxicology screen. More specific tests may include **antinuclear antibody** (ANA), **serum complement levels** (depressed in mixed cryoglobulinemia and lupus), **ANCA** (often directed against proteinase 3 [PR3] in GPA and against myeloperoxidase [MPO] in MPA) and **anti-glomerular basement membrane (GBM)** antibody testing.
- Certain procedures are often crucial for the diagnosis of vasculitides. Specifically, **tissue biopsy** can definitively establish the presence of vasculitis. **Angiography** is useful for vasculitides affecting large- and medium-sized blood vessels. CT and MRI angiography have largely replaced invasive angiography as the study of choice. However, mesenteric or renal artery invasive angiography can assist in patients suspected of having polyarteritis nodosa (PAN) if other imaging modalities are inconclusive.

TREATMENT

While the treatments for ANCA-associated vasculitis will be discussed in their respective sections, management of most vasculitides generally involves **corticosteroids, typically in combination with other immunosuppressive agents**. Other considerations in management specific to a particular vasculitis will be discussed with that particular syndrome.

SPECIAL CONSIDERATIONS

- **Primary large-vessel vasculitides**
  - **GCA or temporal arteritis** represents the most common vasculitis among Caucasians, predominantly affects the elderly, and classically involves the **extracranial branches of the carotid artery**.
    - Respiratory symptoms such as cough, hoarseness, or throat pain represent the initial complaint in up to one-quarter of patients, although CXRs and pulmonary function testing may be normal.
    - Updated 2022 American College of Rheumatology (ACR)/European League Against Rheumatism (EULAR) classification criteria now use a scoring system.[4] It is important to remember that strict scoring systems are made for study enrollment purposes, and additional **clinical judgment** is required.
      - **Age ≥50 is an absolute** requirement.
      - Additional clinical, laboratory, imaging, and biopsy criteria carry different number of points. A score of **≥6 points** is needed for GCA classification.

- **5 points**—positive temporal artery biopsy (**necrotizing arteritis with a predominance of mononuclear cells or a granulomatous process with multinucleated giant cells**[5]) or halo sign on temporal artery ultrasound.
- **3 points** each—sudden visual loss; ESR ≥ 50/CRP ≥10.
- **2 points** each—morning stiffness in shoulders/neck; jaw or tongue claudication; new temporal headache; scalp tenderness; temporal artery that is hard to palpate or has diminished pulse; imaging abnormalities on bilateral axillary vessels; diffuse aortic fluorodeoxyglucose positron emission tomography scan (FDG-PET) activity.
- **Large-vessel GCA** involves the aorta and its major proximal branches and manifests as **arm claudication,** pulselessness, aortitis, aortic aneurysms, or aortic insufficiency. It has been increasingly recognized to be present in as many as 74% of the patients with biopsy-proven GCA.[6]
- **Treatment** approach is based on high-dose steroids with the addition of tocilizumab (anti–IL-6R agent) based on the GIACTA trial that demonstrated superior glucocorticoid-free remission with lower doses of steroids.[7] In the absence of vision loss, steroids are given at 1 mg/kg prednisone equivalent up to 60 mg/d. In the presence of vision loss, pulse-dose steroids should precede the high-dose steroids. Without tocilizumab, **long-term prednisone treatment** (9–12 months) usually leads to symptom resolution in GCA. With tocilizumab, a shorter steroid taper of 6 months is standard,[8] and even shorter steroid regimens in the presence of tocilizumab are being explored.[9]
- **Takayasu arteritis** affects the **aorta and its major branches** and is classically described in young Asian females.
  - Pulmonary manifestations can include mild pulmonary hypertension, fistula formation between branches of the pulmonary artery and bronchial arteries, and nonspecific inflammatory interstitial lung disease.
  - CT or MRI angiography demonstrates **pulmonary artery involvement, most commonly with stenoses and occlusion,** in nearly half of patients.
  - Updated 2022 ACR/EULAR classification criteria now use a scoring system.[10] It is important to remember that strict scoring systems are made for study enrollment purposes, and additional **clinical judgment** is required.
    - **Age ≤60 and evidence of vasculitis** on imaging are **absolute** requirements.
    - Additional clinical and imaging criteria carry different number of points. A score of ≥5 **points** is needed for Takayasu Arteritis classification.
    - **3 points** each—abdominal aorta involvement with renal or mesenteric involvement; three or more arterial territories involved.
    - **2 points** each—angina or ischemic cardiac pain; extremity claudication; vascular bruit; upper extremity pulse reduction; carotid artery pulse reduction or tenderness.
    - **1 point** each—female sex; systolic blood pressure difference between arms ≥20; symmetric involvement of paired arteries; single arterial territory involved.
  - Treatment: **High-dose oral glucocorticoids** (1 mg/kg prednisone equivalent up to 80 mg) combined with a **glucocorticoid-sparing agent** are the foundation of treatment and are weaned over several months. If limb- or

organ-threatening disease is present, initial treatment is with pulse-dose steroids. There is no single superior steroid-sparing agent. Methotrexate and azathioprine (AZA) are the most used nonbiologic disease-modifying antirheumatic drugs (DMARDs) with the biologic therapy most used is a **TNF inhibitor**. Chronic active disease is common, and it may only be detectable by **imaging**. Vascular stenosis and occlusion can require **endovascular** procedures or vascular **surgical** bypass.[7]

- **Primary medium-vessel vasculitides**
  - **PAN** is a necrotizing systemic vasculitis affecting both **medium and small muscular arteries**.
    - Approximately a third are associated with **hepatitis B infection**.
    - Presentation can include skin nodules, mononeuritis multiplex, orchitis, and renal and mesenteric artery branch involvement. It typically does not cause glomerulonephritis, alveolar hemorrhage, or vasculitis of the arterioles, capillaries, or venules.[11]
    - **Pulmonary** involvement is extremely rare in PAN and, if present, a different disease process such as small-vessel vasculitis should be considered.
    - Rare disease processes have been increasingly recognized with clinical overlap with PAN in manifestations and greater pulmonary involvement. Vacuoles, E1 enzyme, X-linked, autoinflammatory, somatic (**VEXAS**) syndrome is more commonly seen in males with vasculitis, chondritis, pulmonary inflammation and hematologic manifestations with features in common with myelodysplastic syndrome.[12] **DADA2** syndrome is most commonly seen in children; however, is increasingly recognized in adults manifesting with systemic vasculitis, early onset stroke, immunodeficiency, and hematologic abnormalities. Pulmonary manifestations can be through opportunistic infections, asthma, bronchiectasis, and pulmonary alveolar proteinosis.[13]
    - Treatment: In nonsevere PAN, high-dose **corticosteroids** are recommended. In severe PAN (organ and life threatening), pulse-dose steroids are followed by high-dose steroids and cyclophosphamide (CYC).
  - **Kawasaki disease** (KD), while primarily a medium-vessel vasculitis, can also affect large and small blood vessels.
    - Usually seen in **children**, this vasculitis has a predilection for the **coronary arteries** and may be associated with a mucocutaneous lymph node syndrome.
    - While pulmonary symptoms are not among the criteria for diagnosis, pulmonary involvement can occasionally occur in KD. These may be misinterpreted as **atypical pneumonia or unresolving pneumonia** with findings ranging from subclinical interstitial micronodular infiltrates to larger inflammatory pulmonary nodules.[14]
    - Treatment typically involves **aspirin** and **IV immunoglobulin (IVIG)**.
    - Multisystem inflammatory syndrome in children (**MIS-C**) is a syndrome resembling KD and associated with persistent fever, elevation of inflammatory markers, multisystem involvement (prominent myocardial involvement), evidence of a recent COVID-19 infection, and absence of other potential etiologies. **Pulmonary** manifestations include respiratory failure in the setting of heart failure, and imaging commonly shows cardiogenic or noncardiogenic pulmonary edema. Accepted treatment includes IVIG and steroids.[15]

- **Behçet disease**
  - Behçet disease is a relapsing multisystem disorder characterized by **recurrent oral ulcerations** and at least two of the following findings: **genital ulcers, ocular involvement including uveitis and retinal vasculitis, cutaneous nodules or pustules, and positive pathergy test.**[16] A more recent scoring system provides better sensitivity for the diagnosis.[17]
  - Vessels of all sizes in both the arterial and venous systems may be affected, although it is most common to have **arterial small vessel or venous involvement.**
  - While cough, dyspnea, or chest pain may represent initial respiratory symptoms, massive hemoptysis may be the most significant complication. Credited as the underlying mechanism in Behçet disease, **immune complex deposition** can lead to lung findings such as **pulmonary artery aneurysms** due to destruction of the elastic lamina or arterial–bronchial fistulae due to erosion of the bronchi.[18] Resultant massive hemoptysis carries an associated mortality of nearly 40%. Pulmonary angiography has given way to CT and magnetic resonance angiography in the diagnosis of Behçet disease.
  - Treatment
    - **Prednisone with azathioprine or CYC** has the most data for pulmonary artery aneurysms, although chlorambucil, colchicine, cyclosporine, and methotrexate in combination with prednisone have been used. More recently, **TNF inhibitors** have shown efficacy when used along with steroids and/or AZA for multiple serious disease manifestations, particularly when inflammation appears to be prominent.[19]
    - Aspirin at 81 mg/d should be considered for the prevention of recurrent venous thrombosis but should be avoided in any patient with known pulmonary involvement, given the risk of hemoptysis.
- **Secondary vasculitides**
  - Both **RA and SLE** are associated with a secondary vasculitis thought to be immune complex mediated. Complications include **rheumatoid nodules in the lungs in RA, pulmonary hypertension, and alveolar hemorrhage in SLE**. While the mortality associated with alveolar hemorrhage in **SLE** is considerable, treatment with the combination of plasmapheresis, pulse-dose steroids, and CYC has demonstrated limited success. More recently, rituximab (RTX) has also been used for immunosuppression. Intrapulmonary recombinant factor VIIa and extracorporeal membrane oxygenation (ECMO) support have also been utilized to support patients through severe phases of illness.[20]
  - **Necrotizing sarcoid granulomatosis** is distinguished from sarcoidosis by its **extensive vasculitis and necrosis**, lack of extrapulmonary involvement, and radiographic findings of pulmonary masses, nodules, and pleural involvement (all less commonly seen in sarcoidosis). The vasculitis may be epithelioid granulomatous (with histiocytes and multinucleated giant cells reminiscent of GCA) or lymphocytic without granuloma formation. Necrotizing sarcoid granulomatosis often features a subacute clinical onset and may include nonspecific respiratory symptoms such as cough, dyspnea, or wheezing. While prognosis is good (with spontaneous resolution seen in some cases), further therapy can include oral corticosteroids (similar to chronic pulmonary sarcoidosis).[21]

Granulomatosis with Polyangiitis

GENERAL PRINCIPLES

- Granulomatosis with polyangitis (GPA) is a multisystem disease primarily involving small- and occasionally medium-sized blood vessels. While GPA was originally described as a variant of PAN, the findings of a **progressive granulomatous process that involved the upper and lower respiratory tract** led the German pathologist Frederick Wegener to believe that he had discovered a unique vasculitic syndrome. Concerns have been raised about Wegener's association with the Nazi regime and, in 2011, the ACR, the American Society of Nephrology, and the EULAR formally changed the name from Wegener's granulomatosis to GPA.[22]
- The Chapel Hill Consensus Conference defined GPA as **"granulomatous inflammation involving the respiratory tract, and necrotizing vasculitis affecting small- to medium-sized vessels."**[1]
- In terms of classification, GPA can be divided into limited and generalized disease.
  - **Limited** GPA is generally accepted to include cases **without kidney involvement** (generally, limited to the upper respiratory tract or the lungs) and reflects pathology mainly due to necrotizing granulomas and not active vasculitis.
  - **Generalized** GPA features pathology characterized by vasculitis and/or with any evidence of end-organ disease or impending organ failure.
- While GPA can occur at any age, ANCA-associated vasculitis typically affects middle-aged and older adults. GPA affects men and women equally but has a predilection for Caucasians.

DIAGNOSIS

Clinical Presentation

The **initial presentation** of GPA may be insidious, with generalized complaints such as malaise, fatigue, weight loss, hearing loss, and upper respiratory symptoms. Soon after, patients may develop symptoms that involve multiple organ systems. Limited GPA tends to feature constitutional symptoms (and may progress to generalized GPA if left untreated), while generalized GPA can involve end-organ disease.

- **Ear, nose, and throat involvement** is present in over 90% of cases of GPA, and may include chronic rhinitis and/or sinusitis, sinus pain, epistaxis, and nasal crusting. Destruction of the nasal cartilage can lead to nasal septal perforation or the saddle-nose deformity. Other manifestations include ulcerations of the oropharynx, gingival hyperplasia, and the rare **strawberry gingival hyperplasia** pathognomonic of GPA.[23]
- Patients can develop symptoms that can be confused with asthma from tracheobronchial ulcerations, intraluminal inflammatory pseudotumor, and bronchomalacia. Scarring from these lesions can lead to significant **airway obstruction**.
- The primary pulmonary manifestations of GPA include **necrotizing granulomas, cavitary lesions, and scattered nodules**. Capillaritis in the lung can lead

to diffuse alveolar hemorrhage (DAH) with an associated mortality of nearly 50%. This clinical presentation may be indistinguishable from Goodpasture syndrome or MPA.
- **Dermatologic** findings in GPA span papules, vesicles, palpable purpura, ulcers, or subcutaneous nodules. **Leukocytoclastic vasculitis** represents the most common manifestation, present in almost one-half of cases of GPA. Other skin lesions such as pyoderma gangrenosum and granulomatous skin lesions have been reported.
- **Nervous system** involvement is thought to be secondary to vasculitis of the vasa nervorum. Most commonly, patients may have **mononeuritis multiplex**, typically a sensorimotor polyneuropathy with asymmetric involvement (i.e., foot or wrist drop). Less commonly, patients may have cranial neuritis, cerebral vasculitis, or granulomatous infiltration.
- **Renal** involvement in GPA due to capillaritis leads to a **pauci-immune crescentic glomerulonephritis** and, if untreated, may lead to end-stage renal failure.

Diagnostic Criteria

- Although the **classic "Wegener triad"** includes necrotizing granulomatous inflammation of the respiratory tract, generalized necrotizing vasculitis of the small arteries and veins, and necrotizing glomerulonephritis, less than one-half of the originally described cases fulfilled these criteria.
- Updated 2022 ACR/EULAR classification criteria now use a scoring system.[24] It is important to remember that strict scoring systems are made for study enrollment purposes rather than for diagnosis and **additional clinical judgment** is required.
  - Clinical, laboratory, imaging, and biopsy criteria carry different number of points. **Criteria should be used in the setting of a small- or medium-vessel vasculitis.** A score of ≥**5 points** is needed for GPA classification.
  - **5 points**—positive test for **c-ANCA** or **anti-PR3** antibodies.
  - **3 points** each—nasal mucosal involvement, septal defect, or perforation.
  - **2 points** each—cartilaginous inflammation of ear, nose, larynx, or trachea; pulmonary nodules, masses, or cavities; extravascular granulomatous inflammation with giant cells on biopsy.
  - **1 point** each—hearing loss; sinusitis or mastoiditis on imaging; renal pauci-immune glomerulonephritis.
  - **−4 points**—Eosinophil count >1000.
  - **−1 point**—Positive p-ANCA or anti-MPO antibodies.
- Eosinophilia and p-ANCA/anti-MPO antibodies carry negative points on the scoring system above. However, they have been well described, even if less common, in the setting of GPA.

Diagnostic Testing

Laboratories

- Initial laboratory data may reveal a leukocytosis, anemia, and/or active urinary sediment with **dysmorphic RBC** and **RBC casts** in small-vessel vasculitis. Limited GPA often shows modest increases in inflammatory markers such as ESR and **CRP**, while generalized GPA can show marked elevations in ESR and CRP.
- **Cytoplasmic ANCA** (c-ANCA, or PR3-ANCA) is most commonly directed against serine proteinase 3, and c-ANCA positivity is prevalent in 70–95% of

generalized GPA and 40–50% of limited GPA (with a specificity as high as 80–100% in all GPA patients). However, serial measurements of c-ANCA have not been shown to reliably assess disease course or predict relapse.[25]
- **Perinuclear ANCA** (p-ANCA) positivity, while quite prevalent in MPA and to a lesser extent, EGPA, is only present in 0–10% of cases of GPA. A definitive positive ANCA test must possess **c-ANCA specificity to PR3** and **p-ANCA specificity to MPO by enzyme-linked immunosorbent assay (ELISA)**. The absence of this result renders this test negative.

Imaging
- **CXR** may reveal lung nodules with or without cavitation, and/or patchy or diffuse opacities. Less commonly, pleural effusions, hilar lymphadenopathy, or diffuse bilateral opacities may be seen.
- **High-resolution CT scanning** of the chest has increased the sensitivity for diagnosis of GPA. CT findings in GPA may include pulmonary nodules with or without cavitations, patchy or diffuse ground-glass (that could represent alveolar hemorrhage) or consolidative opacities, pulmonary microinfarctions, irregular and enlarged peripheral pulmonary arteries, or tracheal or bronchial stenosis.[26]

Diagnostic Procedures
- The histopathologic hallmarks of GPA include **vasculitis, necrosis, and granulomatous inflammation of small- and medium-sized vessels**. While the lung and upper respiratory tracts offer the highest sensitivity and specificity for biopsy sampling, the size of the biopsy specimen as well as any concurrent immunosuppressive therapy may affect the diagnostic value of the biopsy.
- Flexible **fiberoptic bronchoscopy** can aid diagnosis by providing direct visual inspection, obtaining a bronchoalveolar lavage (BAL), and tissue biopsies. Ulcerating tracheobronchitis and mucosal cobblestoning may be seen. Healing can lead to secondary scarring complicated by airway stenosis, obstruction, bronchomalacia, and postobstructive pneumonia. While only 20% of bronchoscopic biopsy samples may be diagnostic of GPA, bronchoscopic and BAL findings, in combination with the appropriate clinical presentation and laboratory data may provide sufficient diagnostic data. Surgical lung biopsy is seldom necessary.
- **Renal biopsy** can commonly provide a definitive answer when combined with the remainder of the clinical data. It typically reveals a focal segmental necrotizing glomerulonephritis that may be indistinguishable from that found in MPA, Goodpasture syndrome, or SLE. However, immunofluorescence microscopy can differentiate GPA and MPA (**pauci-immune crescentic glomerulonephritis**) from the linear fluorescence staining seen in Goodpasture syndrome and the granular pattern of immune deposits found in SLE.

TREATMENT
- The historic mortality associated with untreated GPA was nearly universal, with a mean survival of ~5 months. When steroids were introduced, survival extended by 8 months, however, overall prognosis was unchanged. Therefore, steroids alone are not adequate.

- Traditionally, therapy for GPA was managed according to disease distribution and activity (limited vs. generalized). Updated guidelines utilize **active severe GPA/MPA** (active and life or organ threatening) and **active nonsevere GPA** (active, not life or organ threatening).[27] Treatment can also be divided into **induction and maintenance therapy**.
  - For active severe GPA/MPA induction, pulse-dose methylprednisolone (1 g/d) for 3–5 days with a disease-modifying agent, followed by **high-dose steroids** (1 mg/kg/d).
  - Either **RTX** or **CYC** is recommended. Current guidelines conditionally recommend RTX over CYC as first line.[27]
  - Originally CYC was the only drug that showed improved survival (80%) and significant improvement (90%).[28] CYC IV or PO can be prescribed, with IV more commonly utilized due to decreased cumulative dose and similar outcomes.
  - The **RAVE** trial demonstrated that RTX was not inferior to CYC for induction.[29] While most studies used the weekly RTX dose of 375 mg/m^2 for 4 weeks every 6 months, two doses of 1 g 2 weeks apart are considered equivalent.
  - Once a therapeutic response is achieved, the prednisone may be tapered over 6 months and discontinued if remission persists. **Reduced dose steroid taper** used in the **PEXIVAS** trial is recommended as it offers similar therapeutic benefit and fewer infections.[30] A **remission rate of about 75–90%** can be achieved with this protocol, typically at 2–6 months.
  - If **no remission** is achieved or **relapse** with a severe flare occurs, switching to the other induction agent (RTX or CYC) is recommended.[27]
  - For **active nonsevere GPA,** which often overlaps with limited GPA, **methotrexate** with high-dose **steroids** is the regimen of choice with a favorable side-effect profile and limited toxicity.[27]
  - If **no remission** is achieved or **relapse** occurs, consider switching to a different remission induction agent combined with steroids (RTX, CYC, or AZA).[27]
  - **Plasma exchange (PLEX)** is no longer routinely recommended in AAV based on the **PEXIVAS** trial, where its use did not reduce the incidence of death or ESRD.[30] PLEX may still provide some benefit in patients with severe kidney injury (Cr > 4 or dialysis dependent) or DAH. However, there is no agreement among experts. PLEX should routinely be pursued if double-positive ANCA and anti-GBM are present. Clinical judgment and response to treatment should be used in decision making.
  - **Avacopan** is a novel C5a receptor inhibitor given after the induction treatment and being primarily studied to provide shorter and dose-reduced steroid regimens.[31]
  - **IVIG** can be utilized along with steroids in the setting of infections precluding the standard induction therapy as a temporizing agent, or in the setting of relapse.[32]
- **RTX** at standard or lower dosing 500 mg IV every 6 months is recommended as **maintenance** therapy in severe GPA/MPA regardless of the induction agent. It provided much lower relapse rate compared to AZA in the **MAINRITSAN** study, (5% vs. 29% at 28 months).[33]
- If RTX is not an option, **Azathioprine** can be used as a **second-line maintenance therapy**, as it demonstrated **similar relapse rate** compared to **CYC**.[34]

- Given that the combination of glucocorticoid and additional immunosuppressive therapy has been shown to increase the risk of *Pneumocystis jirovecii*, particularly in AAV, prophylaxis with **trimethoprim-sulfamethoxazole** is now standard. Age-appropriate vaccinations should also be administered.

Microscopic Polyangiitis

GENERAL PRINCIPLES

- MPA is a necrotizing vasculitis that primarily affects small blood vessels. GPA and MPA are virtually the same disease, except that MPA has **no granulomatous pathology**.
- The Chapel Hill Consensus Conference defined MPA as a "**necrotizing vasculitis with few or no immune deposits affecting small vessels**. Necrotizing arteritis of small- and medium-sized arteries may be present. Necrotizing glomerulonephritis is very common, and pulmonary capillaritis often occurs." Notably, granulomatous inflammation is not present in MPA.[1]
- Like GPA, MPA can present at nearly any age with a mean age of onset of 50 years. Men and women are probably affected equally, though studies have suggested a female predominance.

DIAGNOSIS

Clinical Presentation

- The clinical presentation of MPA can be similar to that described above for GPA. The exception is the ear, nose, and throat manifestations, which are seen almost exclusively in GPA.
- **Renal and pulmonary involvements** are the main clinical features of MPA. Pulmonary symptoms can range from mild hemoptysis with transient pulmonary infiltrates seen on CXR to massive hemoptysis with DAH.
- **Pulmonary–renal failure** may be the initial clinical presentation in fulminant MPA, and hemodynamic, respiratory, and/or renal replacement support may be needed.
- Other typical features of small-vessel vasculitis such as cutaneous, peripheral nerve, and gastrointestinal manifestations may also be present.

Diagnostic Criteria

- Updated 2022 ACR/EULAR classification criteria now use a scoring system.[35] It is important to remember that strict scoring systems are made for study enrollment purposes rather than for diagnosis, and **additional clinical judgment** is required.
    - Clinical, laboratory, imaging, and biopsy criteria carry different number of points. Criteria should be used **in the setting of a small- or medium-vessel vasculitis**. A score of **≥5 points** is needed for MPA classification.
    - **6 points**—Positive test for **p-ANCA** or **anti-MPO** antibodies.
    - **3 points** each—Interstitial lung disease on imaging; Pauci-immune glomerulonephritis on biopsy.

- ○ **−4 points**—Eosinophil count >1000.
- ○ **−3 points**—Nasal mucosal involvement or septal defect or perforation.
- ○ **−1 point**—Positive c-ANCA or anti-PR3 antibodies.

Diagnostic Testing

- The initial laboratory workup for MPA is similar to that for GPA. As noted above, while GPA is associated with c-ANCA positivity, MPA is associated with **p-ANCA** positivity, which is present in up to 80% of patients with MPA. The p-ANCA staining needs to be confirmed by ELISA for reactivity to **MPO**.
- Findings on chest imaging (both CXR and CT) are similar to that of GPA.
- Biopsy of affected areas demonstrates necrotizing vasculitis and the typical histology of MPA is **pulmonary capillaritis**. Renal biopsy usually reveals a necrotizing glomerulonephritis indistinguishable from that caused by GPA. However, a key distinction between GPA and MPA is the presence of granulomatous changes on biopsy in GPA.

TREATMENT

Treatment options and recommendations in MPA are the same as for the severe active disease listed under GPA treatment above. Please refer to that section.

Eosinophilic Granulomatosis with Polyangiitis

GENERAL PRINCIPLES

- **Eosinophilic granulomatosis with polyangiitis** (previously known as Churg–Strauss syndrome [CSS]), is a small- to medium-artery vasculitis characterized by **asthma, hypereosinophilia, and necrotizing vasculitis**.
- The Chapel Hill Consensus Conference defined EGPA as an **"eosinophil-rich and necrotizing granulomatous inflammation involving the respiratory tract and necrotizing vasculitis affecting small- to medium-sized vessels, and associated with asthma and blood eosinophilia."**[1]
- Like GPA and MPA, EGPA can present at any age and affects men and women equally.

DIAGNOSIS

Clinical Presentation

- The clinical course of EGPA classically includes **three phases**. While the phases do not have to proceed in order, the ACR has found them to be 95% sensitive and specific for EGPA when coupled with histopathologic evidence of vasculitis.[36,37]
  - ○ The **first, or prodromal, phase** consists of asthma and rhinosinusitis, and can last up to 20 years.
  - ○ The **second, or eosinophilic, phase** is characterized by peripheral and tissue eosinophilia.

- The **third, or vasculitic, phase** is marked by an extensive vasculitis that most commonly involves the **lungs**, but can also affect the dermatologic, nervous, cardiovascular, gastrointestinal, and renal organ systems.
- The hallmark pulmonary manifestation of EGPA is the **prodromal asthma** present in >95% of patients. **Allergic rhinitis, sinusitis, and nasal polyps** are also common. As patients may have been treated with steroids for asthma-type symptoms, the diagnosis of EGPA can be delayed.
- Extrapulmonary manifestations of EGPA
  - **Mononeuritis multiplex,** which affects up to three-quarters of patients, represents the most common extrapulmonary finding.
  - **Dermatologic** findings are also quite common (found in up to two-thirds of patients with EGPA) and may include purpura, livedo reticularis, and subcutaneous nodules.
  - **Cardiovascular** involvement accounts for a significant fraction of the morbidity and mortality of EGPA, and findings may include ECG abnormalities, heart failure, eosinophilic myocarditis, coronary vasculitis, or pericardial effusions.
  - **Renal** involvement, present in one-quarter of EGPA patients and seen far less commonly than in GPA or MPA, typically manifests as a focal segmental necrotizing glomerulonephritis but does not usually result in fulminant renal failure.
  - Eosinophilic or vasculitic involvement of the **gastrointestinal tract** can result in abdominal pain, and other gastrointestinal findings can include pancreatitis, gastrointestinal perforation, or hemorrhage.

Diagnostic Criteria

Updated 2022 ACR/EULAR classification criteria now use a scoring system.[38] It is important to remember that strict scoring systems are made for study enrollment purposes rather than for diagnosis, and **additional clinical judgment** is required.

- Clinical, laboratory, imaging, and biopsy criteria carry different number of points. Criteria should be used **in the setting of a small- or medium-vessel vasculitis**. A score of ≥**6 points** is needed for EGPA classification.
- **5 points**—Eosinophil count >1000
- **3 points** each—Obstructive airway disease; nasal polyps
- **2 points** each—Extravascular eosinophilic predominant inflammation on biopsy
- **1 point** each—Mononeuritis multiplex
- **−3 points**—Positive c-ANCA or anti-PR3 antibodies
- **−1 point**—Hematuria

Differential Diagnosis

In the absence of proven vasculitis, the prodromal phase may be confused with typical asthma, and the eosinophilic phase may be confused with eosinophilic pneumonia, Löffler syndrome, or eosinophilic gastroenteritis.

Diagnostic Testing

Laboratories
- **Peripheral eosinophilia** is characteristic of EGPA and may be present in any phase of the illness.
- ESR and CRP may be elevated in EGPA, especially during active vasculitis.

- Other nonspecific laboratory abnormalities may include a normocytic anemia, leukocytosis, elevated IgE, and a positive but low-titer rheumatoid factor.
- p-ANCA and anti-MPO antibodies may be positive in approximately one-half of patients. **ANCA positivity** is more frequent in the presence of glomerulonephritis, purpura, and peripheral neuropathy. **ANCA-negative** patients more frequently have cardiac and GI involvement.[39]

Imaging
- CXR findings are variable and nonspecific but can include **transient and patchy pulmonary infiltrates**, peripheral parenchymal infiltrates, pulmonary nodules (with cavitation far less frequent than in GPA), or pleural effusions.
- High-resolution CT scanning may reveal bilateral scattered ground-glass opacities and/or bronchial wall thickening, bronchial dilation, pulmonary nodules, and pleural effusions.
- Cardiac MRI may have utility in assessing myocardial involvement in EGPA patients.

Diagnostic Procedures
- **BAL** is often performed and can show a **high percentage of eosinophils** in the setting of active pneumonitis.
- **Tissue biopsy** is helpful in establishing the diagnosis of EGPA and should be performed prior to initiating potentially toxic therapy. As transbronchial lung biopsy is often nondiagnostic, surgical lung biopsy may be required. The typical lung biopsy in EGPA reveals **bronchitis, eosinophilic infiltration, extravascular granulomas, and/or necrotizing vasculitis**.
- Biopsy can be performed on skin, peripheral nerves, lacrimal glands, or kidneys, depending on organ involvement. It classically shows necrotizing, eosinophilic, and/or granulomatous vasculitis and may aid in diagnosis.

TREATMENT

- Treatment options are made based on the severity of the disease and the **five-factor score (FFS)**.
- The FFS assigns one point to each of the five factors and includes **cardiac** involvement, **gastrointestinal** disease, **renal insufficiency** (serum creatinine ≥1.58 mg/dL), **proteinuria ≥1** g/d, and **central nervous system** involvement. The FFS, while designed for prognosis, can be used to guide initial management in EGPA.[40]
- EGPA with a FFS of 0 and nonorgan or life-threatening disease, can be considered a**ctive nonsevere disease**. If FFS is 1 or greater, it is considered **active severe disease**.
- The cornerstone of therapy for EGPA is **glucocorticoids**. Before the use of steroids, patients with EGPA faced a mortality rate of 50% within 3 months of diagnosis.
- In **active nonsevere** disease (FFS of 0) the current recommendation is to treat with high-dose **steroids** and (anti-IL5 agent) **mepolizumab**.[27] If mepolizumab is not available or tolerated, steroids can be combined with methotrexate, AZA, mycophenolate, or RTX.
- In **active nonsevere** disease, if **remission** is achieved, steroids with mepolizumab can be used.

- If no remission is achieved or relapse occurs, consider switching to steroids with a different disease-modifying drug.
- In **active severe** disease (FFS of ≥1) pulse-dose steroids (methylprednisolone 1 g/d × 3–5 days) should be given, followed by high-dose oral steroids and **CYC** or **RTX**. There is a greater historical experience with CYC in this setting, especially in ANCA-negative patients and patients with cardiac, neurologic, and gastrointestinal manifestations.[27]
- In **active severe** disease, if remission is achieved, steroids with RTX, mepolizumab, or other disease-modifying drugs above can be used.
- If **no remission** is achieved or **relapse** with a severe flare occurs, switching to a different induction agent (RTX or CYC) is recommended.[27]
- **Azathioprine and methotrexate** have been used for remission maintenance, but concurrent steroid treatment may be required.[27]
- PLEX and IVIG have been trialed though limited data are available. Their use should be based on clinical judgment. Please see discussion under GPA treatment above.
- At 80–90%, the remission rate for EGPA is comparable to GPA and MPA. However, the relapse rate is somewhat lower, and 5-year survival slightly higher.

REFERENCES

1. Jennette JC, Falk RJ, Bacon PA, et al. 2012 revised International Chapel Hill Consensus Conference Nomenclature of Vasculitides. *Arthritis Rheum.* 2013;65:1–11.
2. Watts RA, Hatemia G, Burns JC, Mohammad AJ. Global epidemiology of vasculitis. *Nat Rev Rheumatol.* 2022;18:22–34.
3. Schwarz MI, Brown KK. Small vessel vasculitis of the lung. *Thorax.* 2000;55:502–510.
4. Ponte C, Grayson PC, Robson JC, et al; DCVAS Study Group. 2022 American College of Rheumatology/EULAR classification criteria for giant cell arteritis. *Ann Rheum Dis.* 2022;81:1647–1653.
5. Hunder GG, Bloch DA, Michel BA, et al. The American College of Rheumatology 1990 criteria for the classification of giant cell arteritis. *Arthritis Rheum.* 1990;33(8):1122–1128.
6. Blockmans D, de Ceunink L, Vanderschueren S, Knockaert D, Mortelmans L, Bobbaers H. Repetitive 18F-fluorodeoxyglucose positron emission tomography in giant cell arteritis: a prospective study of 35 patients. *Arthritis Rheum.* 2006;55:131–137.
7. Maz M, Chung SA, Abril A, et al. 2021 American College of Rheumatology/Vasculitis foundation guideline for the management of giant cell arteritis and Takayasu arteritis. *Arthritis Rheum.* 2021;73:1349–1365.
8. Stone JH, Tuckwell K, Dimonaco S, et al. Trial of tocilizumab in giant-cell arteritis. *N Engl J Med.* 2017;377:317–328.
9. Unizony S, Matza MA, Jarvie A, O'Dea D, Fernandes AD, Stone JH. Treatment for giant cell arteritis with 8 weeks of prednisone in combination with tocilizumab: a single-arm, open-label, proof of concept study. *Lancet Rheumatol.* 2023;5:e736–e742.
10. Grayson PC, Ponte C, Suppiah R, et al; CVAS Study Group. 2022 American College of Rheumatology/EULAR classification criteria for Takayasu arteritis. *Ann Rheum Dis.* 2022;81:1654–1660.
11. Naniwa T, Maeda T, Shimuzu S, Ito R. Hepatitis B virus-related polyarteritis nodosa presenting with multiple lung nodules and cavitary lesions. *Chest.* 2010;138:195–197.
12. Kosmider O, Posseme C, Temple M, et al. VEXAS syndrome is characterized by inflammasome activation and monocyte dysregulation. *Nat Comm.* 2024;15:910.
13. Lee PY, Davidson BA, Abraham RS, et al; DADA2 Foundation. Evaluation and management of deficiency of adenosine deaminase 2: an international consensus statement. *JAMA Netw Open.* 2023;6:e2315894.

14. Singh S, Gupta A, Jindal AK, et al. Pulmonary presentation of Kawasaki disease—A diagnostic challenge. *Periatr Pulmonol.* 2018;53(1):103–107.
15. La Torre F, Taddio A, Conti C, Cattalini M. Multi inflammatory syndrome in children (MIS-C) in 2023. Is it time to forget about it? *Children (Basel).* 2023;10:980.
16. International Study Group for Behçet's Disease. Criteria for diagnosis of Behçet's disease. *Lancet.* 1990;335:1078–1080.
17. International Team for the Revision of the International Criteria for Behçet's Disease (ITR-ICBD). The International Criteria for Behçet's Disease (ICBD): a collaborative study of 27 countries on the sensitivity and specificity of the new criteria. *J Eur Acad Dematol Venereol.* 2014;28:338–347.
18. Ceylan N, Bayraktaroglu S, Erturk SM, Savas R, Alper H. Pulmonary and vascular manifestations of Behcet disease: imaging findings. *Am J Roentgenol.* 2010;194:W158–164.
19. Yazici Y, Hatemi G, Bodaghi B, et al. Behcet syndrome. *Nat Rev Dis Primers.* 2021;7:67.
20. Al-Adhoubi NK, Bystrom J. Sustemic lupus erythematosus and diffuse alveolar hemorrhage, etiology and novel treatment strategies. *Lupus.* 2020;29(4):355–363.
21. Rosen Y. Four decades of necrotizing sarcoid granulomatosis: what do we know now? *Arch Pathol Lab Med.* 2015;139:252–262.
22. Falk RJ, Gross WL, Guillevin L, et al. Granulomatosis with polyangiitis (Wegener's): an alternative name for Wegener's granulomatosis. *Ann Rheum Dis.* 2011;70:704.
23. Knight JM, Hayduk MJ, Summerlin DJ, Mirowski GW. "Strawberry" gingival hyperplasia: a pathognomonic mucocutaneous finding in Wegener granulomatosis. *Arch Dermatol.* 2000;136:171–173.
24. Robson JC, Grayson PC, Ponte C, et al. 2022 American College of Rheumatology/European Alliance of Associations for Rheumatology classification criteria for granulomatosis with polyangiitis. *Ann Rheum Dis.* 2022;81:315–320.
25. Finkielman JD, Merkel PA, Schroeder D, et al; WGET Research Group. Antiproteinase 3 antineutrophil cytoplasmic antibodies and disease activity in Wegener granulomatosis. *Ann Intern Med.* 2007;147:611–619.
26. Ananthakrishnan L, Sharma N, Kanne JP. Wegener's granulomatosis in the chest: high-resolution CT findings. *Am J Roentgenol.* 2009;192(3):676–682.
27. Chung AS, Langford CA, Maz M, et al. 2021 American College of Rheumatology/Vasculitis Foundation Guideline for the management of antineutrophil cytoplasmic antibody–associated vasculitis. *Arthritis Care Res (Hoboken).* 2021;73:1088–1105.
28. Hoffman GS, Kerr GS, Leavitt RY, et al. Wegener granulomatosis: an analysis of 158 patients. *Ann Int Med.* 1992;116:488–498.
29. Stone JH, Merkel PA, Spiera R, et al; RAVE-ITN Research Group. Rituximab versus cyclophosphamide for ANCA-associated vasculitis. *N Engl J Med.* 2010;363:221–232.
30. Walsh M, Merkel PA, Peh C-A, et al; PEXIVAS Investigators. Plasma exchange and glucocorticoids in severe ANCA associated vasculitis. *N Engl J Med.* 2020;382:622–631.
31. Jayne DR, Merkel PA, Schall TJ, Bekker P; ADVOCATE Study Group. Avacopan for the treatment of ANCA associated vasculitis. *N Engl J Med.* 2021;384:599–609.
32. Benavides-Villanueva F, Loricera J, Calvo Rio V, Corrales-Selaya C, Castañeda S, Blanco R. Intravenous immunoglobulin therapy in antineutrophil cytoplasmic antibody-associated vasculitis. *Eur J Intern Med.* 2023;117:78–84.
33. Guillevin L, Pagnoux C, Karras A, et al; French Vasculitis Study Group. Rituximab versus azathioprine for maintenance in ANCA-associated vasculitis. *N Engl J Med.* 2014;371:1771–1780.
34. De Groot K, Rasmussen N, Bacon PA, et al. Randomized trial of cyclophosphamide versus methotrexate for induction of remission in early systemic antineutrophil cytoplasmic antibody-associated vasculitis. *Arthritis Rheum.* 2005;52:2461–2469.
35. Suppiah R, Robson JC, Grayson PC, et al. 2022 American College of Rheumatology/European Alliance of Associations for rheumatology classification criteria for microscopic polyangiitis. *Arthritis Rheumatol.* 2022;74:400–406.

36. Masi AT, Hunder GG, Lie JT, et al. The American College of Rheumatology 1990 criteria for the classification of Churg–Strauss syndrome (allergic granulomatosis and angiitis). *Arthritis Rheum.* 1990;33:1094–1100.
37. Baldini C, Talarico R, Della Rossa A, Bombardieri S. Clinical manifestations and treatment of Churg–Strauss syndrome. *Rheum Dis Clin North Am.* 2010;36:527–543.
38. Grayson PC, Ponte C, Suppiah R, et al; DCVAS Study Group. 2022 American College of Rheumatology/European Alliance of Associations for rheumatology classification criteria for eosinophilic granulomatosis with polyangiitis. *Ann Rheum Dis.* 2022;81:309–314.
39. Emmi G, Bettiol A, Gelain E, et al. Evidence based guideline for the diagnosis and management of eosinophilic granulomatosis with polyangiitis. *Nat Rev Rheumatol.* 2023;19:378–393.
40. Guillevin L, Lhote F, Gayraud M, et al. Prognostic factors in polyarteritis nodosa and Churg–Strauss syndrome. A Prospective study in 342 patients. *Medicine (Baltimore).* 1996;75:17–28.

Pulmonary Embolism and Deep Venous Thrombosis

Elissa Arnold, Sahil Sanghani, and Maanasi Samant

GENERAL PRINCIPLES

- Acute pulmonary embolism (PE) is a commonly diagnosed condition with a morbidity and mortality rate that varies by age, clinical presentation, and the presence of comorbid disease.[1]
- Despite advances in diagnosis and management, PE remains an underdiagnosed condition.
- Untreated PE has a high mortality rate. In some cases, PE can be safely treated at home, while in others, immediate admission to an intensive care unit may be required to prevent death.
- Accurate risk stratification remains a critical component of the initial evaluation of the patient with acute PE.
- Effective, evidence-based approaches exist for the evaluation of patients with suspected PE and the treatment of those diagnosed with PE.

Definition
- Thromboses or blood clots can occur in veins, arteries, or chambers of the heart.
- PE is an embolized thrombus in the pulmonary arterial system.
- Venous thromboembolism (VTE) refers to the presence of deep vein thrombosis (DVT) or PE.

Epidemiology
- The overall annual incidence of PE has been reported to be about 39–115 cases per 100,000.[2] VTE incidence increases sharply after 50 years of age.
- There are differences in mortality between Black and White patients that are thought to be related to social determinants of health and factors external to the hospitalization for PE.[3-5]
- The introduction of contrast-enhanced multidetector helical chest CT scan (PE protocol CT) was associated with a doubling of the incidence of PE.[6,7]
- Autopsy studies suggest that many PEs remain undiagnosed.[8]

Etiology
- The majority of PEs originate from DVTs in the proximal lower extremity, including the iliac, femoral, and popliteal veins.
- DVTs that occur in upper extremities, often secondary to an indwelling catheter, may also cause PE.
- Calf vein DVTs rarely embolize to the lungs, but they can extend proximally after which their risk of embolization increases.
- Only about one-half to three-quarters of the patients diagnosed with PE will have DVT found on venous compression ultrasound of the lower extremities.[9]

TABLE 20-1 RISK FACTORS FOR PULMONARY EMBOLISM

Acquired—Modifiable	Acquired—Nonmodifiable	Inherited
Infection	Malignancy	Facor V Leiden
Hip or knee replacement	Autoimmune disease	Prothrombin gene G20210A
Major trauma	Inflammatory bowel disease	Protein C deficiency
DIC	Heart failure	Protein S deficiency
HIT	Prior VTE	Antithrombin deficiency
Central venous lines	Hospital admission within 90 days	Dysfibrinogenemia
	Spinal cord injury	Hyperhomocysteinemia

DIC, disseminated intravascular coagulation; HIT, heparin-induced thrombocytopenia; VTE, venous thromboembolism.

Risk Factors
- There are extensive predisposing factors for VTE. A method of classifying VTE risk factors uses the categories of inherited, acquired, and idiopathic (Table 20-1).
- Spontaneous (idiopathic) thrombosis, despite the absence of an inherited thrombophilia and detectable autoantibodies, predisposes patients to future thromboses.
- It is not recommended to routinely screen all patients with VTE for inherited thrombophilias, especially in the acute setting, but it may be considered in those presenting with VTE at a young age or without any clear risk factors.

Pathophysiology
- PE can drastically alter oxygenation and gas exchange as well as circulation.
- Vascular obstruction may lead to increased pulmonary vascular resistance (PVR), which if severe enough can lead to acute failure of the right ventricle (RV) and shock. This increase in PVR occurs from direct, physical obstruction, hypoxic vasoconstriction, and PE-related release of vasoconstrictors and inflammatory mediators. Ultimately, RV dilation, hypokinesis, and interventricular septal deviation can lead to impaired left ventricular (LV) filling and reduced cardiac output (CO), resulting in hypotension and shock. This is frequently referred to as the "RV death spiral."
- Pulmonary arterial obstruction may produce hypoxemia via impaired alveolar gas exchange and increased lung dead space ventilation.

DIAGNOSIS
Clinical Presentation
- PE may cause shortness of breath, chest pain (pleuritic), syncope, hypoxemia, hemoptysis, pleural rub, new right-sided heart failure, and tachycardia, but these signs and symptoms are neither sensitive nor specific and vary greatly between patients.

TABLE 20-2 MODIFIED WELLS CRITERIA FOR PULMONARY EMBOLISM

Criterion	Point Value
Symptoms of DVT (leg edema, tenderness)	3.0
Other diagnoses less likely than PE	3.0
Heart rate >100	1.5
Immobilization or surgery within the past 4 weeks	1.5
Prior history of DVT or PE	1.5
Hemoptysis	1.0
Malignancy	1.0

Score	Rate (95% CI)
≤4, PE unlikely	2.3–9.4%
>4, PE likely	27.6–51.6%

DVT, deep venous thrombosis; PE, pulmonary embolism; CI, confidence interval.

With permission from Wells PS, Anderson DR, Rodger, et al. Derivation of a simple clinical model to categorize patient's probability of pulmonary embolism: increasing the models utility with the SimpliRED D-dimer. *Thromb Haemost.* 2000;83:416–420.

- DVT may cause extremity pain and swelling but can also be asymptomatic.
- There are numerous validated tools that combine symptoms, clinical signs, and risk factors to assess pretest probability of PE. One of the most widely utilized for patients presenting through the emergency department is the Wells criteria (Table 20-2).[10]
- Clinical suspicion of DVT or PE should lead to objective testing.
- Vital signs are the most important physical examination findings in PE. Patients with PE often have tachycardia or tachypnea, but they can also present with hypotension and cardiac arrest.
- Other physical examination findings are nonspecific, including rales, prominent S2 and P2 on cardiac auscultation, and elevated jugular venous pressure.

Differential Diagnosis
- Clinicians may underdiagnose PE because it mimics many other diseases.
- The differential is broad and includes pneumonia, acute coronary syndrome, pleuritis, pericarditis, and congestive heart failure.
- In a hypotensive patient, the differential broadens to include sepsis, hypovolemia, cardiac tamponade, and acute myocardial infarction.

Diagnostic Testing
- Pretest probability plays a key role in the workup of patients with suspected PE.
- The incorporation of pretest probability, using scores such as Wells score or Geneva score, with diagnostic tests improves the accuracy of diagnosis.[10–13]
- A proposed diagnostic algorithm for suspected acute PE is presented in Figure 20-1.[2]

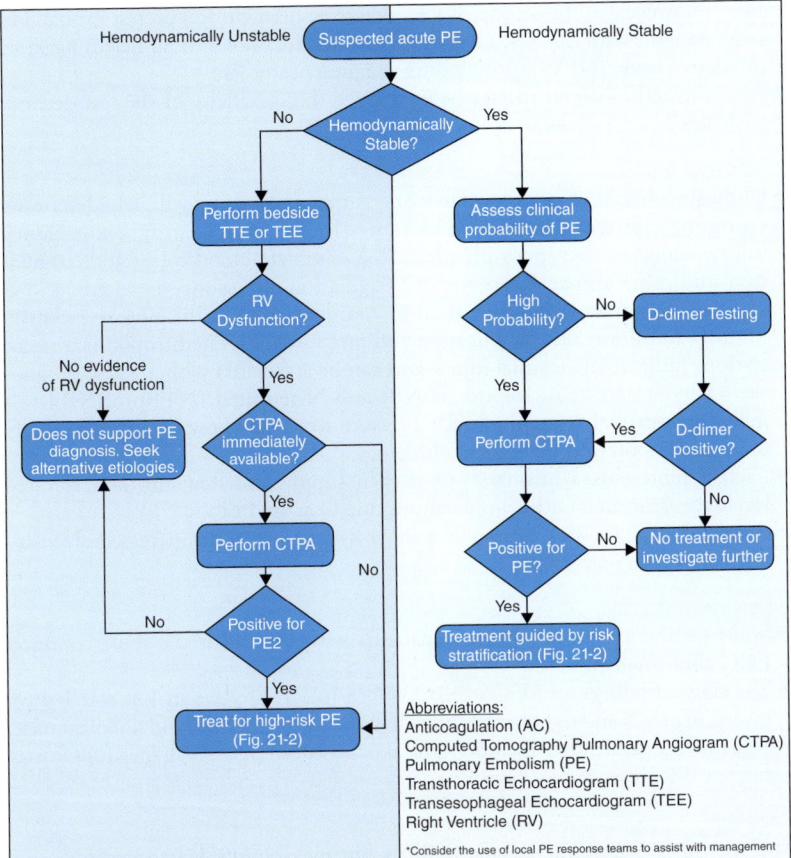

Figure 20-1 Diagnostic evaluation for suspected acute pulmonary embolism (PE). (Adapted from Konstantinides SV, Meyer G, Becattini C, et al. 2019 ESC Guidelines for the diagnosis and management of acute pulmonary embolism developed in collaboration with the European Respiratory Society [ERS]: the Task Force for the diagnosis and management of acute pulmonary embolism of the European Society of Cardiology [ESC]. *Eur Respir J.* 2019;54[3]:1901647.)

D-dimer

- D-dimer and cross-linked fibrin degradation products may increase during PE, but they are nonspecific and have a low positive predictive value (PPV).
- D-dimer should be used after pretest probability has been considered. A negative D-dimer in combination with low pretest probability can exclude almost all

PEs[14]; however, in the setting of a moderate to high clinical pretest probability (e.g., patients with cancer), a negative D-dimer does not have sufficient negative predictive value (NPV) for excluding the presence of PE.
- Age-adjusted D-dimer should be used since the specificity of the test declines with age.[15]

Laboratory Testing
- Clinicians should obtain basic lab work. A metabolic panel will help determine creatinine clearance for anticoagulation selection and identify acute kidney injury, which predicts poor prognosis.[16] A complete blood count and coagulation studies are also necessary for anticoagulation initiation.
- Cardiac biomarkers should be used in conjunction with imaging and clinical findings to inform risk stratification and prognosis. Elevated troponin concentrations indicate myocardial injury and can be associated with a worse prognosis.[17] B-type natriuretic peptide (BNP) and N-terminal (NT)-proBNP levels reflect myocardial stretch and RV pressure overload. Low levels may signify lower likelihood of poor clinical outcomes.[18]
- Lactate represents a mismatch of oxygen supply and demand, and elevated levels are associated with complications due to acute PE.
- Arterial blood gas may or may not show hypoxemia or an increased alveolar–arterial oxygen gradient.

Electrocardiography
- Sinus tachycardia occurs in most patients with PE and is the most common ECG abnormality.
- The classic findings on ECG of S1Q3T3 (S in V1, Q wave in V3, and T-wave inversion in V3) and right bundle branch block are uncommon and not diagnostic.
- Signs of RV strain that include right axis deviation and RV hypertrophy may suggest the presence of a large PE.

Imaging
- CXR usually shows no specific findings but may rapidly help assess for other diagnoses. Classic findings such as Westermark Sign and Hampton Hump rarely occur.
- The most common and important diagnostic modalities for assessing patients with suspected PE include CT and ventilation/perfusion scintigraphy (V/Q scan).
- **Contrast-enhanced CT scan (PE protocol CT),** also known as CT pulmonary angiogram (CTPA) is the gold standard test for evaluating patients for PE, and it may assist with the detection of alternative or concomitant diagnoses.[19]
  - The sensitivity of CT for VTE improves by combining the CTPA results with objective grading of clinical suspicion.
  - The accuracy of CT for diagnosis of PE decreases with poorer scan quality and for smaller and more peripheral clots.
  - CT may also demonstrate evidence of RV dysfunction, including RV enlargement as measured by RV/LV ratio (>0.9) and RV end-diastolic diameter. This has been shown to be a predictor of mortality (all-cause and PE-related) regardless of hemodynamic stability.[20]

- Contraindications to CT include contrast allergy, severe renal dysfunction, or inability to safely travel to the scanner. However, if pretest probability is high enough, CTPA should not be withheld for acute kidney injury, as the benefits of diagnostic and therapeutic information obtained via CTPA generally outweigh the risk of worsening renal function.
- Patients with a contraindication to CT or inadequate CT results should undergo other testing.
- A **ventilation/perfusion or V/Q scan** is useful for diagnosis in conjunction with pretest probability and can sometimes be used in patients with contraindications or indeterminate readings from a PE protocol CT.[21]
  - V/Q scanning remains most useful in a patient with a normal CXR, because nondiagnostic V/Q scans commonly occur in the setting of an abnormal CXR.
  - V/Q scans may be classified as normal, nondiagnostic (i.e., very low probability, low probability, intermediate probability), or high probability for PE.
  - Use of clinical suspicion improves the accuracy of V/Q scanning. A normal or low probability V/Q scan in the setting of a low clinical suspicion adequately rules out PE. A high probability V/Q scan in the setting of a high clinical suspicion adequately confirms PE and no further testing is warranted.
  - In the setting of an indeterminate result, further testing should be done.
- Advantages of CT scan over V/Q scan include more diagnostic results (positive or negative), an assessment of clot burden and chronicity, assessment of RV dysfunction, fewer indeterminate or inadequate studies, and the detection of alternative or concomitant diagnoses, such as dissecting aortic aneurysm, pneumonia, and malignancy.
- **Venous compression ultrasonography** (CUS) is an easily accessible diagnostic modality that can act as a surrogate test for PE if it detects lower extremity proximal DVT and the clinical scenario is highly suggestive of PE.
  - Lower extremity venous CUS is not a first-line modality unless the above testing is not available or indeterminate.
  - If CUS does not detect DVT and clinical suspicion for PE is high, further diagnostic testing should be performed.
- **Transthoracic echocardiography (TTE)** may assess cardiopulmonary reserve and evidence of end-organ damage (RV dysfunction) in patients with PE and has a role in decision making regarding the use of thrombolytic or advanced therapies.
  - Echocardiography may directly visualize a right heart thrombus, an embolism in transit, or a patent foramen ovale with right-to-left shunt.
  - It is also important in evaluating RV function. Echocardiographic findings of RV dysfunction or overload include RV dilation and hypokinesis; increase in RV diameter/LV diameter ratio (>1.0); decreased tricuspid annular plane excursion (TAPSE), pulmonary artery dilation; tricuspid regurgitation; paradoxical septal motion; flattened interventricular septum or shift toward the LV; and McConnell sign, defined by hypokinesis of the free wall of the RV with normal motion of the apex.
  - RV dysfunction has, in prior meta-analysis, been associated with a higher risk of short-term mortality, even in hemodynamically stable patients.[22]

TABLE 20-3 DEFINITIONS OF RISK LEVELS IN ACUTE PULMONARY EMBOLISM (PE)

PE Risk Stratification	Defining Criteria
High risk	Need one of the following: 1. Need for CPR 2. Obstructive shock 3. Persistent hypotension (SBP <90 mm Hg or SBP drop of >40 mm Hg for longer than 15 min, not caused by other etiologies)
Intermediate–high risk	Need all of the following: A. PESI Class III–V or sPESI ≥1 B. RV dysfunction on TTE or CTPA C. Elevated cardiac troponin or BNP levels
Intermediate–low risk	Need one to two of the following: A. PESI Class III–V or sPESI ≥1 B. RV dysfunction on TTE or CTPA C. Elevated cardiac troponin or BNP levels
Low risk	None of the above

CPR, cardiopulmonary resuscitation; SBP, systolic blood pressure; DBP, diastolic blood pressure; PESI, PE severity index; sPESI, simplified PE severity index; TTE, transthoracic echocardiogram; CTPA, computed tomography pulmonary angiogram.

Adapted from Konstantinides SV, Meyer G, Becattini C, et al. 2019 ESC Guidelines for the diagnosis and management of acute pulmonary embolism developed in collaboration with the European Respiratory Society (ERS): the Task Force for the diagnosis and management of acute pulmonary embolism of the European Society of Cardiology (ESC). *Eur Respir J.* 2019;54(3):1901647.

RISK STRATIFICATION

- Classification of acute PE is not based on degree of clot burden alone. Rather, clinicians should perform risk stratification of each patient based on hemodynamics, presence or absence of RV dysfunction and cardiac biomarkers, and underlying comorbidities. This risk stratification predicts risk of early death, either in hospital or 30 days, and is required to determine the appropriate management plan.
- There are multiple risk stratification tools available. One of the most commonly used is from the 2019 European Society of Cardiology (ESC) guidelines on management of PE1. Categories include: high risk, intermediate–high risk, intermediate–low risk, and low risk, with criteria for each category outlined in Table 20-3.[2]

TREATMENT

General Principles

- Clinicians should make their treatment decisions for PE based on confidence in the diagnosis of PE, hemodynamic status, degree of RV dysfunction/injury,

bleeding risk, prognosis, patient preferences, and patient-specific factors that could affect anticoagulant pharmacodynamics and pharmacokinetics.
- The above-defined risk categories provide a framework for management decisions. A proposed management algorithm for confirmed acute PE is presented in Figure 20-2.[2,23]
- If there is high clinical suspicion for PE and diagnostic testing cannot be urgently performed, prompt initiation of empiric anticoagulation should be

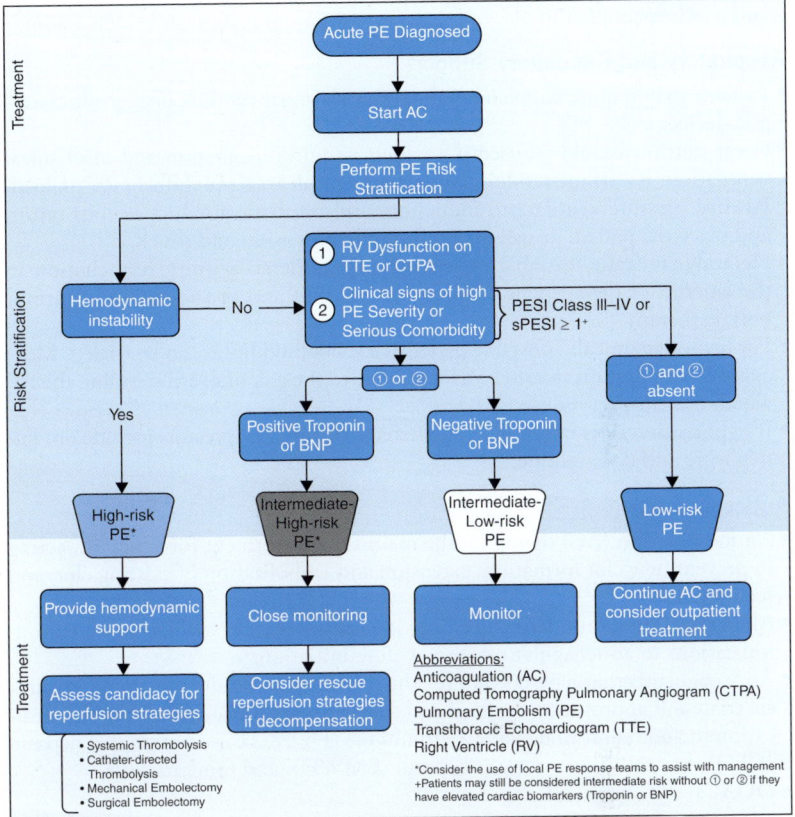

Figure 20-2 Treatment of confirmed acute pulmonary embolism (PE). (Adapted from Konstantinides SV, Meyer G, Becattini C, et al. 2019 ESC Guidelines for the diagnosis and management of acute pulmonary embolism developed in collaboration with the European Respiratory Society [ERS]: the Task Force for the diagnosis and management of acute pulmonary embolism of the European Society of Cardiology [ESC]. *Eur Respir J.* 2019;54[3]:1901647.)

considered if there are no contraindications. If diagnostic testing adequately rules out PE, then anticoagulation therapy should be discontinued and prophylaxis for VTE should be initiated.
- Patients should achieve therapeutic anticoagulant levels soon after PE is diagnosed.
- Consider calculating the PE severity index (PESI) score to determine if a patient is appropriate for outpatient management. Patients who are to be managed outpatient should have low bleeding risk, definite access to their oral anticoagulant, and a follow-up plan in place.

Respiratory and Circulatory Support

- Patients may require supplemental oxygen via nasal cannula or high-flow oxygen devices.
- Great caution should be used if a patient requires intubation and mechanical ventilation. RV failure renders patients susceptible to acute shifts in RV preload. Positive pressure ventilation, induction, and intubation reduce venous return and place the patient at risk for profound hypotension and shock.
- Hemodynamically unstable patients should undergo prompt resuscitation in the emergency department or intensive care unit and consideration of thrombolytic therapy.[24,25]
- For hemodynamically unstable patients, a small fluid bolus can be trialed. More aggressive hydration should be avoided due to the risk of overdistending the RV which may further reduce CO.
- If hypotension does not resolve, suggested first-line vasopressors include norepinephrine and dobutamine.

Anticoagulation

- Anticoagulation (AC) therapy is the mainstay of treatment for acute PE, acting to prevent new clot formation, extension and embolization of existing clot, and recurrence.
- All patients should undergo bleeding risk assessment and evaluation for contraindications to anticoagulant therapy before initiation.
- Anticoagulants that have efficacy for the treatment of PE demonstrated in clinical trials and approval by the food and drug administration (FDA) for this indication include some oral factor Xa inhibitors (DOACs), unfractionated heparin (UFH), low–molecular-weight heparin (LMWH), and fondaparinux.
- **DOACs**
  - Benefits of the use of this class of medications include ease of use and lack of required monitoring.
  - It is appropriate to begin treatment with the DOACs apixaban or rivaroxaban as the sole initial anticoagulant (monotherapy) in patients with low-risk PE without contraindications to DOACs.
  - Bridging parenteral anticoagulation and hospitalization is not always necessary for initiation of DOACs. If there is a delay in obtaining these medications, parenteral therapy should be administered.
- **UFH and LMWH**
  - IV UFH remains the mainstay of anticoagulation for unstable patients, those with high bleeding risk, and those with severe renal failure.

- Use of LMWH or fondaparinux as an initial anticoagulation strategy is recommended for most patients requiring hospitalization.[25,26] Subcutaneous injection is dosed once or twice daily based on body weight. Caution should be used in patients with renal disease because, unlike UFH, LMWH has significant renal clearance. When ready to transition the patient to oral therapy, clinicians should generally select apixaban or rivaroxaban given their ease of use and lack of need for bridging.
- **Warfarin**
  - Warfarin inhibits vitamin K–dependent clotting factors and should be started after initiation of heparin/LMWH/fondaparinux. International normalized ratio (INR) levels should be followed closely in patients on warfarin for PE with a target INR of 2.5 (goal range of 2.0–3.0).
  - Treatment of PE with warfarin requires overlap therapy with a parenteral anticoagulant (UFH, LMWH, or pentasaccharide) for at least 4–5 days and until the INR reaches at least 2.
  - It is important to counsel patients on maintaining stable diets while on warfarin and to be cautious of drug–drug interactions that may lead to rapid INR changes.
- **Duration**
  - Anticoagulation is recommended for 3–6 months for a first-time VTE event.
  - Longer-term anticoagulation is recommended in patients with a second event, a nonmodifiable risk factor, a hypercoagulable state, or malignancy. Longer-term anticoagulation can also be considered in patients with high-risk PE.

PE Response Teams

- Management decisions in acute PE, including the use of thrombolytics, advanced surgical and catheter-directed therapies, and extracorporeal membrane oxygenation (ECMO) are nuanced and influenced greatly by patient factors.
- In recent years, many institutions have developed multidisciplinary PE response teams (PERT), often involving pulmonologists, cardiologists, interventional radiologists, vascular and cardiothoracic surgeons, and hematologists.[2]
- The structure and utilization of these teams are widely variable between institutions. Intermediate and/or high-risk PE should prompt a PERT consult if available.

Thrombolysis

- Systemic thrombolytic therapy should be given in patients with hemodynamic instability due to PE (high-risk PE) if there are no contraindications. The only FDA-approved thrombolytic agent is alteplase, a recombinant tissue-type plasminogen activator (tPA). Other agents used across the world for this include streptokinase, urokinase, reteplase, tenecteplase, and desmoteplase.[24,25]
- The use of thrombolytic agents can lead to more rapid improvement in parameters associated with hemodynamic instability such as PVR and pulmonary arterial pressure.
- Patients with high-risk PE treated with thrombolytics have, on recent meta-analyses, been shown to have reduced mortality.[27]
- Systemic thrombolytic therapy may also be used in patients with PE who develop hemodynamic deterioration, even if they are already on anticoagulation.

- The role of thrombolytic agents in hemodynamically stable patients continues to be investigated.
- The risks of thrombolytic therapy, including major bleeding events and intracranial bleeding, should be weighed carefully, and the patient thoroughly assessed for contraindications.
- Patients who fail to improve with systemic thrombolysis may still be candidates for procedural therapies (described below).

Inferior vena cava (IVC) Filters

IVC filters are net devices placed into the IVC in patients who cannot tolerate anticoagulation in order to help prevent embolism of pelvic or lower extremity DVT.[28–30]

Advanced Therapies

- Catheter-based and surgical management options are determined in consultation with the PERT team (if available), vascular surgery, cardiothoracic surgery, and/or interventional radiology.
- Catheter-directed therapies are sometimes utilized for high-risk and intermediate high-risk PE. Catheter-based lysis involves administration of lower-dose tPA directly into the pulmonary arteries. Patients have faster improvement in RV/LV ratio using this technique but no change in clinical outcomes when compared to patients treated with anticoagulation alone.[31]
- Catheter-based embolectomy involves mechanical breakdown (by a variety of methods) and removal of the clot by fragmentation or thrombus aspiration. Often, a pharmacomechanical approach is used, whereby mechanical techniques are combined with tPA.
- Surgical embolectomy may be an option for patients with high-risk PE in whom thrombolytics are contraindicated or have failed to improve hemodynamics, and those with a visualized clot in transit. This requires an experienced surgeon and often cardiopulmonary bypass.
- Data regarding outcomes following catheter-based therapies and surgical embolectomy is limited and research is still ongoing.
- Mechanical circulatory support via venoarterial (VA) ECMO may be used in patients with hemodynamic collapse or cardiac arrest; it can be used alone or as a bridge to definitive treatment (catheter based or surgical).

Complications of Therapy

- Bleeding is the primary risk of anticoagulation therapy.
    - The use of antiplatelet agents increases the risk of bleeding.
    - If significant bleeding occurs while on anticoagulation therapy, the anticoagulant agent should be stopped immediately, and IVC filter placement should be considered.
- Patients treated with UFH or LMWH are at risk for heparin-induced thrombocytopenia (HIT).
    - HIT leads to increased risk of thrombosis.
    - Clinicians should consider the possibility that HIT has occurred in patients who develop VTE in the setting of absolute or relative thrombocytopenia.
    - Patients receiving UFH or LMWH should undergo monitoring for HIT. Patients with PE and suspected or confirmed HIT should not receive UFH,

LMWH, or warfarin until the HIT has resolved. Such patients should undergo treatment with a parenteral direct thrombin inhibitor such as argatroban or lepirudin.

PROGNOSIS

- The short-term mortality rate for untreated PE may be as high as 5–30%,[5,32,33] and increases with hemodynamic instability.
- The highest risk for death is in the first several hours for those with hemodynamic collapse, but this risk remains elevated for the first several days to week. This timeframe also represents a clinically important one in hemodynamically stable patients with evidence of RV dysfunction (intermediate–high risk), so close observation is suggested.
- Indicators of poor prognosis include hemodynamic instability, signs of RV failure, elevated troponin/BNP, coexisting DVT, RV thrombus, lactic acidosis, and hyponatremia. Hemodynamic stability is the most important factor in prognosis.
- Risk of recurrence in a patient with a clear, transient risk factor is 2.5% per year. This risk increases to about 4.5% per year in patients with no identifiable or nonmalignant persistent risk factors.[34] In patients with malignancy or 2+ recurrent VTE episodes, this risk is even higher.
- Persistent dyspnea and reduced exercise tolerance are frequently present for months to years following PE.

MONITORING AND FOLLOW-UP

- All patients who are diagnosed with acute PE should have close follow-up by a physician, especially regarding anticoagulation management.
- Patients on warfarin for chronic anticoagulation should have close monitoring of INRs.
- Patients should be screened for post–PE-related complications such as post-PE syndrome (persistent symptoms after at least 3–6 months of AC), chronic thromboembolic pulmonary disease, and chronic thromboembolic pulmonary hypertension.[35]

REFERENCES

1. Aujesky D, Obrosky DS, Stone RA, et al. Derivation and validation of a prognostic model for pulmonary embolism. *Am J Respir Crit Care Med.* 2005;172:1041–1046.
2. Konstantinides SV, Meyer G, Becattini C, et al; The Task Force for the diagnosis and management of acute pulmonary embolism of the European Society of Cardiology (ESC). 2019 ESC Guidelines for the diagnosis and management of acute pulmonary embolism developed in collaboration with the European Respiratory Society (ERS): the Task Force for the diagnosis and management of acute pulmonary embolism of the European Society of Cardiology (ESC). *Eur Respir J.* 2019;54:1901647.
3. Schneider D, Lilienfeld DE, Im W. The epidemiology of pulmonary embolism: racial contrasts in incidence and in-hospital case fatality. *J Natl Med Assoc.* 2006;98:1967–1972.
4. Phillips AR, Reitz KM, Myers S, et al. Association between black race, clinical severity, and management of acute pulmonary embolism: a retrospective cohort study. *J Am Heart Assoc.* 2021;10:e021818.

5. Martin KA, Molsberry R, Cuttica MJ, Desai KR, Schimmel DR, Khan SS. Time trends in pulmonary embolism mortality rates in the United States, 1999 to 2018. *J Am Heart Assoc.* 2020;9(17):e016784.
6. Wiener RS, Schwartz LM, Woloshin S. Time trends in pulmonary embolism in the United States: evidence of overdiagnosis. *Arch Intern Med.* 2011;171:831–837.
7. Huang W, Goldberg RJ, Anderson FA, Kiefe CI, Spencer FA. Secular trends in occurrence of acute venous thromboembolism: the Worcester VTE study (1985-2009). *Am J Med.* 2014;127:829–839.e5.
8. Silverstein MD, Heit JA, Mohr DN, Petterson TM, O'Fallon WM, Melton LJ III. Trends in the incidence of deep vein thrombosis and pulmonary embolism: a 25-year population-based study. *Arch Intern Med.* 1998;158:585–593.
9. Kearon C, Ginsberg JS, Hirsh J. The role of venous ultrasonography in the diagnosis of suspected deep venous thrombosis and pulmonary embolism. *Ann Intern Med.* 1998;129:1044–1049.
10. Wells PS, Anderson DR, Rodger M, et al. Derivation of a simple clinical model to categorize patients probability of pulmonary embolism: increasing the models utility with the SimpliRED D-dimer. *Thromb Haemost.* 2000;83:416–420.
11. van Belle A, Büller HR, Huisman MV, et al; Christopher Study Investigators. Effectiveness of managing suspected pulmonary embolism using an algorithm combining clinical probability, D-dimer testing, and computed tomography. *JAMA.* 2006;295:172–179.
12. Le Gal G, Righini M, Roy PM, et al. Prediction of pulmonary embolism in the emergency department: the revised Geneva score. *Ann Intern Med.* 2006;144:165–171.
13. Hendriksen JMT, Geersing GJ, Lucassen WAM, et al. Diagnostic prediction models for suspected pulmonary embolism: systematic review and independent external validation in primary care. *BMJ.* 2015;351:h4438.
14. Kearon C, Ginsberg JS, Douketis J, et al; Canadian Pulmonary Embolism Diagnosis Study (CANPEDS) Group. An evaluation of D-dimer in the diagnosis of pulmonary embolism: a randomized trial. *Ann Intern Med.* 2006;144:812–821.
15. Righini M, Goehring C, Bounameaux H, Perrier A. Effects of age on the performance of common diagnostic tests for pulmonary embolism. *Am J Med.* 2000;109:357–361.
16. Kostrubiec M, Pływaczewska M, Jiménez D, et al. The prognostic value of renal function in acute pulmonary embolism—a multi-centre cohort study. *Thromb Haemost.* 2019;119:140–148.
17. Becattini C, Vedovati MC, Agnelli G. Prognostic value of troponins in acute pulmonary embolism: a meta-analysis. *Circulation.* 2007;116:427–433.
18. Coutance G, Cauderlier E, Ehtisham J, Hamon M, Hamon M. The prognostic value of markers of right ventricular dysfunction in pulmonary embolism: a meta-analysis. *Crit Care.* 2011;15:R103.
19. Stein PD, Hull RD. Multidetector computed tomography for the diagnosis of acute pulmonary embolism. *Curr Opin Pulm Med.* 2007;13:384–388.
20. Meinel FG, Nance JW Jr, Schoepf UJ, et al. Predictive value of computed tomography in acute pulmonary embolism: systematic review and meta-analysis. *Am J Med.* 2015;128:747–759.
21. PIOPED Investigators. Value of the ventilation/perfusion scan in acute pulmonary embolism. Results of the prospective investigation of pulmonary embolism diagnosis (PIOPED). *JAMA.* 1990;263:2753–2759.
22. Sanchez O, Trinquart L, Colombet I, et al. Prognostic value of right ventricular dysfunction in patients with haemodynamically stable pulmonary embolism: a systematic review. *Eur Heart J.* 2008;29:1569–1577.
23. Otepka HC, Yusen RD. Pulmonary embolism. In: Kollef M, Isakow W, eds. *The Washington Manual of Critical Care.* 2nd ed. Lippincott Williams & Wilkins; 2012.
24. Todd JL, Tapson VF. Thrombolytic therapy for acute pulmonary embolism: a critical appraisal. *Chest.* 2009;135:1321–1329.

25. Kearon C, Akl EA, Comerota AJ, et al. Antithrombotic therapy for VTE disease: Antithrombotic Therapy and Prevention of Thrombosis, 9th ed: American College of Chest Physicians evidence-based clinical practice guidelines. *Chest.* 2012;141:e419S–e496S.
26. Garcia DA, Baglin TP, Weitz JI, Samama MM. Parenteral anticoagulants: antithrombotic therapy and prevention of thrombosis, 9th ed: American College of Chest Physicians evidence-based clinical practice guidelines. *Chest.* 2012;141:e24S–e43S.
27. Marti C, John G, Konstantinides S, et al. Systemic thrombolytic therapy for acute pulmonary embolism: a systematic review and meta-analysis. *Eur Heart J.* 2015;36:605–614.
28. PREPIC Study Group. Eight-year follow-up of patients with permanent vena cava filters in the prevention of pulmonary embolism: the PREPIC (Prevention du Risque d'Embolie Pulmonaire par Interruption Cave) randomized study. *Circulation.* 2005;112:416–422.
29. Muriel A, Jiménez D, Aujesky D, et al; RIETE Investigators. Survival effects of inferior vena cava filter in patients with acute symptomatic venous thromboembolism and a significant bleeding risk. *J Am Coll Cardiol.* 2014;63:1675–1683.
30. Mismetti P, Laporte S, Pellerin O, et al. Effect of a retrievable inferior vena cava filter plus anticoagulation vs anticoagulation alone on risk of recurrent pulmonary embolism: a randomized clinical trial. *JAMA.* 2015;313:1627–1635.
31. Kucher N, Boekstegers P, Müller OJ, et al. Randomized, controlled trial of ultrasound-assisted catheter-directed thrombolysis for acute intermediate-risk pulmonary embolism. *Circulation.* 2014;129:479–486.
32. American Lung Association. Learn about pulmonary embolism. Accessed December 30, 2023. https://www.lung.org/lung-health-diseases/lung-disease-lookup/pulmonary-embolism/learn-about-pulmonary-embolism
33. Nijkeuter M, Söhne M, Tick LW, et al; Christopher Study Investigators. The natural course of hemodynamically stable pulmonary embolism: clinical outcome and risk factors in a large prospective cohort study. *Chest.* 2007;131:517–523.
34. Agnelli G, Prandoni P, Becattini C, et al; Warfarin Optimal Duration Italian Trial Investigators. Extended oral anticoagulant therapy after a first episode of pulmonary embolism. *Ann Intern Med.* 2003;139(1):19–25.
35. Klok FA, Ageno W, Ay C, et al. Optimal follow-up after acute pulmonary embolism: a position paper of the European Society of Cardiology Working Group on Pulmonary Circulation and Right Ventricular Function, in collaboration with the European Society of Cardiology Working Group on Atherosclerosis and Vascular Biology, endorsed by the European Respiratory Society. *Eur Heart J.* 2022;43(3):183–189.

Pulmonary Hypertension

21

Matthew Abbott and Murali M. Chakinala

GENERAL PRINCIPLES

Definition
- Pulmonary hypertension (PH) is defined by a **mean pulmonary artery pressure (PAP) >20 mm Hg** at rest.[1,2]
- Discrimination of the type of PH (i.e., precapillary vs. postcapillary vs. combined pre- and postcapillary [CpcPH]) requires additional information about the left heart's filling pressures and the pulmonary vascular resistance (PVR) (Table 21-1).[1]
- Exercise PH is defined by an mPAP/CO slope >3 mm Hg/L/min between rest and exercise.[1]

Classification
- PH is clinically classified into five groups (Table 21-2).[1,2]
- Individuals can have more than one underlying condition leading to a mixed form of PH.
- Pulmonary arterial hypertension (PAH, group 1) patients are risk stratified by assessment of multiple factors, including symptom burden, World Health Organization (WHO) functional class, 6-minute walk distance (6MWD), biomarkers such as B-type natriuretic peptide (BNP or NT-proBNP), echocardiography and hemodynamic parameters that guide therapies and provide a tool to monitor clinical response.[1]

TABLE 21-1 HEMODYNAMIC DEFINITIONS OF PULMONARY HYPERTENSION

Definition	Hemodynamic Profile
Pulmonary hypertension (PH)	mPAP >20 mm Hg
Precapillary PH	mPAP >20 mm Hg, PAWP ≤15 mm Hg, PVR ≥2 WU
Isolated postcapillary PH (IpcPH)	mPAP >20 mm Hg, PAWP >15 mm Hg, PVR ≤2 WU
Combined post- and precapillary PH (CpcPH)	mPAP >20 mm Hg, PAWP >15 mm Hg, PVR ≥2 WU

Reproduced with permission of the © European Society of Cardiology & European Respiratory Society 2025. Humbert M, Kovacs G, Hoeper MM, et al. 2022 ESC/ERS Guidelines for the diagnosis and treatment of pulmonary hypertension. *Eur Respir J.* 2023;61:2200879.

Epidemiology
- The most common type of PH in the developed world is group 2, followed by group 3.
- Group 3 PH tends to correlate with degree of severity of underlying lung disease and/or hypoxemia but exceptions include concomitant conditions having

TABLE 21-2 2022 ESC/ERS CLINICAL CLASSIFICATION OF PULMONARY HYPERTENSION (PH)

Group 1: Pulmonary Arterial Hypertension (PAH)
Idiopathic (IPAH)
  Nonresponders at vasoreactivity testing
  Acute responders at vasoreactivity testing
Heritable
  BMPR2
  ALK-1, endoglin (with or without hereditary hemorrhagic telangiectasia)
  Unknown
Associated with drugs and toxins
Associated with (APAH)
  Connective tissue diseases
  HIV infection
  Portal hypertension
  Congenital heart disease
  Schistosomiasis
PAH with features of venous/capillary involvement (PVOD/PCH)
Persistent pulmonary hypertension of the newborn

Group 2: Pulmonary Hypertension due to Left Heart Disease
Heart failure
  Systolic dysfunction
  Diastolic dysfunction
Valvular disease
Congenital or acquired conditions leading to postcapillary PH

Group 3: Pulmonary Hypertension due to Lung Disease and/or Hypoxia
Chronic obstructive lung disease
Restrictive lung disease
Other pulmonary diseases with mixed restrictive and obstructive pattern
Alveolar hypoventilation disorders
Chronic exposure to high altitude
Developmental abnormalities

Group 4: Pulmonary Hypertension with Pulmonary Artery Obstructions
Chronic thromboembolic pulmonary hypertension (CTEPH)
Other pulmonary artery obstructions (sarcomas, malignant and nonmalignant tumors, arteritis, congenital pulmonary artery stenoses, and hydatidosis)

(continued)

TABLE 21-2	2022 ESC/ERS CLINICAL CLASSIFICATION OF PULMONARY HYPERTENSION (PH) (*Continued*)

Group 5: PH with Unclear and/or Multifactorial Mechanisms
Hematologic disorders: chronic hemolytic anemia, myeloproliferative disorders, splenectomy
Systemic disorders: sarcoidosis, PLCH, LAM, neurofibromatosis, vasculitis
Metabolic disorders: glycogen storage disease, Gaucher disease, thyroid disorders
Chronic renal failure with or without hemodialysis
Pulmonary tumor thrombotic microangiopathy
Fibrosing mediastinitis

BMPR2, bone morphogenic protein receptor, type 2; ALK-1, activin receptor-like kinase 1 gene; PVOD, pulmonary veno-occlusive disease; PCH, pulmonary capillary hemangiomatosis; PLCH, pulmonary Langerhans cell histiocytosis; LAM, lymphangioleiomyomatosis.

Reproduced with permission of the © European Society of Cardiology & European Respiratory Society 2025. Humbert M, Kovacs G, Hoeper MM, et al. 2022 ESC/ERS Guidelines for the diagnosis and treatment of pulmonary hypertension. *Eur Respir J.* 2023;61:2200879.

---

an additive effect, and a discordant degree of PH with the underlying lung disease as measured by spirometry (e.g., chronic obstructive pulmonary disease [COPD] and obstructive sleep apnea [OSA]).
- Prevalence of PAH is estimated to be **48–55 cases per million** with female/male ratio between 2:1 and 3:1. 50–60% of PAH are idiopathic.[1]
- 1-, 2-, and 3-year mortality for PAH is 8%, 16%, and 21%, respectively. Mortality rates differ between PAH subgroups and when stratified by risk assessment.[3]
- Estimated cumulative incidence of chronic PH after acute pulmonary embolism (PE) is 1.0% at 6 months, 3.1% at 1 year, and 3.8% at 2 years with cumulative burden of emboli being a risk factor.[4]

Pathophysiology
- The common finding in all forms of PH is **elevated pressures within pulmonary vessels** as blood flows across the pulmonary circuit.
- **Group 1 PH** (PAH) involves complex mechanisms that progressively narrow and stiffen the pulmonary arterioles.
  - Pathogenesis in PAH may vary with the different etiologies but converges upon **endothelial and smooth muscle cell proliferation and dysfunction** that result in the complex interplay of the following factors:
    - **Vasoconstriction** is caused by overproduction of compounds such as endothelin and insufficient production of prostacyclin and nitric oxide.
    - **Endothelial and smooth muscle proliferation** due to mitogenic properties of endothelin and thromboxane A2 in the setting of low levels of inhibitory molecules, such as prostacyclin and nitric oxide.

- **In situ thrombosis** of small- and medium-sized pulmonary arteries resulting from platelet activation and aggregation.
  - The physiologic consequences of this proliferative vasculopathy are **increased PVR and right ventricle** (RV) **afterload**.
  - Complex origins of PAH include infectious/environmental insults in the setting of predisposing comorbidities and/or underlying genetic predisposition, for example, pathogenic genetic variants of bone morphogenetic protein receptor II (BMPR II), activin receptorlike kinase 1 (ALK1), caveolin-1, among many others.[1,5,6]
  - *BMPR2* gene mutations are found in 75% of familial PAH and 25% of idiopathic pulmonary arterial hypertension (IPAH), while *ALK1* gene mutations, causative of hereditary hemorrhagic telangiectasia (HHT), rarely present with PAH.[1,7]
- Elevated pressures in **groups 2–5** result from several other mechanisms:
  - Elevated downstream pressures on the left side of the heart and pulmonary venous remodeling (group 2).
  - Hypoxemic vasoconstriction, vascular remodeling, and/or parenchymal destruction (group 3).
  - Occlusion of the vasculature by material foreign to the lung (group 4).
  - High flow that exceeds capacitance of the pulmonary circuit, thrombotic occlusion, and/or vasculopathy (group 5).

DIAGNOSIS

Clinical Presentation

An algorithm for evaluating PH is outlined in Figure 21-1.

History

- **Dyspnea with exertion** is the most often reported symptom for patients with PH. Orthopnea and paroxysmal nocturnal dyspnea are important clues of left heart disease and group 2 PH. Symptoms that reflect more advanced disease and secondary RV dysfunction include **fatigue, syncope, peripheral edema, and angina**.
- Hoarseness can develop because of left recurrent laryngeal nerve compression by an enlarging pulmonary artery (i.e., Ortner syndrome).
- **Past medical history** relevant to several organ systems, including the respiratory, cardiovascular, hepatic, rheumatologic, and hematologic systems must be explored.
- Particular emphasis should be placed on prior **cardiac conditions,** including myocardial infarction, heart failure (HF), arrhythmias, rheumatic heart disease, other valvular heart disease, and congenital heart disease.
- **Social history** should focus on prior or current tobacco and alcohol use, as well as illicit or recreational drug use, particularly methamphetamines or cocaine.
- **Family history** should also be explored to exclude a genetic predisposition.
- Risk factors for exposure to **HIV** may disclose an unexpected etiology for PH.
- Careful **medication history** to document use of current or past drugs linked to development of PH is also necessary. This includes anorexigens (e.g., fenfluramine, dexfenfluramine, diethylpropion) and chemotherapeutic agents (e.g., mitomycin, dasatinib).[1]

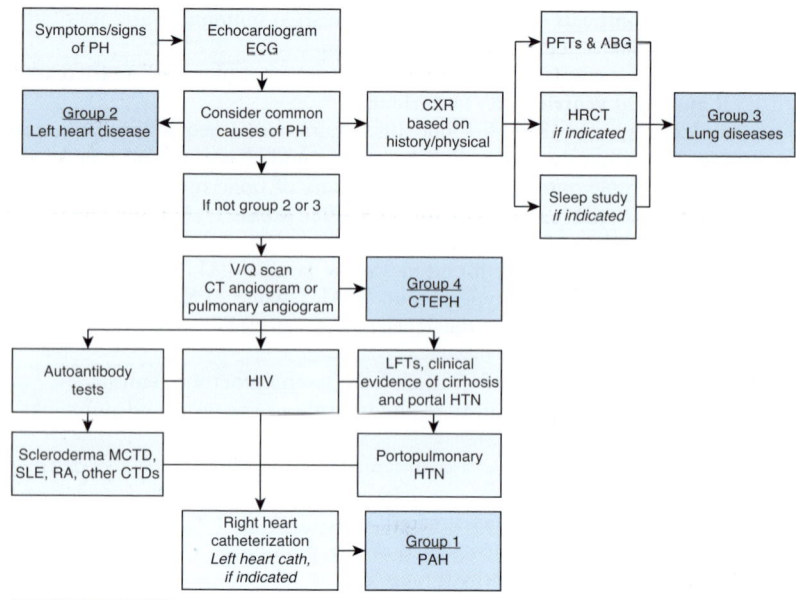

Figure 21-1 Diagnostic approach to pulmonary arterial hypertension. PH, pulmonary hypertension; ECG, electrocardiogram; PFT, pulmonary function tests; ABG, arterial blood gases; HRCT, high-resolution CT; CTEPH, chronic thromboembolic pulmonary hypertension; HTN, hypertension; CTD, connective tissue disease; PAH, pulmonary arterial hypertension.

Physical Examination
- A thorough physical examination to corroborate or refute suspicions of underlying medical problems should be performed; attention should be directed toward the cardiopulmonary examination.
- Auscultatory examination of the heart may reveal an accentuated S2 sound with a **prominent P2** component, systolic ejection murmur at left lower sternal border due to **tricuspid regurgitation,** and diastolic decrescendo murmur (Graham Steell murmur) along the left sternal border due to pulmonary insufficiency. Additional cardiac finding, including continuous murmurs or rumbles and fixed-split S2, may suggest an underlying **congenital cardiac defect**.
- As PH worsens and right HF ensues, resting tachycardia, S3 gallop, elevated jugular venous pulsation of the neck, hepatomegaly, ascites, peripheral edema, diminished peripheral pulses, and cyanosis occur. Presence of these findings, in the absence of clues of left heart disease, should raise suspicion for right HF due to PH.
- **Digital clubbing** indicates underlying conditions such as interstitial lung disease (ILD), bronchiectasis, or congenital heart disease.
- **Telangiectasias** and other skin manifestations (e.g., sclerodactyly, Raynaud phenomenon) may suggest underlying systemic sclerosis (SSc) or HHT.

Diagnostic Criteria
- PH is defined as **mean PAP >20 mm Hg** as determined via **right heart catheterization (RHC)**.[1] PAH requires **normal left ventricular** (LV) **filling pressures** (i.e., pulmonary artery wedge pressure (PAWP) or left ventricular end-diastolic pressure (LVEDP) ≤15 mm Hg) and an **elevated PVR** (≥2 Wood units).
- Pulmonary artery systolic pressure (PASP) can be estimated noninvasively by transthoracic echocardiography (TTE), whereby a **PASP >35 mm Hg (or tricuspid regurgitation jet velocity >2.8 m/s) is considered abnormal and suggestive of PH but is not diagnostic.**[1]

Diagnostic Testing

Laboratories
- Essential laboratory studies to evaluate unexplained PH mirror the studies of a general medical evaluation: **complete blood count** (CBC), **comprehensive metabolic panel** (CMP), **and coagulation studies** may offer diagnostic clues and direct further exploration. A prerenal pattern of blood urea nitrogen (BUN) and creatinine elevations in conjunction with passive congestion of the liver is a sign of advanced right HF and low cardiac output.
- Screening for **collagen vascular disease** with antinuclear antibody (ANA), anticentromere antibody, rheumatoid factor (RF), anti-scl-70 antibody, and antiribonucleoprotein antibody should be completed, as the associated underlying conditions are linked to PAH.
- Thyroid studies, hemoglobin electrophoresis for sickle cell disease, HIV serology, hepatitis serologies, antiphospholipid antibody, or anticardiolipin antibody should also be performed if clinical suspicions exist.
- **Arterial blood gas** can provide invaluable information. Significant resting hypoxemia should raise suspicion for right-to-left shunt, severely reduced cardiac output, or underlying pulmonary disease. **Significant hypercarbia supports a group 3 diagnosis.**

Electrocardiography
- **RV enlargement** is suspected by the presence of an R wave in V1 or an S wave in lead V6 while **RV strain** appears as a triad of S wave in lead I, Q wave in lead III, and inverted T wave in lead III. Other potential findings in cases of PH include right atrial enlargement, right axis deviation, and right bundle branch block.
- LV hypertrophy, left atrial enlargement, left axis deviation, atrial fibrillation, or evidence of prior myocardial infarction provide clues of significant left heart disease that could lead to group 2 PH.

Imaging
- **Transthoracic echocardiography**
  - TTE with Doppler and agitated saline injection serves as an initial test to identify PH.
  - If tricuspid regurgitation is present, Doppler allows for estimation of **PASP**.
  - In combination with PASP, markers of right heart size and function allow for noninvasive assessment of the likelihood of PH. Further, right heart function is an important component of PH risk assessment.

- TTE also identifies potential left-sided cardiac causes of PH and provides estimate of LV systolic and diastolic function.
- The agitated saline (bubble study) may uncover an intracardiac shunt; patent foramen ovale is common in PH and could explain exertional hypoxemia in PH patients, but is not considered causative of PH.
- Presence of a pericardial effusion is a predictor of mortality in PAH.[1]
- **Chest radiograph (CXR)**
  - Features indicative of PH are **enlarged central pulmonary arteries** on frontal views and **RV enlargement** on lateral examination. When PAPs reach systemic levels, pulmonary artery calcifications can be seen.
  - Obliteration of the distal pulmonary arteries leads to tapering of vessels in the peripheral third of the lung parenchyma, referred to as **pruning,** which is classically seen in IPAH.
  - In contrast, prominent pulmonary arteries extending to the periphery of the lung suggest systemic-to-pulmonary shunts and a hypercirculatory state (e.g., atrial or ventricular septal defects).
  - CXR should also be reviewed for **underlying cardiopulmonary diseases,** including ILD, emphysema, or HF.
- **Ventilation/perfusion scan**
  - Provides a sensitive screen for **chronic thromboembolic** disease.
  - While PH due to nonembolic processes, such as IPAH, can display a heterogeneous or mottled perfusion pattern, anatomic perfusion defects of the segmental or lobar level are concerning for thromboembolic disease.
  - Differential diagnosis for an abnormal perfusion scan also includes pulmonary veno-occlusive disease (widespread obstruction of the pulmonary veins due to fibrous tissue), mediastinal fibrosis, or pulmonary vasculitis.
  - Extrapulmonary deposition of perfusion tracer can be seen in right-to-left shunts, including pulmonary arteriovenous malformations (AVMs), hepatopulmonary syndrome, and congenital heart defects.
- **Chest CT**
  - Chest CT can suggest findings of PH, including an enlarged PA diameter (>3 cm) and an enlarged right atrium and RV.
  - Features of chronic thromboembolic disease include eccentric thrombi, intravascular webs, abrupt cut-offs, luminal irregularities leading to atretic vessels and parenchymal "mosaicism." Nevertheless, **VQ scanning remains the preferred screening test.**
  - Chest CT can also identify mediastinal disease leading to PH, (e.g., mediastinal fibrosis or compressive lymphadenopathy).
  - High-resolution chest CT (HRCT) can exclude ILD, if suspicion exists.
- **Cardiac MRI** is useful for evaluating the atrial and ventricular size, morphology, and function. Additionally, flow through the PA and aorta allows for assessment of stroke volume and the ratio between pulmonary and systemic circulations in the presence of anatomic shunts.

Diagnostic Procedures

- **Pulmonary function testing (PFT)**
  - PFT should be inspected for obstructive lung disease while measurement of lung volumes may provide a clue for ILD.

- Diffusing capacity for carbon monoxide (DLCO) is mildly reduced in PH; more severe reductions is a clue for concomitant parenchymal lung disease or PAH with venous/capillary involvement.
- **RHC**[1]
  - **RHC is the gold standard for diagnosing PAH.**
  - Pressure measurements include PA pressures, RV end-diastolic pressure, right atrial pressure (RAP), and PAWP; in particular, the RAP is an important predictor of survival.
  - Cardiac output is determined by either the thermodilution or Fick method. Either can be used but both have drawbacks. Thermodilution is affected by significant tricuspid regurgitation. Fick measurements are often only "assumed" as direct oxygen consumption (VO_2) is infrequently performed in catheterization labs.
  - PVR can be calculated as ([mean PAP – PAWP]/cardiac output), and represents the ratio of pressure decline across the pulmonary circuit to the blood flow through the circuit.
  - An **acute vasodilator challenge** can also be performed to guide the choice of therapeutic agent in group 1 (PAH) patients. A short-acting vasodilator such as **inhaled nitric oxide,** inhaled iloprost, or IV epoprostenol is administered. A **10 mm Hg drop in the mean PAP and a concluding mean PAP <40 mm Hg without systemic hypotension or a decrease in cardiac output** signifies a significant acute hemodynamic response. Exercise RHC may be utilized to evaluate otherwise unexplained dyspnea on exertion in order to diagnose **exercise PH**. An **mPAP/CO slope >3 mm Hg/L/min** is diagnostic for exercise PH but does not discriminate the etiology. PAWP/CO slope >2 mm Hg/L/min is suggestive of underlying cardiac limitation as the cause.
- **Left heart catheterization** (LHC) should be performed to rule out coronary artery disease and/or directly measure the LVEDP when left heart disease is strongly suspected or the PAWP is felt to be unreliable.
- **Polysomnography** should be obtained if there is a concern for OSA or obesity hypoventilation syndrome as a contributing component to PH.
- **Cardiopulmonary exercise testing (CPET)** can show a pattern consistent with PH in the evaluation of exercise intolerance. Such patients typically display a low end-tidal carbon dioxide tension ($P_{ET}CO_2$) and high ventilatory equivalent for carbon dioxide (VE/VCO_2).

TREATMENT

- Management of PH depends on the specific category determined after a comprehensive evaluation.
- A treatment algorithm for PAH (i.e., group 1) is presented in Figure 21-2.[1]

Treatment of Groups 2–4
- **Group 2**
  - PH owing to left heart disease (group 2) should receive **appropriate therapy for underlying causative left heart conditions** with a hemodynamic goal of lowering the PAWP (and LVEDP) as much as possible. Patients with HF with

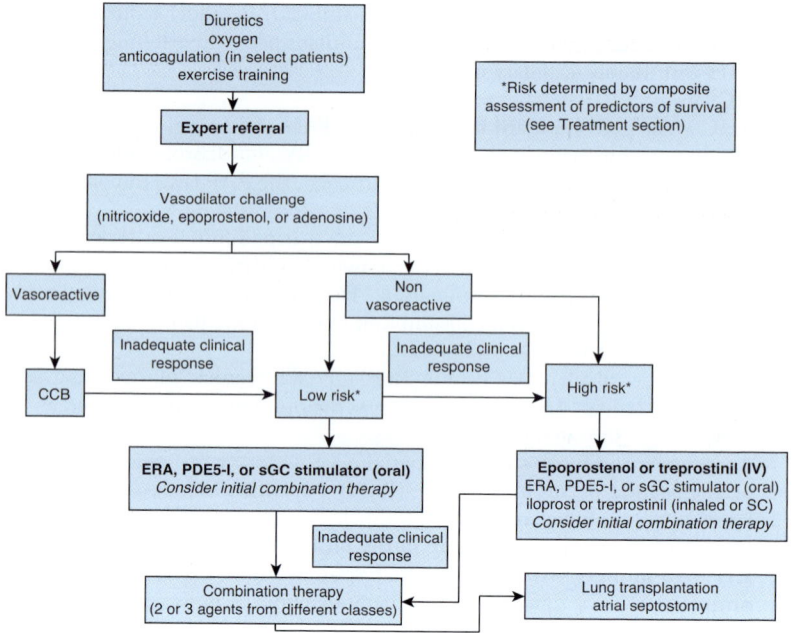

Figure 21-2 Pulmonary arterial hypertension treatment algorithm. Only patients with an acute vasodilator response (see text) should receive CCB treatment. Typical first-line treatment is listed first. Risk determined by variables listed in text. CCB, calcium channel blocker; ERA, endothelin receptor antagonist; PDE-5I, phosphodiesterase-5 inhibitor; sGC, soluble guanylate cyclase.

preserved ejection fraction (HFpEF) often develop secondary PH and should be optimized with SGLT2-inhibitors, afterload reducing agents, and diuretics, while also minimizing myocardial ischemia and tachyarrhythmias.
- Use of chronic NSAIDs can aggravate HF and should be avoided.
- Subset of patients with HFrEF or HFpEF, and CpcPH may benefit from sildenafil (a phosphodiesterase-5 inhibitor, PDE-5I), in terms of exertional capacity, hemodynamics during exercise, and quality of life; however, no multicenter RCT has demonstrated benefit in this population to date.[8–11] Sildenafil should only be considered if PH and PVR remain significantly elevated after optimization of LV filling pressures (i.e., near-normal PAWP or LVEDP) and optimization of LV systolic function.
- Caution should be taken as sildenafil use in patients with PH following intervention for valvular heart disease has been associated with worse outcomes. Additionally, macitentan has been associated with increased risk of fluid retention in PH-LHD with CpcPH.[12]

- **Group 3**
  - PH caused by parenchymal lung diseases (group 3) should be treated with **appropriate therapies for the underlying pulmonary condition**: bronchodilators, pulmonary rehabilitation (obstructive lung disease), immunomodulators (ILDs), and noninvasive ventilation (OSA and/or hypoventilation syndrome).
  - Adequate oxygen saturation (SpO_2 ≥90%) is critical to avoid hypoxic vasoconstriction and cor pulmonale.
  - Most studies have not consistently demonstrated a benefit of PAH-specific therapies; however, **inhaled treprostinil can improve 6MWD and survival from clinical worsening events in patients with PH associated with ILD.**[13–15]
- **Group 4**
  - Group 4 PH (CTEPH) can be cured by pulmonary endarterectomy (PEA) at specialized centers and requires careful screening to determine candidacy and expected hemodynamic response.[1,16]
  - Medical therapy and/or balloon pulmonary angioplasty (BPA) should be considered in patients with inoperable CTEPH (including distal and microvascular disease) or who have persistent or recurrent PH following PEA.[1,16]
  - **Lifelong therapeutic anticoagulation** should be prescribed.[1]

Pharmacologic Therapy for Group 1

- **Vasodilator therapy**
  - Approved PAH therapies have generally been shown to improve short-term exercise capacity, functional classification, hospitalization rate, and time to clinical worsening.
  - Long-term outcomes of prolonging survival are being inferred based on observational data and large-scale contemporary registries.
  - **Calcium channel blockers** (CCBs)[17,18]
    - **CCBs should only be used for treating PAH after demonstrating acute vasoresponsiveness with a short-acting vasodilator** (e.g., nitric oxide) during RHC.
    - **Indiscriminate CCB use can lead to hemodynamic collapse and syncope in patients with advanced right-sided heart failure (RHF) who are not acute vasoresponders.**
    - Chronic CCB therapy, such as **amlodipine, nifedipine, or diltiazem,** can be prescribed at an initial low dose and titrated over several weeks, while monitoring systemic pressures and guarding against aggravation of RHF.
    - **Verapamil should be avoided** due to its negative ionotropic properties.
    - Patients that do not have near normalization of PA pressures with long-term CCB usage should be considered for additional vasodilator/vasomodulator therapies.[1]
  - **Endothelin receptor antagonists** (ERAs)[1,19–23]:
    - ERAs block binding of endothelin-1 to A and/or B receptors on pulmonary artery smooth muscle cells and endothelial cells.
    - Available agents include **bosentan, ambrisentan, and macitentan.**
    - All are teratogenic and bosentan requires monthly laboratory monitoring for hepatotoxicity.

- **PDE-5Is**[1,21,22,24,25]
  - PDE-5Is block phosphodiesterase, which degrades intracellular cyclic guanosine monophosphate (cGMP). The result is pulmonary vasodilation and, ultimately, decreased PAPs.
  - Available agents include **sildenafil and tadalafil**.
  - No specific laboratory monitoring is needed but a potent drug interaction with organic nitrates must be avoided.
- **Soluble guanylate cyclase (sGC) stimulators**
  - **Riociguat** increases the concentration of cGMP and consequently vasodilates, by stimulating sGC directly and by increasing its sensitivity to nitric oxide.[26,27]
  - In general, riociguat is well tolerated but syncope and rare instances of hemoptysis/pulmonary hemorrhage have been reported.
  - Similar trial data suggest that riociguat is effective for CTEPH as well.[28,29]
- **Prostanoids**[1,21,22,30–32]
  - Prostanoids are considered **the most potent, but also the most challenging, class of therapies** due to their complex delivery system and wider therapeutic dosing range.
  - Prostanoids induce vasodilation, inhibit cellular growth, and inhibit platelet aggregation.
  - Commercially available prostanoids include: **epoprostenol** (IV), room temperature stable epoprostenol (IV), **treprostinil** (IV, SC, inhaled, or oral), and **iloprost** (inhaled). **Selexipag** is an oral prostacyclin receptor agonist.
  - Choice of therapy is variable across prescribers and dosing of parenteral agents is highly individualized to the patient and requires great expertise and impeccable nursing.
  - Prostanoids may be used as initial therapy in treatment naïve patients who present in advanced RHF. However, they are most often used as add-on therapies when oral agents provide an ineffective or inadequate treatment response.
  - Several randomized controlled trials of combination therapy have confirmed the benefits of combining prostanoids with an oral agent.[1]
  - Adverse effects include drug-related side effects (e.g., jaw pain, nonpruritic rash, flushing, headache, gastrointestinal side effects, and extremity pain) and delivery system complication (e.g., bloodstream infections, catheter-related thrombosis, inadvertent interruptions of very short-acting continuous medications).

- **Choice of vasodilator therapy**
  - **Initial choice of PAH-specific therapy should be individualized based on risk stratification of an individual, with reliance on several clinical variables.**[1]
  - Multiple risk stratification tools have been validated including the COMPERA registry, the French PH registry, and REVEAL 2.0.[1,33–37] WHO functional class, BNP/NT-proBNP, and 6MWD are consistently utilized in these risk assessment tools.
  - Other potentially worrisome clues are underlying PAH diagnosis (connective tissue disease–associated PAH, porto-PH, and hereditary PAH), presence of pericardial effusion, concomitant renal dysfunction, males >60 years of age,

resting systolic blood pressure (<110 mm Hg), pulse rate (>96 beats/min), and diffusing capacity (<40%).
- Based on these risk assessment tools, individual considered high risk for significant clinical events, including hospitalization or death in the near term, should be strongly considered for parenteral prostanoid therapy (Figure 21-2).[1]
- **Comorbid conditions, social support, and patient's level of sophistication are critical in deciding a therapy, as delivery systems for PAH-specific therapies differ widely.**
- If patients are declining, therapeutic classes are switched or, more likely, a second or third drug from a different therapeutic class is added.
- **Other therapies**
  - **Diuretic therapy**
    - Diuretics critically alleviate RHF and improve symptoms.
    - Often a combination of a loop diuretic, aldosterone antagonist, and/or a thiazide is required.
    - Overdiuresis or too rapid of a diuresis can be poorly tolerated due to preload dependency of the RV and limited ability of the cardiac output to compensate for systemic hypotension.
    - Aggravating chronic renal dysfunction, particularly in an individual with long-standing RHF or intrinsic renal disease, should be avoided.
  - **Inotropic agents** (e.g., dobutamine, milrinone, and epinephrine) improve right heart function and are best suited for short-term use in acutely decompensated states especially when overt organ hypoperfusion is evident.

Other Nonpharmacologic Therapies

- **Supplemental oxygen** should be used to maintain normoxemia and avoid hypoxic vasoconstriction as much as possible. Normoxemia may be impossible to achieve if significant intracardiac right-to-left shunting is present.
- **In-line IV filters** to prevent paradoxical air emboli in patients with significant intracardiac right-to-left shunts should be implemented.
- **Pneumococcal, influenza, and SARS-CoV-2 vaccinations** should be considered to avoid respiratory tract infections.
- Patients should **avoid high-risk behaviors** (e.g., deep **Valsalva** and **high altitudes**) that can acutely decrease RV preload and/or increase RV afterload and worsen RHF.
- Patients should **avoid pregnancy** due to marked hemodynamic alterations that can further strain a compromised RV. Contraception choice is highly variable but choosing methods that do not increase thromboembolic events is recommended.
- Systemic **sympathomimetic agents** with vasoactive properties should be avoided (e.g., over-the-counter decongestant, nicotine, and cocaine).
- Patients should **avoid NSAIDs**, which have multiple counter-productive effects in RHF.

Surgical Management

- **Transplant surgery**[1]
  - Lung transplantation or heart–lung transplantation is reserved for suitable PAH patients who remain in advanced functional classes (III–IV) with

ominous hemodynamics despite maximal medical therapy that includes a parenteral prostanoid.
  - RV recovery after isolated lung transplantation allows for reserving heart–lung transplantation primarily for cases of irreparable complex congenital abnormalities.
  - Median survival after lung transplantation is ~6 years, while conditional median survival in IPAH for those who survive beyond 1 year is 10 years.
  - **Liver transplantation** should be considered on an individual basis in patients with porto-PH if hemodynamics improves to a certain level.
- **Atrial septostomy and Potts Shunt**[1]
  - **Atrial septostomy** is a percutaneously created a right-to-left shunt across the interatrial septum and can increase systemic oxygen transport, in spite of a decrease in systemic arterial oxygen saturation, by increasing cardiac output.
  - Surgically or percutaneously created **Potts shunts** (from the left pulmonary artery to the descending aorta) can also off-load the pulmonary circulation and improve systemic delivery of blood flow in patients whose PA pressures are at a suprasystemic level.
  - The indications are rare but can be explored in cases of refractory RHF (e.g., recurrent syncope, severe ascites, or poor systemic end-organ perfusion).
- **Septal defect closure**[1]
  - Septal defect closure is feasible in carefully selected cases of intracardiac defects to prevent or minimize progression of PAH.
  - Requirements for closure include significant net left-to-right shunting (pulmonary/systemic flow ratio ≥1.5) and low PVR (PVR <5 Wood units).

Lifestyle/Risk Modification

- **Fluid and sodium restriction** should be employed for individuals with RHF.
- **Exercise training** and **pulmonary rehabilitation** have been shown to improve 6MWD, WHO functional class, and quality of life. Exercise may improve right heart function and hemodynamics; however, further studies are needed.[38,39]

REFERRAL

The field of PH is rapidly evolving with a better understanding of its pathophysiology and development of numerous pharmacologic options. Given its complex nature, most patients suspected of having PAH should be evaluated in a specialized PH center.

MONITORING/FOLLOW-UP

- PAH remains incurable and patients require close monitoring to detect deteriorating RV function and clinical progression.
- Patients with a favorable profile can be evaluated every 3–6 months while more unstable patients should be seen every 1–3 months.
- While no consensus exists for monitoring PAH patients, most centers utilize composite clinical variables (WHO functional class), exercise measures (e.g., 6MWD), and periodic objective RV assessments (e.g., echocardiography, catheterization, BNP, cardiac MRI).

OUTCOME/PROGNOSIS

- Prognosis in PAH has improved considerably over the last 20 years due to better disease recognition, numerous treatment options, and more aggressive treatment strategies.
- **Patients are still at significant risk for disease progression and individuals in intermediate and high-risk categories (based on validated risk assessment tools) are still at significant risk for mortality and significant clinical events, including hospitalization.**[1]

REFERENCES

1. Humbert M, Kovacs G, Hoeper MM, et al; ESC/ERS Scientific Document Group. 2022 ESC/ERS Guidelines for the diagnosis and treatment of pulmonary hypertension. *Eur Heart J.* 2022;43:3618–3731.
2. Simonneau G, Montani D, Celermajer DS, et al. Haemodynamic definitions and updated clinical classification of pulmonary hypertension. *Eur Respir J.* 2019;53:1801913.
3. Chang KY, Duval S, Badesch DB, et al; PHAR Investigators. Mortality in pulmonary arterial hypertension in the modern era: Early insights from the pulmonary hypertension association registry. *J Am Heart Assoc.* 2022;11:e024969.
4. Pengo V, Lensing AWA, Prins MH, et al; Thromboembolic Pulmonary Hypertension Study Group. Incidence of chronic thromboembolic pulmonary hypertension after pulmonary embolism. *N Eng J Med.* 2004;350:2257–2264.
5. Newman JH, Wheeler L, Lane KB, et al. Mutation in the gene for bone morphogenetic protein receptor II as a cause of primary pulmonary hypertension in a large kindred. *N Eng J Med.* 2001;345:319–324.
6. Soubrier F, Chung WK, Machado R, et al. Genetics and genomics of pulmonary arterial hypertension. *J Am Coll Cardiol.* 2013;62:D13–D21.
7. Trembath RC, Thomson JR, Machado RE, et al. Clinical and molecular genetic features of pulmonary hypertension in patients with hereditary hemorrhagic telangiectasia. *N Engl J Med.* 2011;345:325–334.
8. Guazzi M, Samaja M, Arena R, Vicenzi M, Guazzi MD. Long-term use of sildenafil in the therapeutic management of heart failure. *J Am Coll Cardiol.* 2007;50:2136–2144.
9. Lewis GD, Shah R, Shahzad K, et al. Sildenafil improves exercise capacity and quality of life in patients with systolic heart failure and secondary pulmonary hypertension. *Circulation.* 2007;116:1555–1562.
10. Wu X, Yang T, Zhou Q, Li S, Huang L. Additional use of a phosphodiesterase 5 inhibitor in patients with pulmonary hypertension secondary to chronic systolic heart failure: a meta-analysis. *Eur J Hear Fail.* 2014;16:444–453.
11. Guazzi M, Vicenzi M, Arena R, Guazzi MD. Pulmonary hypertension in heart failure with preserved ejection fraction: a target of phosphodiesterase-5 inhibition in a 1-year study. *Circulation.* 2011;124:164–174.
12. Vachiéry JL, Tedford RJ, Rosenkranz S, et al. Pulmonary hypertension due to left heart disease. *Eur Respir J.* 2019;53:1801897.
13. Nathan SD, Barbera JA, Gaine SP, et al. Pulmonary hypertension in chronic lung disease and hypoxia. *Eur Respir J.* 2019;53(1):1801914.
14. Waxman A, Restrepo-Jaramillo R, Thenappan T, et al. Inhaled treprostinil in pulmonary hypertension due to interstitial lung disease. *N Engl J Med.* 2021;384:325–334.
15. Nathan SD, Tapson VF, Elwing J, et al. Efficacy of inhaled treprostinil on multiple disease progression events in patients with pulmonary hypertension due to parenchymal lung disease in the INCREASE trial. *Am J Respir Crit Care Med.* 2022;205:198–207.

16. Kim NH, Delcroix M, Jais X, et al. Chronic thromboembolic pulmonary hypertension. *Eur Respir J.* 2019;53:1801915.
17. Rich S, Kaufmann E, Levy PS. The effect of high doses of calcium-channel blockers on survival in primary pulmonary hypertension. *N Engl J Med.* 1992;327:76–81.
18. Sitbon O, Humbert M, Jaïs X, et al. Long-term response to calcium channel blockers in idiopathic pulmonary arterial hypertension. *Circulation.* 2005;111:3105–3111.
19. Rubin LJ, Badesch DB, Barst RJ, et al. Bosentan therapy for pulmonary arterial hypertension. *N Engl J Med.* 2002;346:896–903.
20. Galiè N, Olschewski H, Oudiz RJ, et al; Ambrisentan in Pulmonary Arterial Hypertension, Randomized, Double-Blind, Placebo-Controlled, Multicenter, Efficacy Studies (ARIES) Group. Ambrisentan for the treatment of pulmonary arterial hypertension: results of the ambrisentan in pulmonary arterial hypertension, randomized, double-blind, placebo controlled, multicenter, efficacy (ARIES) study 1 and 2. *Circulation.* 2008;117:3010–3019.
21. Galiè N, Manes A, Negro L, Palazzini M, Bacchi-Reggiani ML, Branzi A. A meta-analysis of randomized controlled trials in pulmonary arterial hypertension. *Eur Heart J.* 2009;30:394–403.
22. He B, Zhang F, Li X, et al. Meta-analysis of randomized controlled trials on treatment of pulmonary arterial hypertension. *Circ J.* 2010;74:1458–1464.
23. Pulido T, Adzerikho I, Channick RN, et al; SERAPHIN Investigators. Macitentan and morbidity and mortality in pulmonary arterial hypertension. *N Engl J Med.* 2013;369:809–818.
24. Galiè N, Ghofrani HA, Torbicki A, et al; Sildenafil Use in Pulmonary Arterial Hypertension (SUPER) Study Group. Sildenafil citrated therapy for pulmonary arterial hypertension. *N Engl J Med.* 2005;353:2148–2157.
25. Galiè N, Brundage BH, Ghofrani HA, et al; Pulmonary Arterial Hypertension and Response to Tadalafil (PHIRST) Study Group. Tadalafil therapy for pulmonary arterial hypertension. *Circulation.* 2009;119:2894–2903.
26. Ghofrani HA, Galiè N, Grimminger F, et al; PATENT-1 Study Group. Riociguat for the treatment of pulmonary arterial hypertension. *N Engl J Med.* 2013;369:330–340.
27. Rubin LJ, Galiè N, Grimminger F, et al; PATENT-1 Study Group. Riociguat for the treatment of pulmonary arterial hypertension: a long-term extension study (PATENT-2). *Eur Respir J.* 2015;45:1303–1313.
28. Ghofrani HA, D'Armini AM, Grimminger F, et al; CHEST-1 Study Group. Riociguat for the treatment of chronic thromboembolic pulmonary hypertension. *N Engl J Med.* 2013;369:319–329.
29. Simonneau G, D'Armini, Ghofrani HA, et al. Riociguat for the treatment of chronic thromboembolic pulmonary hypertension: a long-term extension study (CHEST-2*).* *Eur Respir J.* 2015;45:1293–302.
30. Barst RJ, Rubin LJ, Long WA, et al; Primary Pulmonary Hypertension Study Group. A comparison of continuous intravenous epoprostenol (prostacyclin) with conventional therapy for primary pulmonary hypertension. *N Engl J Med.* 1996;334:296–301.
31. Simonneau G, Barst RJ, Galiè N, et al; Treprostinil Study Group. Continuous subcutaneous infusion of treprostinil, a prostacyclin analogue, in patients with pulmonary arterial hypertension: a double-blind, randomized, placebo-controlled trial. *Am J Respir Crit Care Med.* 2002;165:800–804.
32. Olschewski H, Simonneau G, Galiè N, et al; Aerosolized Iloprost Randomized Study Group. Inhaled iloprost for severe pulmonary hypertension. *N Engl J Med.* 2002;347:322–329.
33. Kylhammar D, Kjellström B, Hjalmarsson C, et al. A comprehensive risk stratification at early follow-up determines prognosis in pulmonary arterial hypertension. *Eur Hear J.* 2017;39:4175–4181.

34. Hoeper MM, Kramer T, Pan Z, et al. Mortality in pulmonary arterial hypertension: prediction by the 2015 European pulmonary hypertension guidelines risk stratification model. *Eur Respir J*. 2017;50:1700740.
35. Boucly A, Weatherald J, Savale L, et al. Risk assessment, prognosis and guideline implementation in pulmonary arterial hypertension. *Eur Respir J*. 2017;50:1700889.
36. Benza RL, Gomberg-Maitland M, Elliott CG, et al. Predicting survival in patients with pulmonary arterial hypertension: the REVEAL Risk Score Calculator 2.0 and comparison with ESC/ERS-based risk assessment strategies. *Chest*. 2019;156:323–337.
37. Benza RL, Kanwar MK, Raina A, et al. Development and validation of an abridged version of the REVEAL 2.0 risk score calculator, REVEAL Lite 2, for use in patients with pulmonary arterial hypertension. *Chest*. 2021;159:337–346.
38. Grünig E, Eichstaedt C, Barberà JA, et al. ERS statement on exercise training and rehabilitation in patients with severe chronic pulmonary hypertension. *Eur Respir J*. 2019;53:1800332.
39. Grünig E, MacKenzie A, Peacock AJ, et al. Standardized exercise training is feasible, safe, and effective in pulmonary arterial and chronic thromboembolic pulmonary hypertension: results from a large European multicentre randomized controlled trial. *Eur Hear J*. 2020;42:2284–2295.

Pleural Diseases

22

Praveen R. Chenna and
Brandt Lydon

GENERAL PRINCIPLES

- The pleural lining is a serous membrane covering the lung parenchyma, chest wall, diaphragm, and mediastinum.
- The pleural membrane covering the surface of the lung is known as the visceral pleura, the parietal pleura cover the remaining structures.
  - In between the visceral and parietal pleura of each lung is the pleural space, a potential space that contains a thin layer of fluid of approximately 10 mL in volume.
  - The parietal pleura secretes approximately 2400 mL of fluid daily, which is reabsorbed by the visceral pleura.[1]

Definition
- A pleural effusion is excessive accumulation of fluid in the pleural space.
  - A hemothorax refers to a pleural effusion that is comprised mainly of blood.
  - Chylothorax is a collection of chyle within the pleural space.
  - An empyema refers to infected fluid within the pleural space.
- A pneumothorax is a collection of gas in the pleural space.[2]
  - Primary spontaneous pneumothorax occurs when there is no obvious underlying lung disease.
  - Secondary spontaneous pneumothorax is a complication of underlying lung disease.

Epidemiology
- More than one million cases of pleural effusion occur annually in the US.
- Incidence of pneumothorax varies widely by gender, country, and race.

Etiology
- Pleural effusions have a variety of causes and are listed below; see Table 22-1.
  - Empyema is generally caused by extension of an infection of the lung or surrounding tissue.
    - Common microbial pathogens are *Staphylococcus aureus*, *Streptococcus* species, and *Haemophilus influenza*.
    - Empyemas are frequently polymicrobial in cases where aspiration is suspected.
  - The three major grouped causes of chylothorax are malignancy (50% of cases), trauma (25%), and idiopathic (15%). Other causes account for 10%.[3]
    - 75% of chylous effusions related to malignancy are due to lymphomas related to obstruction of pleural lymphatics.

TABLE 22-1 CAUSES OF PLEURAL EFFUSION

Transudates
Infections
  Bacteria
  TB
  Fungi
  Parasites
  Viruses
  Mycoplasma
Neoplasms
  Metastatic carcinoma
  Lymphoma
  Leukemia
  Mesothelioma
  Bronchogenic carcinoma
  Chest wall tumors
Intra-abdominal disease/GI
  Abdominal surgery
  Pancreatitis
  Meigs syndrome
  Intrahepatic abscess
  Incarcerated diaphragmatic hernia
  Subdiaphragmatic abscess
  Esophageal rupture
  Endoscopic variceal sclerotherapy
  Hepatitis
Collagen vascular diseases
  SLE
  Rheumatoid arthritis
  Drug-induced lupus
  Sjögren syndrome
  Granulomatosis with polyangiitis
  Churg–Strauss syndrome
  Immunoblastic lymphadenopathy
Drug-induced pleural disease
  Nitrofurantoin
  Dantrolene
  Methysergide
  Bromocriptine
  Procarbazine
  Amiodarone
Pulmonary infarction
  Miscellaneous
    Dressler syndrome (postcardiac injury)
    Sarcoidosis
    Yellow nail syndrome
    Trapped lung
    Radiation therapy
    Electrical burns
    Iatrogenic injury
    Ovarian hyperstimulation syndrome
    Chronic atelectasis
    Asbestos exposure
    Familial Mediterranean fever
    Urinoma
Idiopathic
  Lipid laden
    Chylous
    Pseudochylous
Trauma

Exudates
Increased hydrostatic pressure
  Congestive heart failure
  Constrictive pericarditis
  Superior vena caval obstruction
Decreased oncotic pressure
  Cirrhosis
  Nephrotic syndrome
  Hypoalbuminemia
  Peritoneal dialysis
Miscellaneous
  Acute atelectasis
  Subclavian catheter misplacement
  Myxedema
  Idiopathic

GI, gastrointestinal; SLE, systemic lupus erythematosus.

- Trauma as a causative factor of chylothorax includes any cardiothoracic surgical procedure. It may take place 1–2 weeks postsurgery for the chylothorax to become apparent.
- In a number of cases, chylothorax results from transdiaphragmatic leakage of chylous ascites. Causes of chylous ascites include nephrotic syndrome, hypothyroidism, and cirrhosis.
  - Hemothorax may result from trauma or iatrogenesis, and rarely are spontaneous.
- Secondary pneumothorax is often seen in chronic obstructive pulmonary disease (COPD), acquired immunodeficiency syndrome (AIDS), cystic fibrosis, tuberculosis, sarcoidosis, pulmonary fibrosis, asthma, Marfan disease, lymphangioleiomyomatosis, Pulmonary Langerhans cell histiocytosis, trauma, or any disease with pulmonary cavity formation.[4]

Pathophysiology
- Pleural effusions can be categorized as transudates or exudates.
  - Transudates result primarily from passive fluid shifts that occur as a result of changes in the hydrostatic and oncotic pressures of the circulation.
  - Exudates imply an active pleural process such as inflammation of the pleura or underlying lung tissue.
  - There are numerous causes of both transudates and exudates (see Table 22-1).
- Primary spontaneous pneumothorax is thought to result from the rupture of subpleural apical blebs.[5]
- Secondary pneumothorax results from rupture of already pathologic lung architecture.

Risk Factors
- Risk factors for pleural effusion reflect those of the underlying causative disease.
- Primary spontaneous pneumothoraces are more common in tall, thin males, and recur 50% of the time.

DIAGNOSIS

- Diagnosis of a pleural disease is based on history, physical examination, and radiographic imaging.
- Differentiation into a specific pathologic entity is based on imaging as well as laboratory studies of the pleural fluid if present.

Clinical Presentation
- Symptom onset may be chronic, subacute, or acute depending on the rapidity with which the pleural pathology developed.
- If the effusion or pneumothorax is very large in nature, it may cause mass effect and even cardiac tamponade, resulting in a life-threatening condition.

History
- Dyspnea is the primary symptom of pleural disease, and pain may also be present.
  - Pain is generally pleuritic in nature.
  - Referred pain to the abdomen and ipsilateral shoulder are possible.

- Other symptoms depend on the specific etiology of the pleural disease:
  - Empyema may be associated with fevers, chills, and malaise.
  - Hemothorax may present with signs and symptoms of anemia.
  - Chylothorax contains large amounts of fat, protein, and lymphocytes, which accounts for nutritional and immunologic deficiencies observed when they are chronic in nature.

Physical Examination
- Decreased expansion on inspiration, dullness to percussion, and decreased or absent breath sounds on auscultation are all consistent with a pleural effusion. However, the exam finding that correlates best with presence of pleural effusion is asymmetric chest wall expansion.
- Asymmetric chest wall, decreased breath sounds, decreased tactile fremitus, and hyperresonance to percussion are all consistent with a large pneumothorax.

Diagnostic Criteria
There are no clinical criteria to definitively diagnose a pleural effusion or pneumothorax and radiographic imaging is generally needed.

Differential Diagnosis
The differential diagnosis for pleural effusion or pneumothorax includes other causes of dyspnea including pulmonary edema, pneumonia, atelectasis, thromboembolic disease, or interstitial lung disease.

Diagnostic Testing
Radiographic imaging and laboratory testing of pleural fluid are the two most useful diagnostic modalities for diagnosing pleural disease.

Imaging
- Chest radiograph is generally the first imaging study obtained when a patient presents with a suspected pleural effusion or pneumothorax.
  - On a posteroanterior chest film, blunting of the costophrenic angle or blurring of the diaphragmatic margin suggests the presence of a pleural effusion. Generally, 200–500 mL of fluid is needed to generate this finding.
  - A lateral decubitus film of the affected side can reveal an effusion of approximately 100 mL and allows for assessment of a free flowing versus loculated effusion.[6]
- CT is more sensitive than radiography and can detect the presence of even a very small amount of fluid or air in the pleural space as well as the presence of loculations in the pleural fluid.
- Ultrasound is a modality that is increasingly being used to image the pleural space. Ultrasound can detect fluid or air and provides qualitative information regarding pleural fluid.
  - Ultrasound findings such as fluid echogenicity and the presence or absence of septations within the pleural space may change management and predict clinical outcome.
  - Ultrasound guidance is often used to direct treatments such as drainage of fluid or chest tube insertion.

Diagnostic Procedures
- Thoracentesis should be performed for diagnosis in cases of pleural effusion of unknown etiology.[7]
- Therapeutic thoracentesis can lead to symptom relief.[8]
  - Thoracentesis should generally be performed after ultrasound localization to decrease risk of complications.
  - CXR should be performed after the procedure to rule out a complicating pneumothorax.

Laboratories
- Categorization of pleural fluid as transudative or exudative assists with diagnosis and therapeutic management.[9]
  - Light criteria compare levels or protein and lactate dehydrogenase in the effusion with those in the patient's serum to determine whether inflammation or fluid shift is responsible for the effusion. If one of the three criteria is met, the effusion is defined as an exudate (Table 22-2).[10]
  - Heffner criteria has similar sensitivity for identifying exudative pleural effusions when compared to Light criteria and do not require concomitant serum values for comparison (Table 22-2).[11]
- Other useful studies to differentiate the type of pleural effusion include pH, glucose, cell count, gram stain, culture, and triglycerides. Hematocrit should be sent if hemothorax is suspected.
  - Empyema can be diagnosed by a positive gram stain or culture.[12] Empyema is also characterized by a low pH and glucose.
  - Hemothorax is defined by a pleural hematocrit/serum hematocrit of >0.5.
  - Chylothorax is diagnosed by pleural triglycerides >110 mg/dL or by the presence of chylomicrons. If chylothorax is suspected, and triglycerides are 50–110 mg/dL, a lipoprotein electrophoresis can confirm the presence of chylomicrons.

TABLE 22-2 CRITERIA FOR DEFINING AN EFFUSION

Light criteria for exudative effusion (one or more of the following)	Heffner criteria for exudative effusion (one or more of the following)
Pleural fluid protein to serum protein ratio of >0.5	Pleural fluid protein >2.9 g/dL
Pleural fluid LDH to serum LDH ratio of >0.6	Pleural fluid cholesterol >45 mg/dL
Pleural fluid LDH >2/3 serum upper limit of normal	Pleural fluid LDH >45% of upper limits of normal serum value

Adapted from Light RW. Clinical manifestations and useful tests. In: Light RW. *Pleural diseases*, 4th ed. Lippincott Williams and Wilkins; 2001:42–86; and Heffner JE, Brown LK, Barbieri CA. Diagnostic value of tests that discriminate between exudative and transudative pleural effusions. *Chest.* 1997;111:970–980.

TABLE 22-3	HELPFUL FEATURES OF THE PLEURAL FLUID OF EXUDATIVE EFFUSIONS
Malignancy	Fluid cytology positive for malignant cells
Tuberculosis	Pleural fluid is lymphocytic Positive AFB stain is very rare Pleural fluid is sanguineous
Connective tissue disease	Pleural fluid usually lymphocytic and will often have ANA positivity
Pancreatitis	Increased amylase
Infection	Gram stain and culture often reveal specific infection Empyema is accompanied by very low glucose and pH, and a markedly elevated LDH
Drug related	Eosinophilic fluid
Chylothorax	Milky fluid, triglyceride level >110 mg/dL
Hemothorax	Sanguineous fluid Hematocrit of pleural fluid is >50% of peripheral blood

AFB, acid-fast bacilli; ANA, antinuclear antibody; LDH, lactate dehydrogenase.

- Malignant pleural effusion is diagnosed by a positive fluid cytology, and though highly specific it is not sensitive.
- See Table 22-3 for other pleural fluid laboratory values associated with specific pleural effusions.

TREATMENT

- Generally, treatment of a pleural effusion depends on the etiology.
  - Transudative pleural effusions are most appropriately managed by treating the underlying cause. Symptomatic treatment may involve drainage of the effusion.
  - Exudative pleural effusions should be evaluated for an underlying cause.
    - Treatment may involve drainage of the effusion or even pleurodesis to prevent reaccumulation of fluid.
    - Treatment of recurrent malignant pleural effusions (and occasionally benign effusions such as hepatic hydrothorax) will sometimes involve placement of a tunneled pleural catheter.
- Treatment of pneumothorax generally involves draining the air from the pleural space by insertion of a chest tube; see Figure 22-1.

Medications

- Pleural effusions can sometimes be treated with medications depending on the cause.
- Parapneumonic effusions and empyema are treated with antibiotics in conjunction with fluid drainage.[13]

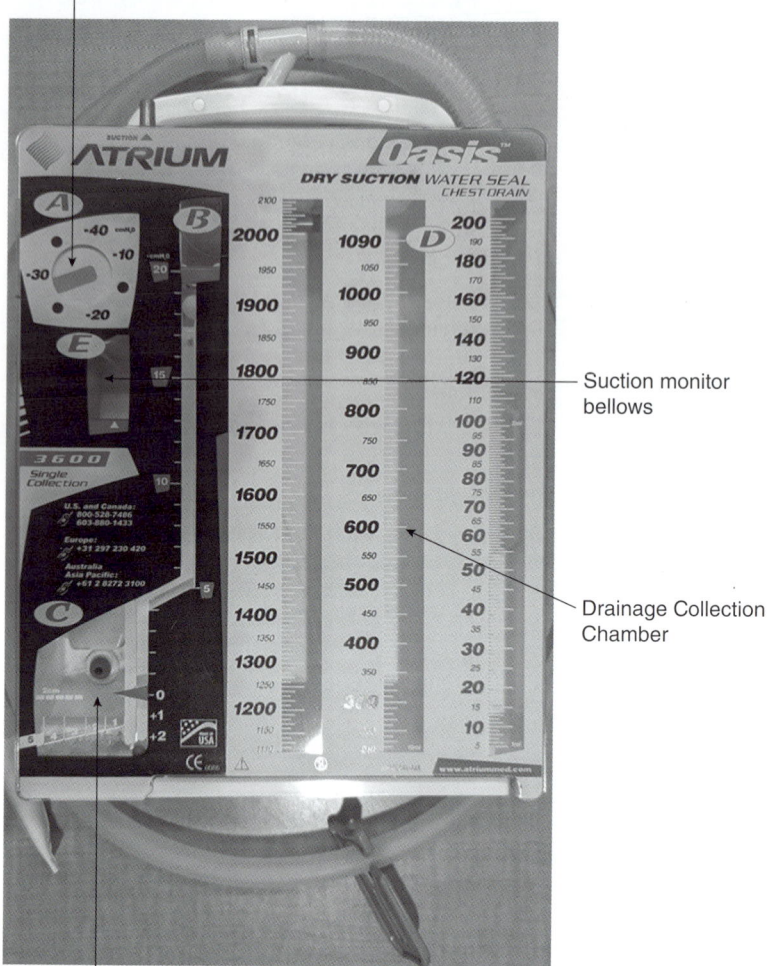

Figure 22-1 An example of a pleural fluid drainage chamber. This is based on the three-chamber design, with a drainage collection chamber, a water seal chamber, and a suction chamber. These are all contained within the single device. This allows air and pleural fluid drainage to exit, but not re-enter the pleural cavity. It also allows for the application and titration of suction to the pleural cavity.

- Transudative pleural effusions can sometimes be treated effectively with diuretics.
- There is no medical treatment for pneumothorax.

Other Nonpharmacologic Therapies
- Pleurodesis involves instillation of a sclerosing agent into the pleural space to cause scarring and restriction of the space itself. This is generally performed for recurrent malignant effusion, recurrent pneumothorax once the lung has re-expanded, and occasionally chylothorax.
- When other modalities fail, total parenteral nutrition with complete bowel rest can cause chylothoraces to resolve as oral intake results in chyle formation. Medium-chain triglyceride diets have been tried as chyle is derived from long-chain triglycerides in the diet, though this has yielded mixed results.
- If the pneumothorax is <15% of the hemithorax volume, it is safe to observe. High oxygen content (e.g., 100% nonrebreather mask) administration increases the rate of pleural air reabsorption by increasing the nitrogen gradient between the air in the pneumothorax and the pleural capillaries.
- In cases of persistent pneumothorax secondary to bronchopleural fistula, fiberoptic bronchoscopy with placement of endobronchial valves causing atelectasis of the distal lung can be placed in a segmental or subsegmental bronchus if the bronchopleural fistula has been localized to one location.

Surgical Management
- For pleural effusions:
  - Chest tube insertion is often indicated for large pleural effusions.
  - Other indications for chest tube insertion include empyema, chylothorax, and hemothorax.
  - As discussed, thoracentesis can be used as a therapeutic modality.
  - Undifferentiated exudative pleural effusion
    - In patients with exudative effusion for whom thoracentesis has not yielded a diagnosis (especially if malignancy is expected), medical thoracoscopy is indicated.
    - Medical thoracoscopy (pleuroscopy) utilizes a single incision and introduction of a rigid or simi-rigid pleuroscope into the pleural space for visualization of the pleural surfaces and biopsy.[14]
    - Diagnostic yield is comparable to that of video-assisted thoracic surgery (VATS) for malignancy, including mesothelioma, and can be performed under moderate sedation and local anesthesia.
  - Malignant pleural effusion
    - Tunneled pleural catheter is used for recurrent malignant pleural effusion and occasionally hepatic hydrothorax not amenable to diuresis.
    - This catheter can be drained at home once every other day with attachment of a bottle.
    - In our experience approximately 50% of effusions are permanently drained by way of autopleurodesis allowing for removal of the tunneled pleural catheter.
  - Empyema: In cases where chest tube drainage does not effectively drain an empyema and there is continued evidence of infection, VATS with decortication is often indicated.

- Hemothorax
  - Requires surgical stabilization in 30% of penetrating injuries and 15% of blunt injuries.
  - Initial output of >1500 mL of blood, or continued chest tube output or >200 mL of blood over 2 hours requires surgical intervention.
  - Clotted blood in the pleural space may require VATS to prevent development of empyema or fibrothorax.[15,16]
- Chylothorax
  - For persistent chylothorax, surgical interventions include thoracic duct ligation via video-assisted thoracoscopic surgery in conjunction with pleurectomy or pleurodesis.[17]
  - For patients who are not a surgical candidate or who would prefer to avoid surgery, lymphangiography with embolization of the thoracic duct is an option.[18]
  - Pleuroperitoneal shunting is also occasionally performed, though obviously not in cases in which the pleural disease is secondary to chylous ascites.
  - Early surgical intervention for chylothorax should be considered when chest tube output is >1500 mL/d, or in a patient with malnourishment or immune compromise.
- Pneumothorax
  - Treated with chest tube insertion if they are large, symptomatic, under tension, recurrent, or bilateral. In extreme circumstances where a large pneumothorax is causing cardiovascular collapse, immediate needle decompression is indicated by inserting a needle in the 2nd intercostal space in the midclavicular line.
  - For recurrent pneumothorax, VATS may be indicated with endoscopic stapling and removal of the bulla or fistula, particularly if there is a bronchopleural fistula.[19]

SPECIAL CONSIDERATIONS

- The etiology of pleural effusions can often be discerned by their appearance.
  - A serous effusion is more likely to be transudative, while an exudative effusion is more likely to have other appearances.
  - If the fluid appears bloody, a hemothorax should be suspected.
  - Pus indicates an empyema.
  - Milky white and opalescent pleural fluid is indicative of a chylothorax.
- In cases of massive hemothorax requiring surgical intervention, clamping the chest tube may result in tension hemothorax and cardiovascular collapse.
- Chylothorax is nonirritating and bacteriostatic, thus secondary infection is extremely rare.

COMPLICATIONS

- Disease recurrence.
- Cardiovascular compromise in extreme cases.
- Other complications are disease specific.

REFERRAL

- Interventional pulmonology may be consulted for the placement of chest tubes, tunneled pleural catheters, or endobronchial valve placement.
- Surgical consultation may be needed as per the above section on surgical management.

REFERENCES

1. Sahn SA. State of the art. The pleura. *Am Rev Respir Dis*. 1988;138:184–234.
2. Sahn SA, Heffner JE. Spontaneous pneumothorax. *N Engl J Med*. 2000;342:868–874.
3. Doerr CH, Miller DL, Ryu JH. Chylothorax. *Semin Respir Crit Care Med*. 2001; 22:617–626.
4. Fraser RS, Muller NL, Colman NC, Pare PD. Pneumothorax. In: Fraser RS, Paré PD, eds. *Fraser and Pare's Diagnosis of Diseases of the Chest*. 4th ed. WB Saunders, 1999: 2781–2794.
5. Jantz MA, Pierson DJ. Pneumothorax and barotraumas. *Clin Chest Med*. 1994;15:75–91.
6. Woodring JH. Recognition of pleural effusion on supine radiographs: how much fluid is required? *AJR Am J Roentgenol*. 1984;142:59–64.
7. Kennedy L, Sahn SA. Noninvasive evaluation of the patient with a pleural effusion. *Chest Surg Clin North Am*. 1994;4:451–465.
8. Feller-Kopman D, Berkowitz D, Boiselle P, Ernst A. Large volume thoracentesis and the risk of re-expansion pulmonary edema. *Ann Thorac Surg*. 2007;84:1656–1661.
9. Light RW, Macgregor MI, Luchsinger PC, Ball WC Jr. Pleural effusions: the diagnostic separation of transudates and exudates. *Ann Intern Med*. 1972;77:507–513.
10. Light RW. Clinical manifestations and useful tests. In: Light RW. *Pleural diseases*. 4th ed. Lippincott Williams and Wilkins; 2001:42–86.
11. Heffner JE, Brown LK, Barbieri CA. Diagnostic value of tests that discriminate between exudative and transudative pleural effusions. Primary Study Investigators. *Chest*. 1997; 111:970–980.
12. Light RW. A new classification of parapneumonic effusions and empyema. *Chest*. 1995; 108:299–301.
13. Light RW, Girard WM, Jenkinson SG, George RB. Parapneumonic effusions. *Am J Med*. 1980;69:507–512.
14. Rahman NM, Ali NJ, Brown G, et al. Local anesthetic thoracoscopy: British Thoracic Society Pleural Disease Guideline 2010. *Thorax*. 2010;65:ii56–ii60.
15. Jacoby RC, Battistella FD. Hemothorax. *Semin Respir Crit Care Med*. 2001;22(6): 627–630.
16. Light RW, Broaddus VC. Pneumothorax, chylothorax, hemothorax, and fibrothorax. In: Murray RF, Nadel JA, eds. *Textbook of respiratory medicine*. 3rd ed. Elsevier Science, 2000: 2043–2055.
17. Yeam I, Sassoon C. Hemothorax and chylothorax. *Curr Opin Pulm Med*. 1997;3:310–314.
18. Itkin M, Chen EH. Thoracic duct embolization. *Semin Intervent Radiol*. 2011;28:261–266.
19. Miller AC, Harvey JE. Guidelines for the management of spontaneous pneumothorax. Standards of Care Committee, British Thoracic Society. *BMJ*. 1993;307:114–116.

Sleep-Disordered Breathing

Tonya D. Russell

GENERAL PRINCIPLES

Sleep-disordered breathing (SDB) is comprised of multiple different entities:

- Obstructive sleep apnea (OSA)
- Central sleep apnea (CSA)
- Sleep-related hypoventilation of which obesity hypoventilation (OHV) is a common form.

Definitions[1]
- An **apnea** is defined as ≥90% decrease in airflow as measured by an oral–nasal thermal sensor, lasting at least 10 seconds in duration.
- A **hypopnea** is a ≥30% decrease in airflow as measured by nasal pressure lasting at least 10 seconds in duration and associated with a ≥3% desaturation or arousal (Medicare requires a 4% desaturation).
- A **respiratory effort-related arousal** (RERA) is a sequence of breaths lasting at least 10 seconds associated with increased respiratory effort or change in airflow which is associated with an arousal, but does not meet criteria for hypopnea. The scoring of RERAs is optional.
- The **apnea–hypopnea index** (AHI) is the number of apneas and hypopneas per hour of sleep.
- The **respiratory disturbance index** (RDI) is the number of apneas, hypopneas, and RERAs per hour of sleep.
- **Sleep-related hypoventilation** is defined by meeting one of two parameters for ≥10 minutes during sleep:
  - An increase in arterial PCO_2 to >55 mm Hg OR
  - An increase in arterial PCO_2 by ≥10 mm Hg from baseline to a level >50 mm Hg
  - PCO_2 can be arterial, transcutaneous, or end tidal

Classification
- Apneas can be obstructive, central, or mixed in nature.[1]
  - **Obstructive apneas** are associated with continued or increased respiratory effort.
  - **Central apneas** have no respiratory effort. Central apneas can have a Cheyne–Stokes breathing (CSB) pattern if there are ≥3 consecutive central apneas or hypopneas with a crescendo–decrescendo respiratory pattern between the events. The event cycle must be ≥40 seconds and the central apnea–hypopnea index (CAHI) must be ≥5 during at least 2 hours of monitored sleep.

- **Mixed apneas** have no airflow and a lack of respiratory effort during the first part of the event, but resumption of respiratory effort during the latter part of the event.
- Hypopneas can electively be scored as obstructive or central in nature.[1]
  - **Obstructive hypopneas** are scored when any of the following are present during the event: snoring, increased flattening of the nasal pressure, and respiratory effort demonstrating thoracic–abdominal paradox.
  - **Central hypopneas** are scored when all the parameters associated with an obstructive hypopnea are absent during the event.
- Severity of sleep apnea is based on AHI or RDI: normal–AHI/RDI <5, mild–AHI/RDI ≥5 and <15, moderate–AHI/RDI ≥15 and <30, severe–AHI/RDI ≥30.[2]

Epidemiology

- OSA is the most common form of SDB. OSA associated with daytime sleepiness (OSA-hypopnea syndrome) occurs in 2–4% of the general population.[3]
- This percentage likely underestimates current prevalence due to the increasing prevalence of obesity in the United States and the strong association between obesity and OSA.
- Sleep-related hypoventilation can also be associated with multiple different etiologies. The prevalence of OHV in obese patients referred to sleep centers has been reported to be as high as 20%.[4] In patients with a body mass index (BMI) ≥50 who are hospitalized, approximately 50% of patients have evidence of hypoventilation.[5]

Etiology

- OSA occurs due to narrowing of the upper airway either due to excessive soft tissue or structural abnormalities.
- CSA can have a variety of causes including stroke, brain tumor, congestive heart failure, and use of positive airway pressure (PAP) to treat OSA (treatment-emergent CSA).[6]
- Sleep-related hypoventilation can also be due to a variety of causes including morbid obesity, severe OSA, neuromuscular disease with respiratory muscle weakness, thoracic cage abnormality, diaphragmatic paralysis, or severe obstructive lung disease.

Pathophysiology

- In OSA, narrowing of the upper airway leads to recurrent desaturations and/or arousals.
- In CSA, direct effects on the medullary respiratory centers (stroke or brain tumor) can trigger respiratory events. In addition, central apneas may be due to increased sensitivity to small changes in carbon dioxide levels (congestive heart failure and treatment-emergent central apneas).
- In OHV, any of three factors may contribute to the development of hypoventilation: severe OSA, impairment of respiratory mechanics due to morbid obesity, and leptin resistance contributing to decreased ventilatory response.[7]

Risk Factors

- Risk factors for OSA include obesity, macroglossia, micrognathia, retrognathia, neck circumference >17 inches in men and >16 inches in women, enlarged tonsils, increasing age, male gender, postmenopausal state in women, family history, use of alcohol or sedatives, and medical conditions affecting upper airway muscle tone such as hypothyroidism.[8,9]
- Risk factors for CSA include use of PAP (treatment-emergent), heart failure with reduced ejection fraction, stroke, high altitude, and opioid use.[10]
- Risk factors for sleep-related hypoventilation include severe OSA, respiratory muscle weakness, morbid obesity, severe obstructive lung disease, thoracic cage abnormalities, high altitude, and use of respiratory suppressant medications.[11]

Prevention

- OSA: Weight loss, avoidance of alcohol or sedatives, and treatment of underlying medical conditions that affect upper airway muscle tone can help improve or potentially prevent the development of OSA. Weight loss alone may not be sufficient to prevent OSA if there are also craniopharyngeal structural abnormalities present.
- CSA: Medical treatment of reduced ejection fraction, avoiding overtitration of PAP in OSA, and avoiding opioid medications can help improve or prevent the development of CSA.
- Sleep-related hypoventilation: Significant weight loss and avoidance of respiratory suppressant medications may help improve or prevent the development of hypoventilation.

Associated Conditions

- Conditions associated with OSA and OHV include hypertension, atrial fibrillation, coronary artery disease, stroke, diabetes mellitus, metabolic syndrome, and pulmonary hypertension. Patients can also be at increased risk for motor vehicle collisions due to sleepiness.[7,12,13]
- Conditions associated with CSA include congestive heart failure and stroke, although CSA is less common than OSA in patients recovering from stroke.[14,15]

DIAGNOSIS

Clinical Presentation

History

When obtaining the history, the presence or absence of the following symptoms should be elicited: daytime sleepiness, unrefreshing sleep, witnessed apneas, awakening gasping, loud snoring, morning headaches, nocturia, and decreased ability to concentrate.

Physical Examination

- The physical examination to evaluate for OSA focuses on the upper airway. The presence or absence of the following features should be ascertained: obesity, macroglossia, micrognathia, retrognathia, neck circumference (>17 inches in men and >16 inches in women), enlarged tonsils, and crowded posterior oropharynx.

Diagnosis

- Physical examination findings that would elicit concern for CSA include those associated with underlying medical conditions that predispose to CSA, such as congestive heart failure or stroke.
- The physical examination for OHV should focus on many of the same areas as for OSA and include morbid obesity. In addition, examination findings related to complications from OHV, such as right heart failure may be present.

Diagnostic Criteria

- OSA as defined by the International Classification of Sleep Disorders requires the presence of obstructive events associated with either an AHI/RDI ≥15 or an AHI/RDI ≥5 along with symptoms (daytime sleepiness, fatigue, insomnia, awakening gasping, persistent snoring, or witnessed apneas).[16]
- CSA as defined by the International Classification of Sleep Disorders requires ≥5 central events per hour of sleep (with the CAHI representing >50% of total AHI) associated with symptoms (daytime sleepiness, disrupted sleep, awakening short of breath, or witnessed apneas). CSB may or may not be present with CSA. In order to diagnose CSB, the respiratory criteria as previously defined must be met along with the presence of symptoms as above or an associated medical condition (atrial flutter, congestive heart failure, or neurologic condition).[16]
- OHV as defined by the International Classification of Sleep Disorders[16] must meet all the following criteria: BMI >30, daytime hypoventilation with $PaCO_2$ ≥45 mm Hg, and no other cause for the hypoventilation. OHV can be diagnosed based off awake criteria, but ideally polysomnogram (PSG) should be performed to assess the contribution of OSA and to monitor transcutaneous CO_2 levels.

Differential Diagnosis

- OSA, CSA, and OHV can present with similar symptoms although CSA is not typically associated with snoring. Therefore, any of the forms of SDB are in the differential diagnosis for patients presenting with daytime sleepiness, fatigue, disrupted sleep, and awakening with shortness of breath.
- Consider other causes of daytime sleepiness: periodic limb movement disorder, narcolepsy, and idiopathic hypersomnia.

Diagnostic Testing

Laboratories

- Thyroid-stimulating hormone should be measured when hypothyroidism suspected.
- Serum bicarbonate ≥27 mEq/L should raise concern for hypoventilation.[17] Arterial blood gas (ABG) should be done to confirm $PaCO_2$ if serum bicarbonate is elevated or hypoventilation is suspected.

Diagnostic Procedures

- **PSG: Split-night PSG** involves the first 2 hours of sleep being recorded to determine severity of underlying SDB. PAP is initiated if prespecified AHI criteria are met after 2 hours of sleep is obtained, and at least 3 hours of time is left for PAP titration.[2] **All-night polysomnogram (ANPSG)** is performed if SDB

is mild to moderate during baseline to allow determination of severity of SDB in different stages of sleep and sleeping positions. **PAP titration** is performed if the diagnosis of SDB is already made.
- **Home sleep apnea testing (HSAT)** can be used in patients in which there is a high suspicion for moderate to severe OSA. It should not be used in patients in whom there is concern for CSA or hypoventilation.[2]

TREATMENT
Medications
- Modafinil and armodafinil are approved for patients with OSA and residual sleepiness despite adequate use of continuous positive airway pressure (CPAP).[18] Proper adherence to and functioning of PAP therapy should be ascertained before starting mediation. Side effects from these medications include headache, nervousness/anxiety, dizziness, and nausea. Rare severe dermatologic and systemic hypersensitivity reactions have been reported. Lower doses should be used in the elderly. These medications can decrease the effectiveness of hormonal contraceptives. These medications are not recommended for use in pregnancy due to animal models demonstrating developmental toxicity. Women of childbearing age should be warned of these risks before starting on these medications and should be advised to use birth control other than hormonal contraceptives.[19,20]
- In CSA, medical therapy for congestive heart failure should be provided if present.

Nonpharmacologic Therapies
- OSA
  - PAP should be used in patients with significant OSA associated either with symptoms impairing quality of life or hypertension. **Auto-titrating positive airway pressure (APAP)** can be implemented without a PAP titration study in patients without significant comorbid conditions.[21]
  - Positional therapy can be used if respiratory events occur mainly in supine position (sleep belt or sleep shirt).
  - Oral appliances are an option for patients who have mild OSA or are intolerant of PAP. A custom, titratable device should be made by a qualified dentist. Ideally, a repeat sleep study should be performed with the device in place to determine efficacy as oral appliances are less effective in treating OSA than PAP.[22]
  - Hypoglossal nerve stimulation can significantly improve AHI. It is an option for patients with moderate to severe OSA who are intolerant of PAP.[23]
- CSA
  - CPAP should be tried as first-line therapy for CSA in the setting of congestive heart failure. Bilevel positive airway pressure (BiPAP) with a backup rate may be used for central apneas not responsive to CPAP.[4]
  - Adaptive/auto-servo ventilation (ASV) may also be used in the setting of CSA. The device is equipped with an algorithm for titrating inspiratory positive airway pressure (IPAP) to help stabilize significant respiratory variations that can occur in CSA. However, ASV should not be used in patients with an ejection fraction <45% due to increased mortality in this patient population when using ASV.[4,24,25]

- OHV
  - CPAP should be used as the initial treatment in patients with OHV who also have severe OSA. Hospitalized patients who have evidence of OHV should be initiated on noninvasive ventilation prior to discharge with expedited outpatient sleep study for confirmation of diagnosis and PAP titration.[5]
  - Nocturnal ventilation via tracheostomy may be necessary if no optimal setting can be found for noninvasive ventilation or if a patient cannot tolerate noninvasive ventilation.

Lifestyle/Risk Modification

- Lifestyle modification emphasizing weight loss, and avoidance of alcohol and sedatives which may decrease upper airway muscle tone, can be beneficial in OSA/OHV.
- Avoidance of medications that act as respiratory suppressants can also be beneficial in CSA and other forms of sleep related hypoventilation.

REFERENCES

1. American Academy of Sleep Medicine. *The AASM Manual for the Scoring of Sleep and Associated Events: Rules, Terminology, and Technical Specifications, Version 3*. American Academy of Sleep Medicine; 2023.
2. Kapur VK, Auckley DH, Chowdhuri S, et al. Clinical practice guidelines for diagnostic testing for adult obstructive sleep apnea: an American Academy of Sleep Medicine clinical practice guideline. *J Clin Sleep Med*. 2017;13:479–504.
3. Senaratna CV, Perret JL, Lodge CJ, et al. Prevalence of obstructive sleep apnea in the general population: a systematic review. *Sleep Med Rev*. 2017;34:70–81.
4. Mokhlesi B, Masa JF, Brozek JL, et al. Evaluation and management of obesity hypoventilation syndrome: an Official American Thoracic Society Clinical Practice Guideline. *Am J Respir Crit Care Med*. 2019;200:e6–e24.
5. Nowbar S, Burkart KM, Gonzales R, et al. Obesity-associated hypoventilation in hospitalized patients: prevalence, effects, and outcome. *Am J Med*. 2004;116:1–7.
6. Aurora RN, Chowdhuri S, Ramar K, et al. The treatment of central sleep apnea syndromes in adults: practice parameters with an evidence-based literature review and meta-analyses. *Sleep*. 2012;35:17–40.
7. Masa JF, Pépin JL, Borel JC, Mokhlesi B, Murphy PB, Sánchez-Quiroga MÁ. Obesity hypoventilation syndrome. *Eur Respir Rev*. 2019;28(151):180097.
8. Gottlieb DJ, Punjabi NM. Diagnosis and management of obstructive sleep apnea: a review. *JAMA*. 2020;323:1389–1400.
9. Epstein LJ, Kristo D, Strollo PJ Jr, et al. Clinical guideline for the evaluation, management and long-term care of obstructive sleep apnea in adults. *J Clin Sleep Med*. 2009;5:263–276.
10. Randerath W, Verbraecken J, Andreas S, et al. Definition, discrimination, diagnosis, and treatment of central breathing disturbances during sleep. *Eur Respir J*. 2017;49:1600959.
11. Böing S, Randerath WJ. Chronic hypoventilation syndromes and sleep-related hypoventilation. *J Thoracic Dis*. 2015;7:1273–1285.
12. Knauert M, Naik S, Gillespie MB, Kryger M. Clinical consequences and economic costs of untreated obstructive sleep apnea syndrome. *World J Otorhinolaryngol Head Neck Surg*. 2015;1:17–27.
13. Jennum P, Ibsen R, Kjellberg J. Morbidity prior to a diagnosis of sleep-disordered breathing: a controlled national study. *J Clin Sleep Med*. 2013;9:103–108.
14. Constanzo MR, Khayat R, Ponikowski P, et al. Mechanisms and clinical consequences of untreated central sleep apnea in heart failure. *J Am Coll Cardiol*. 2015;65:72–84.

15. Schütz SG, Lisabeth LD, Hsu CW, Kim S, Chervin RD, Brown DL. Central sleep apnea is uncommon after stroke. *Sleep Med.* 2021;77:304–306.
16. American Academy of Sleep Medicine. *International Classification of Sleep Disorders.* 3rd edition, text revision. American Academy of Sleep Medicine; 2023.
17. Macavei VM, Spurling KJ, Loft J, Makker HK. Diagnostic predictors of obesity-hypoventilation syndrome in patients suspected of having sleep disordered breathing. *J Clin Sleep Med.* 2013;9:879–884.
18. Sukhal S, Khalid M, Tulaimat A. Effect of wakefulness-promoting agents on sleepiness in patients with sleep apnea treated with CPAP: a meta-analysis. *J Clin Sleep Med.* 2015; 11:1179–1186.
19. Robertson P Jr, Hellriegel ET, Arora S, Nelson M. Effect of modafinil on the pharmacokinetics of ethinyl estradiol and triazolam in healthy volunteers. *Clin Pharmacol Ther.* 2002;71:46–56.
20. Krystal A, Attarian H. Sleep medications and women: a review of issues to consider for optimizing the care of women with sleep disorders. *Curr Sleep Medicine Rep.* 2016; 2:218–222.
21. Patil SP, Ayappa IA, Caples SM, Kimoff RJ, Patel SR, Harrod CG. Treatment of adult obstructive sleep apnea with positive airway pressure: an American Academy of Sleep Medicine Clinical Practice Guideline. *J Clin Sleep Med.* 2019;15:335–343.
22. Ramar K, Dort LC, Katz SG, et al. Clinical practice guideline for the treatment of obstructive sleep apnea and snoring with oral appliance therapy: an update for 2015. *J Clin Sleep Med.* 2015;11:773–827.
23. Strollo PJ, Soose RJ, Maurer JT, et al. Upper-airway stimulation for obstructive sleep apnea. *NEJM.* 2014;370:139–149.
24. Aurora RN, Bista SR, Casey KR, et al. Updated adaptive servo-ventilation recommendations for the 2012 AASM guideline: "the treatment of central sleep apnea syndromes in adults: practice parameters with an evidence-based literature review and meta-analyses." *J Clin Sleep Med.* 2016:12:757–761.
25. Cowie MR, Woehrle H, Wegscheider K, et al. Adaptive servo-ventilation for central sleep apnea in systolic heart failure. *NEJM.* 2015;373:1095–1105.

Interstitial Lung Disease

24

Andrew Peters and
Mary Clare McGregor

GENERAL PRINCIPLES

Classification and Epidemiology

- Interstitial lung disease (ILD) describes a heterogeneous group of over 200 diseases affecting the pulmonary interstitium with varying degrees of involvement of the pleural space, airways, and pulmonary vasculature.[1]
- The estimated prevalence of ILD in the US is approximately 180 per 100,000 males and 220 per 100,000 females.[2]
- Various subgroups of ILD have been described including idiopathic interstitial pneumonias (IIP), connective tissue disease (CTD)-related ILD, hypersensitivity pneumonitis (HP), pneumoconioses, and more. However, there is currently no universal classification system that encompasses all ILDs.
- One classification scheme based loosely on etiology and disease association is presented in Table 24-1[3,4]; note that this table is not comprehensive, and the categories will likely change in both terminology and concept over time as we learn more about these diseases.

TABLE 24-1 CLASSIFICATION OF INTERSTITIAL LUNG DISEASES

A. Known etiologies

Connective tissue disease	Scleroderma
	Rheumatoid arthritis
	Polymyositis/dermatomyositis
	Antisynthetase syndrome
	Sjögren syndrome
Vasculitis	Granulomatosis with polyangiitis (GPA)
	Eosinophilic granulomatosis with polyangiitis (EGPA)
	Microscopic polyangiitis
	Goodpasture syndrome[a]
Pneumoconioses	Asbestosis
	Coal worker's pneumoconiosis
	Silicosis
	Berylliosis
	Many others

(*continued*)

TABLE 24-1 CLASSIFICATION OF INTERSTITIAL LUNG DISEASES (Continued)

Hypersensitivity pneumonitis	Bird fancier's lung (pigeons, parakeets, others) Farmer's lung (moldy hay) Hot tub lung Many others
Drug induced	Chemotherapeutic agents (bleomycin, methotrexate, busulfan, others) Amiodarone Nitrofurantoin Many others
B. Unknown etiologies	
Major idiopathic interstitial pneumonias (IIPs)	Idiopathic pulmonary fibrosis (IPF) Idiopathic nonspecific interstitial pneumonia (NSIP) Cryptogenic organizing pneumonia (COPD) Acute interstitial pneumonia (AIP) Respiratory bronchiolitis-interstitial lung disease (RB-ILD)[a] Desquamative interstitial pneumonia (DIP)[a]
Rare IIPs	Idiopathic lymphoid interstitial pneumonia (LIP) Idiopathic pleuroparenchymal fibroelastosis (PPFE)
Unclassifiable IIPs	
Others	Interstitial pneumonia with autoimmune features (IPAF) Familial pulmonary fibrosis Sarcoidosis Lymphangioleiomyomatosis (LAM) Pulmonary Langerhans cell histiocytosis (PLCH)[a] Pulmonary alveolar proteinosis (PAP)[a] Acute eosinophilic pneumonia[a] Chronic eosinophilic pneumonia Pulmonary alveolar microlithiasis Combined pulmonary fibrosis and emphysema (CPFE)[a]
C. Hereditary diseases with diffuse lung involvement	Tuberous sclerosis Neurofibromatosis Hermansky–Pudlak syndrome Gaucher disease Niemann–Pick disease

[a]These diseases are strongly but not exclusively associated with tobacco smoking.

- Since ILDs differ greatly in presentation, clinical course, and response to therapy, establishing an accurate diagnosis is essential for determining the optimal management strategy.

Etiology and Pathogenesis
- As above, ILD encompasses numerous diseases, which have varying pathophysiology.
- In general, environmental and heritable factors play a role in the pathogenesis of many ILDs, with numerous environmental exposures and genetic modifiers of disease susceptibility having been elucidated, but the complex interactions between these factors and disease development remain poorly understood.
- Alveolar epithelial cell injury is a hallmark of ILD. The source of injury may be extrinsic, as in cases of HP, pneumoconiosis, or radiation pneumonitis; alternatively, the insult may arrive via the circulation, as suspected in CTD, vasculitis, or drug-induced lung disease.
- In particular, recurrent or persistent lung injury from various mechanisms appears to provoke a maladaptive tissue repair response which leads to disruption of lung architecture and function, manifesting on tissue biopsy as inflammation and/or fibrosis.[5]
- Short telomere length is known to be associated with idiopathic pulmonary fibrosis (IPF) and possibly some other fibrotic ILDs; these may implicate accelerated cellular aging and stem cell exhaustion as mechanisms of disease in some ILDs.[6]

DIAGNOSIS
Overview of Diagnosis
- Establishing an accurate diagnosis in ILD is a complex process that requires expertise in integration of clinical, physiologic, laboratory, radiographic, and histopathologic data.
- **Expert multidisciplinary discussion** (MDD) by a specialist team including pulmonologists, thoracic surgeons, radiologists, and pathologists has become the gold standard for ILD diagnosis, rather than histopathology or any other single test.
- Accordingly, clinicians encountering suspected ILD in a community setting should strongly consider referral to a tertiary center where ILD MDD is available.
- An algorithm illustrating general principles in the evaluation of ILD is presented in Figure 24-1.[7,8]

Clinical Presentation
History
- A comprehensive history will often guide or narrow the differential diagnosis in ILD.
- **Exertional dyspnea** is the most common presenting symptom, though breathlessness can also occur at rest in severe disease. The time course of dyspnea is variable: some ILDs present with rapid onset of symptoms (e.g., acute interstitial pneumonia [AIP], acute eosinophilic pneumonia [AEP]), while others are slow and insidious over months to years (e.g., IPF, nonspecific interstitial pneumonia [NSIP], sarcoidosis) or waxing and waning (e.g., HP if the inciting exposure is intermittent).[1]

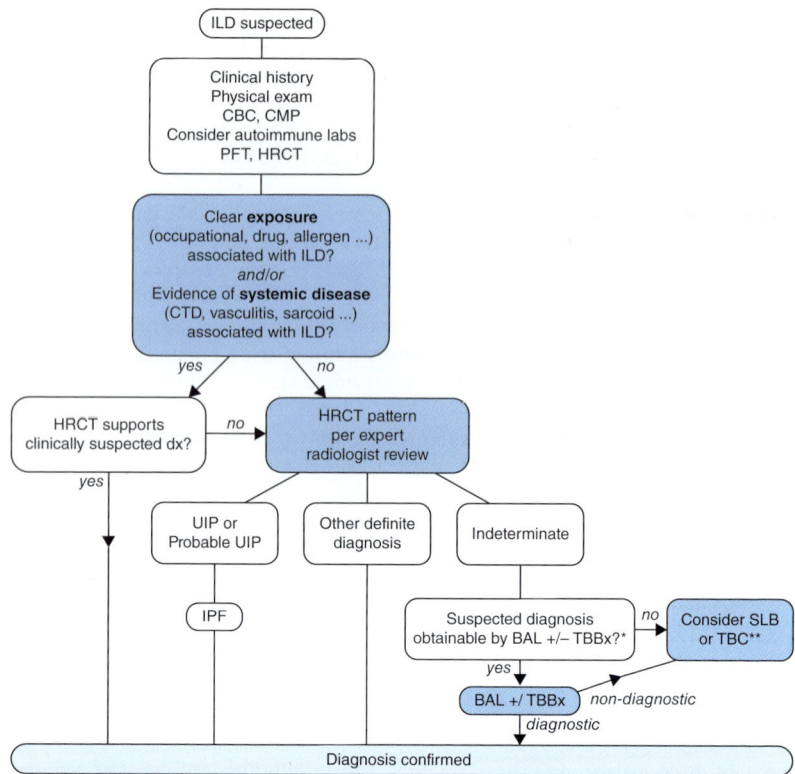

Figure 24-1 Evaluation of suspected interstitial lung disease. Examples of suggested autoimmune laboratory testing, and of diagnoses obtainable by bronchoalveolar lavage and/or transbronchial biopsy, are detailed further in the text.

- **Cough,** typically nonproductive, is a frequent complaint.
- **Wheezing** is infrequent; when present, it may suggest an ILD involving the airways (e.g., HP, Respiratory bronchiolitis-interstitial lung disease [RB-ILD], sarcoidosis) or a comorbid non-ILD airways disease (e.g., chronic bronchitis or asthma).
- **Hemoptysis** is infrequent but can occur in ILDs associated with vasculitis, CTD, and/or diffuse alveolar hemorrhage (including Goodpasture syndrome, microscopic polyangiitis, and granulomatosis with polyangiitis [GPA]).[9]
- **Chest pain** is unusual.
  ○ When present it may suggest diseases with pleural inflammation (e.g., systemic lupus erythematosus [SLE], rheumatoid arthritis), pneumothorax

(lymphangioleiomyomatosis [LAM], Pulmonary Langerhans cell histiocytosis [PLCH]), or sarcoidosis.
- Coronary artery disease may go overlooked in patients with advanced lung disease and limited functional capacity and should be considered especially in the presence of atherosclerotic cardiovascular disease risk factors.
- **Symptoms of CTD** (e.g., inflammatory arthritis, muscle weakness, Raynaud phenomenon, rash, dysphagia, and sicca) should be reviewed in all patients presenting with ILD.
- **Constitutional symptoms** such as fevers, chills, weight loss, night sweats, and fatigue occur with variable frequency. Unintentional weight loss may be caused by advanced lung disease itself ("pulmonary cachexia") but should also raise concern for malignancy; certain ILDs are associated with increased risk of lung malignancies including IPF, lymphoid interstitial pneumonia (LIP), and asbestosis.
- Some ILDs have strong **age and demographic** associations: for example, LAM is almost exclusive to young women; CTD-related ILD has a mild female predominance and typically presents in the third to fifth decades of life; and IPF is more common in elderly males.
- **Past and current medical histories** may reveal systemic conditions associated with ILD including CTD, vasculitis, and other autoimmune diseases (Table 24-1).
- **Social history** should be reviewed with particular attention to inhaled substances and occupational/environmental exposures.
  - Cigarette smoking has an integral causal relationship with diseases including RB-ILD, desquamative interstitial pneumonia (DIP), and PLCH.[10]
  - Other inhaled recreational drugs have also been implicated in ILD.
  - A thorough occupational history over the patient's entire lifetime should be reviewed, since the time between exposure and disease onset may span many years.
  - Nonoccupational environmental exposures including pets, hobbies, and recreational activities should also be elicited.
  - Finally, a detailed travel and residential history should be obtained.
- **Family history** may prompt diagnosis of heritable ILDs such as familial pulmonary fibrosis (FPF), Hermansky–Pudlak syndrome, and lysosomal storage disorders.
- **Therapeutic agent history** may reveal exposures associated with ILD.
  - This includes not only prescription drugs, but also over-the-counter medications, herbal supplements, radiation therapy, and other forms of medical therapy.
  - ILD may develop years after the initial exposure, so review of previous treatments is important, not just a current medication list.

Physical Examination

- **Pulmonary** examination in fibrotic ILDs is classically characterized by bilateral fine inspiratory crackles. Digital clubbing may be present.
- **Cardiovascular** examination in advanced disease may reveal signs of pulmonary hypertension and cor pulmonale including elevated jugular venous pressure, hepatojugular reflux, accentuated second heart sound, and pitting edema.

- The remainder of the multi-system physical exam should be conducted with attention to findings of systemic diseases associated with ILD, particularly **CTDs, sarcoidosis, and vasculitis**.[1] Examples of pertinent findings include episcleritis, lymphadenopathy, hepatosplenomegaly, synovitis, joint deformities, muscle weakness, peripheral neuropathy, sclerodactyly, and various rashes.

Diagnostic Testing

Laboratory Testing
- Laboratory testing for ILDs should be directed by history and physical examination findings.
- **General testing** should include complete blood count with differential, renal and liver chemistries.
- **Testing for autoimmune diseases** is recommended during the initial evaluation of ILD without otherwise apparent etiology, even without overt extrapulmonary CTD symptoms. This may include[11]:
  ○ Antinuclear antibodies (ANA) and extractable nuclear antigens (ENA)
  ○ Rheumatoid factor (RF) and anticyclic citrullinated peptide antibodies (anti-CCP)
  ○ Creatine kinase (CK), aldolase, and myositis panel
  ○ Scl-70 and anticentromere antibodies
  ○ Double-stranded DNA antibodies
  ○ Antineutrophil cytoplasmic antibodies and urinalysis (to evaluate for vasculitis)
- We do **not** recommend routine use of the following tests:
  ○ Angiotensin-converting enzyme (ACE) levels have both poor sensitivity and specificity for the diagnosis of sarcoidosis.
  ○ Serum tests for antibodies against various allergens ("HP panels") provide only evidence of exposure, not causation; the presence of specific circulating antibodies does not confirm that the exposure is responsible for the disease. Furthermore, commercially available panels often test for common environmental antigens rather than novel or rare exposures.

Physiologic Testing
- **Pulmonary function tests** (PFTs) in ILDs most commonly show a restrictive pattern, but this finding alone is not sensitive or specific for ILD.[8]
- A mixed obstructive-restrictive or predominantly obstructive pattern may narrow the differential diagnosis toward ILDs with small airways involvement including sarcoidosis, HP, and smoking-related ILDs (PLCH, RB-ILD, DIP).[9]
- Normal or relatively preserved lung volumes and spirometry are seen in combined pulmonary fibrosis and emphysema (CPFE).
- Diffusion capacity for carbon monoxide (DLCO) is reduced in almost all forms of ILD.
- PFTs are the most commonly used tool to monitor disease progression in ILD and are routinely obtained at both the initial presentation and regular follow-up intervals.
- The **6-minute walk test with oxygen assessment** is also valuable as a measurement of exercise capacity, disease progression, and/or response to therapy.

Imaging

Chest Radiography
- CXR is often the initial test to reveal ILD, but rarely confirms a specific diagnosis.
- Radiographic findings of ILD are often incidental, and sometimes predate clinical presentation by many years; thus, reviewing old films may shed light on the disease course.
- The prototypical CXR finding of fibrotic ILDs is the presence of coarse interstitial (reticular) markings, but numerous other patterns can appear, all of which are better characterized on high-resolution computed tomography (HRCT) as discussed further below.
- Some CXR findings that may guide the initial ILD differential diagnosis include:
- **Distribution of disease**
    - Upper-zone predominant diseases include sarcoidosis, silicosis, and PLCH; upper-zone predominance can also be suggestive of HP but is not always present.
    - Lower-zone predominant diseases include asbestosis, IPF/usual interstitial pneumonia (UIP), DIP, NSIP, scleroderma, and chronic aspiration.
    - Peripheral predominant diseases include COP and chronic eosinophilic pneumonia (CEP).
- **Pleural disease** is found in relatively few ILDs including CTD (effusion and/or thickening), asbestosis (plaques and/or calcifications), and LAM (pneumothorax and chylous effusions).
- **Volume loss** is seen in IPF and other fibrotic ILDs, while **preserved or large lung volumes** are seen in a narrower set of diseases including LAM, PLCH, and CPFE.
- Some ILDs are notable for discordance between radiographic findings and clinical severity. For example, patients with IPF may have severe symptoms despite relatively mild radiographic fibrosis, while patients with sarcoidosis and pneumoconiosis may be asymptomatic despite marked radiographic abnormalities.

High-Resolution Computed Tomography
- High-resolution chest CT is perhaps the single most powerful tool in the modern evaluation of ILD; in many cases, its accuracy has replaced the need for tissue biopsy.
- However, an important caveat is that most evidence for the high accuracy of HRCT in ILD diagnosis comes from experienced thoracic radiologists at academic centers and may not be achievable in community settings where this resource is not available.
- Phenomena described on HRCT in ILD may include (far from an exhaustive list)[1]:
    - **Honeycombing** represents end-stage fibrosis that can occur in multiple types of ILD including IPF, HP, sarcoidosis, and scleroderma.
    - **Ground-glass opacities** are also found in numerous ILD types including NSIP, HP, AIP, pulmonary alveolar proteinosis (PAP), and eosinophilic pneumonias.
    - **Nodules** may occur in conditions including vasculitis, sarcoidosis, pneumoconiosis, rheumatoid arthritis, and malignancy.[9]

- **Cysts** are a distinctive feature of several diseases including LAM, PLCH, LIP, and DIP.
- **"Crazy paving,"** which refers to superimposed ground-glass opacities and interlobular septal thickening, is classically associated with PAP but can also be seen in other conditions including AIP and Goodpasture syndrome.[12]
- Some characteristic HRCT findings of selected ILDs are described further at the end of this section.
- HRCTs should also be carefully reviewed for coexisting thoracic pathology such as lung cancer, right ventricular and/or pulmonary artery enlargement (which can be seen in ILD-related pulmonary hypertension), and esophagogastric abnormalities (systemic sclerosis and/or chronic aspiration).
- Though patients with ILD often undergo multiple HRCTs over time in response to clinical changes, the routine use of serial HRCT as a tool for monitoring disease progression is not recommended.

Lung Sampling
Overview
- For the vast majority of patients with ILD, HRCT and other noninvasive studies plus expert MDD are sufficient to establish a diagnosis; tissue sampling is reserved for selected patients, with the exact indications remaining controversial.
- In general, invasive sampling is appropriate when a suspected diagnosis is amenable to confirmation by the proposed sampling technique and/or the diagnosis is truly indeterminate, the patient is fit to tolerate the procedure, and the result would alter management.

Bronchoalveolar Lavage
- Bronchoalveolar lavage (BAL) samples bronchial and alveolar epithelial secretions by instilling sterile saline into the distal lung units and retrieving the fluid for analysis including cell count and differential, microbiologic studies, and histopathology.
- BAL is performed via fiberoptic bronchoscopy (FOB), and the target site is usually guided by HRCT.
- ILDs that can be diagnosed definitively by BAL include eosinophilic pneumonias (>25% eosinophils), PAP (milky white fluid with positive periodic acid-Schiff staining), and pneumoconioses (asbestos or silica in fluid).[12,13]
- Lymphocyte predominance in BAL fluid is a nonspecific finding but can shift the differential diagnosis toward certain entities including HP, sarcoidosis, NSIP, organizing pneumonia (OP), and drug-induced ILD.[13]
- BAL can also be useful to exclude infectious processes from the differential diagnosis.

Transbronchial Forceps Biopsy
- Traditional transbronchial lung biopsy (TBBx) is performed by the use of flexible forceps inserted via bronchoscopy to obtain small samples of peripheral lung tissue.
- Though still fairly safe, risks of pneumothorax and bleeding are higher with TBBx than with FOB/BAL alone and may preclude safe TBBx in patients with significant hypoxemia and/or coagulopathy.

- ILDs amenable to diagnosis by TBBx include sarcoidosis, berylliosis, PAP, and lymphangitic carcinomatosis.[8]
- The major limitation of TBBx is the small size of the biopsy specimens, which cannot adequately capture the patchy and heterogeneous pathology that characterizes many ILDs.
- In particular, TBBx cannot be used to diagnose IPF and most other IIPs; interstitial fibrosis when noted on TBBx specimens is nonspecific and not distinguishable between different types of fibrotic ILD.

Surgical Lung Biopsy
- Surgical lung biopsy (SLB) is considered when noninvasive diagnostics remain indeterminate and tissue confirmation of a specific ILD diagnosis would alter management.
- When feasible, video-assisted thoracoscopic surgery (VATS) is preferable over an open thoracotomy approach, as the former results in similar diagnostic yield with less morbidity and shorter hospital stays.
- As with BAL and TBBx, SLB should be guided by HRCT to target areas of the lung with abnormal findings. Diagnostic yield is further improved by selecting areas of active disease with relatively preserved lung architecture (rather than dense fibrosis or honeycombing), by sampling more than one lobe of the lung, and by obtaining specimens >2 cm in diameter.[14]
- Relative contraindications to SLB include end-stage disease with honeycombing, major cardiovascular disease, advanced age, and severe hypoxemia.
- Notably, SLB can sometimes provoke a postoperative ILD exacerbation, which must be weighed in the risk/benefit consideration of whether to pursue the surgery.

Transbronchial Cryobiopsy
- Transbronchial cryobiopsy (TBC) is a newer bronchoscopic technique in which an area of peripheral lung is rapidly frozen using a flexible cryoprobe and then extracted.[15]
- This provides larger and more architecturally intact biopsy specimens than those obtained by TBBx, which can be sufficient to confirm diagnoses of IPF and other IIPs.[7]
- Both diagnostic yield and risk/morbidity of TBC are greater than that of TBBx, but less than SLB.
- Head-to-head evidence comparing TBC with SLB is lacking; some experts now prefer TBC, but this is controversial.
- Currently, SLB remains the gold standard for tissue sampling in ILD, but TBC is likely a reasonable alternative for selected patients at high-volume centers with expertise in the procedure.

Diagnostic Features of Selected Diseases
A full review of each condition under the umbrella of ILD is beyond the scope of this chapter, but several diagnostic entities of particular interest are highlighted below.

Idiopathic Pulmonary Fibrosis
- Most common form of ILD, comprising 25–35% of all patients with ILD; typically affects patients over 60 years old and has a strong male predominance.

- Has a relentlessly progressive course; median survival is 2–5 years after diagnosis.
- IPF is defined by radiographic and/or histopathologic evidence of usual UIP without an apparent underlying cause such as CTD or drug exposure.[16]
- Histopathologic features of UIP include patchy dense fibrosis with architectural distortion, predominance of subpleural and paraseptal involvement, fibroblastic foci, and the absence of incongruous features such as granulomas, OP, and hyaline membranes.
- HRCT features of UIP include honeycombing with or without traction bronchiectasis, irregular interlobular septal thickening, and reticular opacities, in a subpleural and basilar predominant distribution.
- The finding of a UIP pattern on HRCT has high concordance with UIP on histopathology. Accordingly, when the HRCT result is classified by an experienced radiologist as "definite" or "probable" UIP and alternate causes have been excluded, a lung biopsy is unnecessary; if the HRCT pattern is indeterminate, SLB or TBC can be considered.[16]
- Last, a genomic classifier assay to predict UIP using TBBx samples (which otherwise cannot be used to diagnose UIP via conventional histopathology) is now available.
  - The test is fairly specific (92%), but not sensitive (68%), for histologic UIP.[7]
  - There are currently no guidelines regarding use of the genomic classifier. We suggest it may be useful in settings where TBBx but not SLB/TBC is feasible; where expert pathologist and/or radiologist review is unavailable; and/or where diagnosis remains indeterminate despite conventional testing.

Nonspecific Interstitial Pneumonia
- NSIP is a common radiographic and histopathologic pattern of ILD that is often associated with CTD but can also result from other underlying conditions or exposures or be idiopathic.
- HRCT features include relatively symmetric and bilateral ground-glass opacities, subpleural sparing, fine reticulations, traction bronchiectasis, and volume loss.
- Two subtypes have been described, **cellular** (characterized by predominance of inflammatory infiltrate and little or no fibrosis) and **fibrotic**; the cellular type has a better prognosis and is more apt to respond to immunosuppressive therapy.[17]

Organizing Pneumonia
- OP is a nonspecific pattern of alveolar inflammation that occurs as a result of diverse insults including bacterial or viral pneumonia, drugs, inhalational injury, and autoimmune disease. Idiopathic OP is termed cryptogenic organizing pneumonia (COP).
- COP classically presents similarly to infectious pneumonia but does not improve with antibiotics.
- HRCT findings include patchy ground-glass or consolidative opacities with a subpleural and/or peribronchovascular distribution.
- Histopathologic findings include patchy interstitial inflammation without fibrosis but with collagenous granulation tissue in both the alveolar lumens and distal small airways (hence the condition's former name "bronchiolitis obliterans organizing pneumonia").

Hypersensitivity Pneumonitis
- Also known as **extrinsic allergic alveolitis,** HP is an inflammatory immune-mediated process caused by repeated inhalation of an inciting agent in a sensitized host.
- Antigens known to provoke HP include avian proteins ("bird fancier's lung") and nontuberculous mycobacteria encountered in hot tubs ("hot tub lung"), but there are hundreds of other documented causes; in many cases a culprit exposure is never identified.
- HRCT features are variable but include bilateral ground-glass opacity, mosaic attenuation, centrilobular nodules, and air trapping; distribution may be diffuse or mildly upper-zone predominant; fibrosis may or may not be present.[18]
- HP was historically classified as "acute" or "chronic" according to the tempo of disease but is now classified by **fibrotic** and **nonfibrotic** phenotypes on HRCT.

Combined Pulmonary Fibrosis and Emphysema
- CPFE refers to the presence of both interstitial fibrosis of any type—most commonly UIP, but not exclusively—and significant emphysema.[19]
- It remains unclear whether CPFE represents a truly distinct syndrome, or two separate concurrent disease processes (fibrotic ILD plus emphysema).
- CPFE is associated with high rates of lung cancer and pulmonary hypertension, often seemingly disproportionate to the extent of fibrosis and emphysema.
- On PFT, spirometry and lung volumes may be normal or relatively preserved because the effects of fibrosis and emphysema on these parameters "cancel out," but DLCO will be markedly reduced.
- Consequently, unlike other fibrotic ILDs, spirometry and lung volumes are not reliable measures of disease severity or progression in CPFE.

Progressive Pulmonary Fibrosis
- Progressive pulmonary fibrosis (PPF) is not a single disease, but a syndrome that can occur in many different types of ILD.
- This recently defined entity captures the observation that a subset of patients across a wide variety of underlying ILD types (i.e., HP and NSIP) share a clinically similar phenotype of progressively worsening fibrosis.
- PPF is defined as any non-IPF ILD with radiology evidence of pulmonary fibrosis meeting at least two of the following three criteria over the course of 1 year[7]:
  - Worsening respiratory symptoms
  - Decline in forced vital capacity (FVC) by ≥5% predicted and/or DLCO by ≥10% predicted
  - Progression of fibrosis by HRCT

Connective Tissue Disease-Related Interstitial Lung Disease and Interstitial Pneumonia with Autoimmune Features
- CTD-ILD is a general term encompassing any ILD secondary to a CTD; the CTD most commonly associated with ILD is systemic sclerosis, followed by rheumatoid arthritis and inflammatory myopathies, but essentially all CTDs confer some risk of ILD.[11]
- CTD-ILD can manifest in diverse radiographic and histopathologic patterns including NSIP (most common overall), UIP (relatively associated with rheumatoid arthritis), OP, and more. Pleural, airway, and pulmonary vascular

involvement (i.e., pulmonary arterial hypertension) also occur to varying degrees depending on the underlying CTD type.
- In some cases, ILD is the earliest or only manifestation of a CTD, with extrapulmonary symptoms being subtle or absent at the time of diagnosis.
- Recently, the category "interstitial pneumonia with autoimmune features" has been introduced to describe patients who have ILD plus findings suggestive of a systemic autoimmune process, but do not meet criteria for a defined CTD syndrome.
- The classification criteria for IPAF require at least one element from at least two of three domains, which are reproduced in part here[20]:
  - Clinical: signs/symptoms including digital fissuring, digital ulcerations, inflammatory arthritis, palmar telangiectasia, Raynaud phenomenon, digital edema, and rash on the digital extensor surfaces.
  - Serologic: ANA titer ≥1:320; RF greater than twice the upper limit of normal; abnormal autoantibodies including CCP, dsDNA, SS-A, SS-B, RNP, Smith, Scl-70, Jo-1, MDA-5.
  - Morphologic: HRCT and/or biopsy evidence of NSIP, OP, or LIP; or unexplained pleural, pericardial, airways, or pulmonary vascular disease.

Eosinophilic Pneumonias
- AEP is characterized by acute presentation with severe hypoxemia and diffuse radiographic infiltrates that improve dramatically in response to corticosteroids.
- CEP is a slow and progressive disease with distinctive HRCT findings of bilateral ground-glass and/or consolidative opacities in a "reverse bat wing" (peripheral and upper-zone predominant) distribution.
- In both AEP and CEP, diagnosis is confirmed by an elevated eosinophil percentage in BAL fluid (>25%); peripheral blood eosinophil count is often normal.

Sarcoid Interstitial Lung Disease
- Sarcoidosis is a systemic inflammatory granulomatous disease with diverse manifestations in multiple organ systems, one of which can be ILD.
- Thoracic manifestations of sarcoidosis on HRCT include perilymphatic nodules, middle and upper lung zone predominant fibrosis, and symmetric hilar/mediastinal adenopathy.[21]

Cystic Lung Diseases
- Several types of ILD are characterized by the radiographic finding of pulmonary cysts and can be diagnosed via distinctive HRCT features combined with clinical history; some of these conditions include[22]:
  - LAM
    - Rare condition that predominantly affects young women and can be either sporadic or associated with tuberous sclerosis complex (TSC).
    - The characteristic HRCT finding is numerous uniform thin-walled cysts with otherwise normal lung parenchyma.
    - Associated conditions include spontaneous pneumothorax, chylothorax, and renal angiomyolipomas.[23]
  - PLCH is strongly associated with smoking; HRCT features include numerous irregularly shaped cysts and centrilobular nodules with a middle and upper lung zone predominance.

- LIP is a benign lymphoproliferative disorder with HRCT features including scattered thin-walled cysts associated with small solid or ground-glass nodules; in about 5% of cases, transformation to lymphoma can occur.

TREATMENT
Overview of Treatment
- A full review of treatments for the various ILDs is beyond the scope of this chapter.
- In general, if a causative agent is suspected (e.g., drugs, occupational exposures, and cigarette smoke), withdrawal and avoidance of the agent is imperative.
- Pharmacologic treatments for some ILDs include **immunosuppressive** and **antifibrotic** therapy.
- Nonpharmacologic therapies include supplemental oxygen, pulmonary rehabilitation, and lung transplantation in selected patients.
- Comorbidities including coronary artery disease, pulmonary hypertension, gastroesophageal reflux disease, and thromboembolic disease should be optimized.

Immunosuppressive Therapy
- Immunosuppression is a mainstay of treatment for many ILDs including CTD-ILDs, idiopathic NSIP, OP, some forms of HP, eosinophilic pulmonary syndromes, and sarcoidosis.[24]
- Acute exacerbation of IPF (AE-IPF) is also sometimes treated with a limited course of corticosteroids, although the safety and efficacy of this practice is controversial.[7]
- The anticipated benefit of immunosuppression varies depending on the specific ILD diagnosis and other case-specific factors; in general terms, patients with evidence of significant acute inflammation (e.g., ground-glass opacities on HRCT) will have a better therapeutic response to immunosuppression than those with significant fibrosis.
- **Corticosteroids** are typically used as initial therapy and, in some cases, may achieve disease remission as monotherapy.
- When long-term immunosuppression is needed, a **steroid-sparing agent** is added. Options used in multiple autoimmune ILD types include the oral antimetabolites azathioprine and mycophenolate, and the chemotherapeutic agents cyclophosphamide and rituximab.[24] Selection depends on the underlying disease, comorbidities, and shared decision-making.
- **Methotrexate** is commonly used in sarcoidosis and occasionally in other types of ILD (despite its historical association as a cause of ILD).[24]
- **mTOR inhibitors** (sirolimus or everolimus) are used in selected cases of LAM.[23]
- The calcineurin inhibitor **tacrolimus** is used in some cases of myositis-associated ILD.[24]
- Patients on chronic corticosteroid therapy at least 20 mg prednisone-equivalent daily for over 4 weeks, especially if combined with another immunosuppressant, should be prescribed *Pneumocystis jirovecii* prophylaxis.

Antifibrotic Therapy
- Two antifibrotic agents, **nintedanib** (tyrosine kinase inhibitor) and **pirfenidone** (multiple mechanisms), have become standard therapies for IPF.

- Both drugs slow progression of disease (as measured by PFT) in IPF, though studies to date have not demonstrated reversal of fibrosis.
- More recent evidence suggests that nintedanib also confers similar benefits in PPF due to other ILD types.[25] Current guidelines recommend nintedanib in PPF if there is disease progression despite initial standard therapy or observation, but not at initial presentation.[7]
- Gastrointestinal side effects are common, with diarrhea frequently occurring with nintedanib and nausea frequently occurring with pirfenidone. These side effects are generally manageable with supportive care, but in a minority of patients necessitate discontinuation of the medication.

Other Pharmacologic Therapies
- Inhaled treprostinil (prostacyclin analogue) has been shown to improve exercise capacity in ILD-associated group III pulmonary hypertension.[26]
- Medical management of comorbid GERD with proton pump inhibitors or H2 receptor antagonists may slow progression of fibrotic ILD, though this is debated.[7]
- Granulocyte colony–stimulating factor (G-CSF) is used in selected cases of PAP, along with whole-lung lavage via bronchoscopy.[12]
- Though commonly prescribed, there is little role for inhaled bronchodilators and/or inhaled corticosteroids in ILD, unless comorbid airways disease is present.

Nonpharmacologic Therapies
- Supplemental oxygen should be prescribed if there is resting or exertional hypoxemia (SpO_2 ≤88%), which should be assessed at routine clinic visits.
- Patients with significant physiologic impairment should be referred for pulmonary rehabilitation.
- Smoking cessation is imperative regardless of the etiology of ILD.
- Lung transplantation is an option for selected patients with severe disease and few comorbidities.

Advance Care Planning and Palliative Care
- Many ILDs, particularly IPF and other forms of PPF, confer a poor prognosis with rapid disease progression, limited survival despite standard therapies (especially if lung transplantation is not an option), and high symptom burden.
- Clinicians should engage patients with ILD in advance care planning discussions regarding their goals and preferences around medical treatment during severe illness; when appropriate depending on the patient's goals, palliative care and/or hospice services should be offered.

CONCLUSIONS
- ILD comprises a wide spectrum of diseases accounting for a considerable portion of everyday pulmonary practice.
- The pathogenesis of many ILDs remains poorly understood and requires further investigation to facilitate development of novel therapies.
- Management of ILD requires comprehensive integration of clinical, physiologic, radiographic, and histopathologic data to make an accurate diagnosis and determine the optimal course of treatment.

REFERENCES

1. Raghu G, Brown KK. Interstitial lung disease: clinical evaluation and keys to an accurate diagnosis. *Clin Chest Med.* 2004;25:409–419.
2. Jeganathan N, Sathananthan M. The prevalence and burden of interstitial lung diseases in the USA. *ERJ Open Res.* 2021;8:00630–02021.
3. Society BT, Committee SO. The diagnosis, assessment and treatment of diffuse parenchymal lung disease in adults. Introduction. *Thorax.* 1999;54:S1–S14.
4. Travis WD, Costabel U, Hansell DM, et al. An official American Thoracic Society/European Respiratory Society statement: Update of the international multidisciplinary classification of the idiopathic interstitial pneumonias. *Am J Respir Crit Care Med.* 2013; 188:733–748.
5. Wuyts WA, Agostini C, Antoniou KM, et al. The pathogenesis of pulmonary fibrosis: a moving target. *Eur Respir J.* 2013;41:1207–1218.
6. Adegunsoye A, Newton CA, Oldham JM, et al. Telomere length associates with chronological age and mortality across racially diverse pulmonary fibrosis cohorts. *Nat Commun.* 2023;14:1489.
7. Raghu G, Remy-Jardin M, Richeldi L, et al. Idiopathic pulmonary fibrosis (an update) and progressive pulmonary fibrosis in adults: An Official ATS/ERS/JRS/ALAT Clinical Practice Guideline. *Am J Respir Crit Care Med.* 2022;205:e18–e47.
8. Deconinck B, Verschakelen J, Coolen J, Verbeken E, Verleden G, Wuyts W. Diagnostic workup for diffuse parenchymal lung disease: schematic flowchart, literature review, and pitfalls. *Lung.* 2013;191:19–25.
9. Frankel SK, Cosgrove GP, Fischer A, Meehan RT, Brown KK. Update in the diagnosis and management of pulmonary vasculitis. *Chest.* 2006;129:452–465.
10. Caminati A, Cavazza A, Sverzellati N, Harari S. An integrated approach in the diagnosis of smoking-related interstitial lung diseases. *Eur Respir Rev.* 2012;21:207–217.
11. Fischer A, du Bois R. Interstitial lung disease in connective tissue disorders. *Lancet.* 2012;380:689–698.
12. Borie R, Danel C, Debray MP, et al. Pulmonary alveolar proteinosis. *Eur Respir Rev.* 2011;20:98–107.
13. Meyer KC, Raghu G, Baughman RP, et al. An official American Thoracic Society clinical practice guideline: the clinical utility of bronchoalveolar lavage cellular analysis in interstitial lung disease. *Am J Respir Crit Care Med.* 2012;185:1004–1014.
14. Hariri LP, Roden AC, Chung JH, et al. The role of surgical lung biopsy in the diagnosis of fibrotic interstitial lung disease: perspective from the Pulmonary Fibrosis Foundation. *Ann Am Thorac Soc.* 2021;18:1601–1609.
15. Maldonado F, Danoff SK, Wells AU, et al. Transbronchial cryobiopsy for the diagnosis of interstitial lung diseases: CHEST Guideline and Expert Panel Report. *Chest.* 2020; 157:1030–1042.
16. Raghu G, Remy-Jardin M, Myers JL, et al. Diagnosis of idiopathic pulmonary fibrosis. An official ATS/ERS/JRS/ALAT Clinical Practice Guideline. *Am J Respir Crit Care Med.* 2018;198:e44–e68.
17. Kligerman SJ, Groshong S, Brown KK, Lynch DA. Nonspecific interstitial pneumonia: radiologic, clinical, and pathologic considerations. *Radiographics.* 2009;29:73–87.
18. Selman M, Pardo A, King TE Jr. Hypersensitivity pneumonitis: insights in diagnosis and pathobiology. *Am J Respir Crit Care Med.* 2012;186:314–324.
19. Cottin V, Selman M, Inoue Y, et al. Syndrome of combined pulmonary fibrosis and emphysema: An Official ATS/ERS/JRS/ALAT Research Statement. *Am J Respir Crit Care Med.* 2022;206:e7–e41.
20. Fischer A, Antoniou KM, Brown KK, et al. An official European Respiratory Society/American Thoracic Society research statement: interstitial pneumonia with autoimmune features. *Eur Respir J.* 2015;46:976–987.

21. Criado E, Sánchez M, Ramírez J, et al. Pulmonary sarcoidosis: typical and atypical manifestations at high-resolution CT with pathologic correlation. *Radiographics.* 2010;30: 1567–1586.
22. Raoof S, Bondalapati P, Vydyula R, et al. Cystic lung diseases: algorithmic approach. *Chest.* 2016;150:945–965.
23. McCarthy C, Gupta N, Johnson SR, Yu JJ, McCormack FX. Lymphangioleiomyomatosis: pathogenesis, clinical features, diagnosis, and management. *Lancet Respir Med.* 2021; 9:1313–1327.
24. Mathai SC, Danoff SK. Management of interstitial lung disease associated with connective tissue disease. *BMJ.* 2016;352:h6819.
25. Flaherty KR, Wells AU, Cottin V, et al. Nintedanib in progressive fibrosing interstitial lung diseases. *New Eng J Med.* 2019;381:1718–1727.
26. Waxman A, Restrepo-Jaramillo R, Thenappan T, et al. Inhaled Treprostinil in pulmonary hypertension due to interstitial lung disease. *New Eng J Med.* 2021;384:325–334.

Occupational Lung Disease

25

Adam Anderson

INTRODUCTION

- The workplace contains a wide range of materials and conditions that can potentially aggravate pre-existing conditions or cause pulmonary disease in susceptible hosts. Table 25-1 lists some relatively common potentially hazardous agents.
- Diagnosis of workplace-related pulmonary disease requires a high index of suspicion because there may be no clear temporal relationship between an exposure and the subsequent development of signs and symptoms, which may be non-specific and fleeting.
- Obtaining a detailed occupational history from a patient with a possible workplace-related pulmonary disease is an essential part of the diagnostic evaluation.[1]
  - The occupational history is a comprehensive list of the activities and environments of all remunerative or volunteer work the patient has ever performed, including short-term/temporary/military jobs and hobbies, which is compiled to identify all exposures (Table 25-2).
  - Assessment of the home environment, especially during childhood, emphasizing biomass fuel exhaust, radon, and mineral dust exposures may also be important.
- General management principles
  - The patient should **avoid further exposure** to the offending agent. This intervention may involve a change in job responsibilities and patients should be made aware of the fact.
  - Supportive care measures which will depend upon individual patient requirements:
    - Supplemental oxygen
    - Pulmonary rehabilitation
    - Tobacco cessation
    - Bronchodilators
    - Age-appropriate vaccinations
  - Because disease can progress even after exposure has ended, serial imaging and pulmonary function tests (PFTs) are recommended in the first years after retirement.
  - Issues of impairment, disability, and workers' compensation frequently arise with a diagnosis of workplace-related pulmonary disease.
  - Impairment refers to an objectively determined abnormality of functional assessment.
  - Disability implies inability to perform certain tasks owing to impairment.
  - The disability certification process often involves multiple agencies and procedures that vary from state to state.
  - For assistance with definitions and criteria, the American Medical Association Guides to the Evaluation of Permanent Impairment is a valuable resource.[2]

TABLE 25-1 POTENTIALLY HAZARDOUS AGENTS IN THE WORKPLACE

Gases/vapors
Carbon monoxide
Formaldehyde
Hydrochloric acid
Sulfuric acid
Sodium hydroxide
Bleach
Hydrogen sulfide
Ethylene oxide
Nitrogen dioxide
Ozone
Phosgene
Smoke
Sulfur dioxide
Fumes from welding and metal processing
Acids/alkalis
Ammonia
Chlorine

Biologic agents
Bacteria
Fungi
Molds
Rickettsia
Spores

Inorganic dusts
Asbestos
Silica
Coal mine dust
Nickel
Talc
Beryllium

Organic dusts
Cotton dust
Wood dust

Solvents
Benzene
Carbon tetrachloride
Methanol
Chloroform
Trichloroethylene
Xylene

Metals
Aluminum
Arsenic
Cadmium
Cobalt
Iron
Lead
Mercury
Chromium

Other
Plastics
Vinyl chloride
Acrylonitrile
Styrene
Dyes
Petrochemicals
Creosote
Asphalt and tar
Poisons
Insecticides
Herbicides
Products of combustion
Biomass fuel
Diesel exhaust

Asbestos-Associated Lung Disease

GENERAL PRINCIPLES

- Asbestos is composed of hydrated silicates with varying combinations of other elements such as sodium, magnesium, and iron.

TABLE 25-2 SAMPLE OCCUPATIONAL HISTORY

1. **List all jobs you have ever held and the dates of employment beginning with the very first one.**
2. For each job identify:
   a. Chemicals/dusts or other substances you may have been exposed to? Nature of exposure risk: contact/inhalation/ingestion?
   b. Protective equipment:
      1. Was equipment available? Did you use it? Describe.
      2. Was the equipment fit tested?
      3. Did you use the equipment as instructed? When? What percentage of the time? Under what circumstances did you not use it?
   c. Air quality:
      1. What kind of active ventilation was provided? What was the maintenance schedule?
      2. Were there strong odors/taste in the air?
      3. Could you see haze/dust in the air?
      4. Did your eyes burn/water?
   d. Facilities for washing/showering present?
   e. Were uniforms provided? Did you wear them? Were they washed at home? By whom?
   f. Did you eat, drink, or smoke in the workplace?
   g. Procedures for accidental exposure?
   h. Your symptoms:
      1. Date of onset?
      2. Relationship to exposure: Worse at beginning/end of shift/week? Better after weekend off/vacation?
      3. Do you blow dust from your nose or cough it up?
   i. Coworkers with similar symptoms? Other problems?
   j. Were there animals/insects in the workplace?
   k. Is the workplace damp? Is there standing water?
   l. Any usual event such as spills, excessive exposure, or fires?
3. **Other exposures:**
   a. Smoking history?
   b. Alcohol history?
   c. Chemicals used at home in housekeeping/hobbies/lawn care/automobile maintenance?
   d. Animals at home: pets, livestock, birds?

- Asbestos can be classified according to the shape of its fibers: amphibolites which are linear fibers or serpentines which are curly fibers.
- Asbestos fibers can damage lung parenchyma and pleura, causing both benign and malignant disease by complex processes that are incompletely understood.[3,4]

- Fibers can be suspended in air and inhaled.
- Inhaled fibers penetrate deeply into the lungs and cellular structures.
- Fibers are incompletely cleared.
- All asbestos-containing materials can cause fibrosis, lung cancer, and diffuse malignant mesothelioma.
- Clinical and radiographic manifestations of disease may be delayed for decades.
- Asbestos was widely used in construction and manufactured products until 1975. Routes for exposure include:
  - The manufacture of asbestos-containing products.
  - Removal of floor tiles, insulated pipes, roofing materials, brake linings, and other asbestos-containing materials currently in place.
  - Employment in the construction, maintenance, textile, or roofing industries.

DIAGNOSIS

- The exposure history may be essential to making the diagnosis. The patient should have a history of exposure to asbestos fibers and a suitable latency period before development of symptoms or radiographic findings.
  - Pleural effusions >1 year
  - Pleural plaques >10 years
  - Asbestosis, lung cancer, malignant pleural mesothelioma (MPM) >20 years
- The presentation, examination, PFTs, and radiologic findings can be nonspecific.[3]
  - Patients may complain of cough, persistent progressive dyspnea, and sometimes chest discomfort.
  - Late inspiratory crackles may be heard on auscultation and clubbing may be seen in some cases.
  - PFTs show decreased lung volumes, especially total lung capacity (TLC) and decreased forced vital capacity (FVC), along with decreased diffusing capacity of the lung for carbon monoxide (DLCO).
  - Impairment of gas exchange is most sensitively determined by arterial blood gas (ABG) analysis conducted at rest and during exercise.
  - CT is more sensitive than CXR for detecting subtle findings as well as for characterizing pleural processes.[5–7]
  - Special studies such as bronchoalveolar lavage or tissue biopsy may be necessary to find asbestos fibers if exposure requires documentation.
- **Asbestosis**
  - The presence of asbestos fibers may result in a persistent inflammatory process culminating in diffuse interstitial fibrosis, with distortion of the lung parenchyma. Diffuse interstitial fibrosis usually develops no sooner than 20 years after the first and heavy exposure.
  - CT scan shows multiple abnormalities: curving subpleural lines, parenchymal banding, short peripheral lines, and honeycombing in advanced disease.
  - Both bilateral pleural plaques and parenchymal processes must be present to make the diagnosis.

- **Pleural disease**[5–7]
    - Pleural disease may result from translocation of fibers into the pleural space to stimulate an inflammatory and fibrotic response.
    - Pleural thickening
        - Fibrosis of the visceral pleura with adhesions to the parietal pleura occurs, obliterating the pleural space and extending into lung parenchyma.
        - CXR shows widely distributed plaques that do not spare the apices or the costophrenic angles.
        - Plaques are invariably asymptomatic.
    - Rounded atelectasis
        - Pleural thickening may entrap a section of lung, causing atelectasis and associated volume loss.
        - CXR shows thickened pleura surrounding a section of atelectatic lung with a so-called comet tail extending in the direction of the hilum.
    - Pleural effusion
        - This is the earliest clinical phenomenon, occurring as early as 1 year, but more typically, longer than 10 years after exposure.
        - Patients may complain of chest pain and breathlessness.
        - CXR usually shows a unilateral effusion, but it may be bilateral, either synchronous or metachronous.
        - Thoracentesis yields an exudative, sometimes bloody effusion. Fibers are not often found in pleural fluid.
- **MPM**
    - MPM is a malignant process of the parietal surface of the thoracic and/or abdominal cavities that invades heart and lung by direct extension.
    - Almost all MPM in the US is due to asbestos exposure. Exposure may have been apparently minimal, indirect, and not occupational. For example, helping a parent to clean work clothes as a child or being present during a ship refitting.
    - Exposure almost always occurs >20 years before clinical manifestations.
    - Radiographic findings include lobulated growth over the parietal pleural surface.[5]
    - There is no curative treatment. The prognosis for this malignancy is grim but combined surgical and chemotherapeutic regimens show some therapeutic promise.
- There is an association of asbestos-related lung disease and **lung cancer**.[3,4,6–9]
    - Asbestos has been classified by the International Agency for Research on Cancer (IARC) as **group 1, carcinogenic to humans**.[10] Exposure to asbestos, both in amphibole or serpentine forms, clearly is associated with increased lung cancer risk.
    - **Tobacco smoking additively, and possibly synergistically, increases lung cancer risk** in persons who have even short-term exposure to asbestos. Therefore, tobacco cessation is imperative.
    - Because asbestos exposure has been associated with a substantial increased risk for lung cancer and early diagnosis may improve outcome, CT surveillance may be employed with expected outcome benefit.

Coal Dust-Associated Pulmonary Disease

GENERAL PRINCIPLES
- Coal is ranked according to its carbon content, which is determined by the geologic setting in which it was formed.
- Coal dust is primarily carbon but silica, kaolin, mica, metal dusts, and other potentially harmful contaminants may also be present.
- The amount and nature of exposure during coal mining depends upon the rank of coal, quality of dust control measures, and the individual's work responsibilities.
  - Exposure is greatest working underground at the coal face.
  - Above-ground workers who operate drills or transport coal may also have sufficient exposure to produce disease in a susceptible host.
- The prevalence of coal dust–associated pulmonary disease among workers with 25 years or more of exposure is over 10%, with some areas in Appalachia exceeding 20%.[11]

DIAGNOSIS
- The spectrum of clinical manifestations is wide. Patients may be asymptomatic with mild radiographic abnormalities or severely disabled with obvious and advanced radiographic abnormalities.
- **Coal workers' pneumoconiosis**
  - The hallmark symptom is shortness of breath.
  - Persistent late inspiratory crackles are heard on examination.
  - PFTs may show a restrictive ventilatory defect, with impaired O_2 exchange. Obstructive ventilatory defects are rarely due to coal mine dust and difficult to distinguish from the more common tobacco-associated disease in smoking miners.
  - CXR shows small nodular opacities in the upper lobes in the early stages, which become more numerous and confluent as disease progresses.
- **Progressive massive fibrosis**
  - Patients complain of shortness of breath and cough.
  - PFTs may show both obstructive and restrictive ventilatory defects.
  - CXR shows coalescence of nodules >12 mm in size.
- **Chronic obstructive pulmonary disease** (COPD) **phenotype**[12,13]
  - Rarely, never-smoking miners present with cough, expectoration, and/or wheezing with manifestations of airflow obstruction on physical examination and confirmed by PFTs.
  - CXR is free of interstitial changes.
  - If no other cause for this clinical presentation is found (e.g., bronchiectasis, asthma, chronic exposure to biomass fuel combustion smoke, cystic fibrosis, α1-antitrypsin deficiency) it should be attributed to coal dust.
- **Industrial bronchitis:** This diagnosis is associated with a clinical picture of cough during times of exposure that resolves with cessation of coal mine dust exposure. No other associated impairment is seen.
- There is no specific association between coal mining and lung cancer, though there is some possible uncertainty in this regard.[14] As with the general

population, when miners are exposed to multiple carcinogens, including radon gas and cigarette smoke, they are at increased risk for lung cancer.

Silica-Associated Lung Disease

GENERAL PRINCIPLES

- Silica (SiO_2), in its amorphous form, is noncrystalline and relatively nontoxic if inhaled. In its crystalline form, most commonly occurring as quartz, it can cause pulmonary toxicity if inhaled.[15–17]
- A detailed occupational history may be necessary to determine all possible routes of silica exposure.
  - Found in soil and rock, it is a hazard for tunnelers, sandblasters, millers, and foundry workers.
  - It is also found in manufactured materials as diverse as plaster and toothpaste.
- Workers who believe they worked under safe conditions may still have significant potential risk of developing disease regardless of the chronology of exposure.

DIAGNOSIS

- **Acute silicosis**
  - Acute silicosis may develop within weeks to months after exposure to very high concentrations of silica in small particles of airborne dust, such as may occur when sandblasting, rock drilling, tunneling, or quartz milling in an unprotected manner.
  - Patients develop dyspnea, hypoxemia, and possible respiratory failure, which may be lethal.
  - PFTs show restrictive and/or obstructive ventilatory defects, usually with impaired oxygen gas exchange.
  - Radiographic findings include abundant ground-glass infiltrates seen on both CXR and CT.
  - A subset of acute silicosis patients develop silicoproteinosis, which mimics pulmonary alveolar proteinosis radiographically and pathologically.
- **Accelerated silicosis**
  - Accelerated silicosis develops 2–10 years after heavy exposure.
  - Patients complain of progressive exertional dyspnea and cough.
  - Patients may have restrictive and/or obstructive ventilatory defects.
  - CXR and CT show multiple small nodules in the upper and midzone regions of the lungs.
- **Chronic silicosis**
  - Chronic silicosis develops after ≥10 years of exposure to relatively low concentrations of silica.
  - Patients report progressive exertional dyspnea and cough.
  - Patients may have restrictive and/or obstructive ventilator defects.
  - CXR and CT demonstrate multiple small nodules in the upper and midzone regions of the lungs, becoming larger and more diffusely distributed with

disease progression. Characteristic eggshell calcification may outline enlarged hilar and mediastinal lymph nodes.
- Progressive massive fibrosis results from enlargement and confluence of nodules.
- Progression may continue after cessation of exposure.
* Patients with silicosis are **prone to infection with both tuberculous and nontuberculous mycobacteria**. Patients who are tuberculin skin test or interferon gamma release assay (IGRA) positive should be treated appropriately.
* The IARC has classified silica as **group 1, carcinogenic to humans**.[18]
  - This classification has been somewhat controversial as not all studies have shown a clear relationship between exposure to silica and the development of cancer. In many studies, smoking history and other confounding factors must be taken into account.
  - It should be stated, however, that silica exposure, especially with silicosis, **likely increases the risk for malignancy**.[19–22]
  - Abnormalities seen on CXR should be followed closely, and any findings concerning for malignancy should be evaluated with chest CT and tissue diagnosis as appropriate.

Workplace- and Environment-Associated Bronchial Reactivity

GENERAL PRINCIPLES

* Occupational asthma is characterized by variable airflow limitation and/or airway hyperresponsiveness attributable to the workplace environment, although the syndrome can develop outside the workplace as well.
* IgE-mediated immunologic mechanisms are not necessarily responsible.
* Individual variability in genetic susceptibility to disease, symptom presentation, and response to therapy, in addition to the differences in apparently similar workplaces produce a very diverse clinical picture.
* It is challenging to differentiate occupational asthma versus a pre-existing asthma phenotype aggravated by the workplace.
* In almost all settings, there is **substantial individual variation of the dose–response and the type of symptoms that result**.
  - Several workers may experience apparently similar exposures in an industrial spill but not all are adversely affected.
  - Workers with either retrospectively identified or extremely quiescent atopy may have a greater susceptibility to develop latency-associated occupational asthma of any sort (immunologic and nonimmunologic), especially with repeated exposures.[23]
* **Nonantigenic chemicals** such as hydrochloric acid, sulfuric acid, diacetyl sodium hydroxide, chlorine, other inorganic acids, alkalis, and low–molecular-weight irritants can induce this syndrome either immediately after a single massive exposure, or, more slowly, after multiple, less intense exposures. Chronic exposure to formaldehyde, pesticides, insecticides, solvents, isocyanates (toluene diisocyanate, methylene diphenyl diisocyanate, hexamethylene diisocyanate), and cleaners can produce similar clinical responses.[24]

- Consideration should also be given to **immunologic agents** such as cotton, textile dust exposures, animal, insect, or shellfish allergies; western red cedar dust in the lumber industry; wheat or rye dusts in the baking industry; or other food industry exposures to garlic dust, cinnamon, and mushrooms.
- Flour and isocyanates are the most common culprits in the developed world.[25]

DIAGNOSIS

- The patient complains of some combination of breathlessness, cough, expectoration, wheezing, and chest tightness.
- Persistent bronchial reactivity is manifested over time by different symptom patterns triggered by irritants differing from the initial etiologic agent.
- In general, irritant triggers include extremes of temperature and humidity, ambient tobacco smoke, perfumes, colognes, hairspray, cooking fumes, products of combustion, and cleaning materials.
- The physical examination may be normal; intermittently, wheezing may be heard on auscultation.
- PFTs are often normal at baseline but may demonstrate airflow obstruction with or without improvement after bronchodilator administration.
  - Methacholine challenge test is generally considered diagnostic for the presence of bronchial reactivity.[26,27]
  - Specific inhalation challenge is sometimes necessary.[27]
  - In some cases, airflow limitation may be demonstrated years after exposure.[28]
  - If only small airways dominant disease is present, such as occurred among first responders to the World Trade Center disaster, conventional methacholine test may be normal. In such cases, the only measurable abnormality identifiable may be through the use of impedance oscillometry (IOS).[29,30]
- CXR is typically normal.
- Provocative laryngoscopy to exclude paroxysmal vocal fold motion is sometimes necessary.

TREATMENT

- Environmental
  - Environmental control is foremost; patients should not return to the workplace without proper respiratory protection, which can be difficult to achieve.[27]
  - Patients must be fastidious in their avoidance of other non–workplace-associated triggers, both allergic and irritant.
- Pharmacologic
  - Treatment with β2 agonists and inhaled corticosteroids should be the first-order approach to blunt the effect of inadvertent breaches in environmental control.
  - Anticholinergics and systemic steroids seem less successful.
  - Advanced therapies including desensitization and biologics can be considered in refractory cases, especially if concern for concomitant asthma.
- Reports to patients and third parties
  - Because of the nature of reversible or partially reversible airflow obstruction, and because appropriate treatment may preclude an individual's return to the workplace, the physician may be faced with difficulty in explaining the apparent

inconsistency between no measurable impairment on PFTs and the presence of disability owing to dysfunction that develops when returning to the workplace.
- Although this situation is well understood by the worker, others may be less accepting.
- Family and social problems: because regularly occurring irritants in the household may trigger symptoms, a former wage earner may be unable to return to work and also limited household chores.
- Special cases
  - **World Trade Center disaster**[29–31]
    - Many first responders exposed to the mixed dusts and fumes at the site developed persistent and chronic respiratory symptoms.
    - Symptoms were triggered by a wide variety of exposures.
    - Most had poor response to traditional bronchodilator and anti-inflammatory treatment.
    - Spirometry may be normal and small airway abnormalities may only be found through the use of frequency dependence of compliance and IOS.
  - **Popcorn lung**[32]
    - In 2002, workers in popcorn factories developed pulmonary symptoms that were sometimes disabling.
    - Those who mixed butter flavoring were most frequently affected. Inhalation of flavoring compounds (diacetyl) was identified as the causative agent.
    - CT images were consistent with bronchiolitis obliterans (BO).
    - Treatment requires avoidance of diacetyl and standard therapy for BO.
  - **Biomass fuel combustion fumes**
    - Biomass products such as wood, coal, charcoal, or agricultural residue are often used to fuel cook stoves in many parts of the world, including North America.[33]
    - Never-smoking homemakers and children are most frequently exposed.
    - The clinical picture resembles COPD.
    - When studying COPD epidemiology, biomass fume exposure must be considered as well as genetic propensity, α1-antitrypsin deficiency, and workplace exposures.

Hypersensitivity Pneumonitis

GENERAL PRINCIPLES

- Hypersensitivity pneumonitis (HP) (also known as extrinsic allergic alveolitis) develops when susceptible hosts become sensitized and are repeatedly exposed to a myriad of offending antigens (Table 25-3) that can be found in virtually any environment.
- Although many persons may be exposed to a particular antigen, few develop disease.[34,35]
- Multiple exposures may be necessary to become sensitized.
- Smokers may be less prone to developing the disease.[34,35]
- Previously HP was differentiated into acute, subacute, and chronic disease. This system did not adequately differentiate between phenotypes and suggested a progressive process.

TABLE 25-3 HYPERSENSITIVITY PNEUMONITIS—CAUSATIVE AGENTS

Organisms
  Bacteria
    Thermophilic actinomycetes
      Moldy hay, grain, compost
      Air conditioners, humidifiers
    Mycobacterium avium complex–contaminated water
    Mixed bacteria/fungi-contaminated metal-working fluids
  Fungi
    Aspergillus species—moldy malt dust
    Alternaria species—moldy wood dust
    Cryptostroma corticale—wet maple bark
    Pullularia species—moldy redwood dust
    Trichosporon cutaneum—Japanese house mold
  Amoebae
    Naegleria gruberi–contaminated ventilation system
    Acanthamoeba castellanii–contaminated ventilation system

Animal proteins
  Bovine/porcine protein
  Rat urinary protein—rat urine
  Oyster/mollusk shell protein—shell dust
  Animal fur protein
  Fish meal dust
  Birds (pigeons, doves, domestic pet birds)

Plants
  Soybean hulls
  Coffee bean dust
  Lycoperdon species (puffball mushrooms)

Chemicals and manufactured products
  Amiodarone
  Procarbazine
  Toluene diisocyanate—paints, plastics
  Diphenylmethane diisocyanate—paints, plastics
  Phthalic anhydride—plastics
  Trimellitic anhydride—plastics
  Nylon flock

- An updated classification system has been proposed including nonfibrotic and fibrotic phenotypes.[34,35]

DIAGNOSIS

- A high level of clinical suspicion is necessary for diagnosis.
- A detailed social history is required to identify possible antigens. Questionnaires, though unvalidated, are available to assist in a comprehensive exposure history.[34,35]

- A causative antigen is only found in roughly half of cases.[36]
- Patient presentation and radiographic studies can vary according to the stage of the disease.
- Findings are not pathognomonic. HP should be considered when symptoms improve with avoidance of the suspected agent and recur or worsen with re-exposure.
- Generic symptoms of dyspnea and cough are most common.
- Examination may reveal crackles or mid-inspiratory squeaks consistent with bronchiolitis.
- **Farmer's lung**
  - Disease results from exposure to the several possible antigens, most commonly *Saccharopolyspora rectivirgula* and *Thermoactinomyces vulgaris*, which are found in moldy hay.
  - Spores become airborne and are inhaled by susceptible persons.
  - The risk of disease is increased by weather conditions conducive to mold growth, frequent and heavy exposures to hay, and poor-quality ventilation in the workplace.
- **Bird Fancier's disease**
  - Several possible exposure environments exist though predominately with domesticated birds or bird feather products (down pillows, comforters, etc.).
  - The extent and duration of exposure may increase the risk of development.

Diagnostic Testing

- Laboratory evaluation is not helpful as elevations in erythrocyte sedimentation rate (ESR), C-reactive protein (CRP), and immune globulin levels are nondiagnostic.
- Precipitin tests are of limited utility.[34,35]
  - Specific tests do not exist for all potential antigens and both test reagents and testing procedures vary widely in quality.
  - A positive result shows only that the patient has had sufficient exposure to develop an immunologic response but is not proof the particular antigen is responsible for the disease.
- PFTs may show decreased TLC, decreased DLCO, and oxygen desaturation with exercise.
- Inhalation challenge, in which the expected offending agent is inhaled in a similar fashion to that used in a methacholine challenge, is not necessary for diagnosis. Such testing is usually most useful if symptoms appear promptly after exposure and improve after removal from offending agents.[34–37]
- All patients with suspicion of HP should receive a **high-resolution CT (HRCT)** including thin-sections (~1-mm images) and both inhalation and exhalation images.
- In **nonfibrotic HP,** HRCT may show ground-glass opacification, mosaic attenuation, centrilobular nodules and/or air trapping without requiring a zonal distribution.[34,35]
- HRCT findings in **"typical" fibrotic HP** are irregular linear opacities/coarse reticulation with lung distortion; traction bronchiectasis and honeycombing may be present but do not predominate. The distribution can be random, mid-lung zone predominant or relative sparing of the lower lung zones. The "three-density sign" is sometimes used that shows a mixture of ground-glass opacities, mosaic attenuation, and normal lung attenuation in a lobular distribution.[34,35]

- **Bronchoalveolar lavage** may show a lymphocyte predominance.
- Lung biopsies are sometimes needed for definitive diagnosis. The yield of transbronchial biopsies is low, while cryobiopsy and ultimately surgical lung biopsy provide greater information.
- A multi-disciplinary discussion with pulmonology, radiology, and pathology helps guide discussions in diffuse parenchymal lung disease.[38]

TREATMENT

- If identified, removal/avoidance of antigen exposure is essential to prevent progression.
- Supportive measures include smoking cessation, bronchodilators if PFTs show a reactive airway component to the disease, supplemental oxygen if needed, and pulmonary rehabilitation.
- Corticosteroids and other immunosuppressants can be considered for non-fibrotic phenotypes. The dose and duration of therapy may depend on whether a causative antigen is found and avoidance is possible.
- Antifibrotics may serve a role in fibrotic HP or progressive disease.[39]

Toxic Lung Injury

SILO FILLER'S DISEASE

- Workers who upload silage without appropriate ventilation and protective gear can develop pulmonary injury from **exposure to nitrogen oxides**.
- Patients may present with moderate breathlessness and cough, or respiratory failure with pulmonary edema.
- Survivors of the toxin-induced process may have permanent lung injury characterized by airway obstruction and/or an interstitial process causing impairment of oxygen gas exchange and a restrictive abnormality.

CHRONIC BERYLLIUM DISEASE

- Chronic beryllium disease (CBD) is a granulomatous pulmonary process also known as **berylliosis**.
- Workers may be exposed to beryllium aerosols in the manufacture of nuclear weapons, viscose rayon, electronics, and when employed by dental laboratories.
- Not all persons with beryllium sensitization develop CBD.
- Diagnosis requires prior exposure, a positive beryllium lymphocyte proliferation test and compatible biopsy with noncaseating granulomas or mononuclear cell interstitial infiltrates.
- Studies have shown a disconnect between disease severity and intensity of exposure, beryllium sensitization, and the development of disease. The odds of developing beryllium sensitization and CBD are differentially distributed by HLA-DPB1 genotype.[40]

REFERENCES

1. Goldman RH, Peters JM. The occupational and environmental health history. *JAMA.* 1981;246:2831–2836.
2. American Medical Association. *Guides for the Evaluation of Permanent Impairment.* 6th ed. American Medical Association; 2023.
3. Levin SM, Kann PE, Lax MB. Medical examination for asbestos-related disease. *Am J Ind Med.* 2000;37:6–22.
4. Kamp DW. Asbestos-induced lung diseases: an update. *Transl Res.* 2009;153:143–152.
5. Roach HD, Davies GJ, Attanoos R, Crane M, Adams H, Phillips S. Asbestos: when the dust settles—an imaging review of asbestos-related disease. *Radiographics.* 2002;22:S167–S184.
6. Chapman SJ, Cookson WOC, Musk AW, Lee YCG. Benign asbestos pleural diseases. *Curr Opin Pulm Med.* 2003;9:266–271.
7. Ross RM. The clinical diagnosis of asbestosis in this century requires more than a chest radiograph. *Chest.* 2003;124:1120–1128.
8. Pairon JC, Andujar P, Rinaldo M, et al. Asbestos exposure, pleural plaques, and the risk of death from lung cancer. *Am J Respir Crit Care Med.* 2014;190:1413–1420.
9. Weiss W. Asbestosis: a marker for the increased risk of lung cancer among workers exposed to asbestos. *Chest.* 1999;115:536–549.
10. IARC Working Group on the Evaluation of Carcinogenic Risks to Humans. 2012. *Arsenic, metals, fibres and dusts.* Lyon (FR): International Agency for Research on Cancer. (IARC Monographs on the Evaluation of Carcinogenic Risks to Humans, No. 100C.)
11. Blackley DJ, Halldin CN, Laney AS. Continued increase in prevalence of coal workers' pneumoconiosis in the United States, 1970–2017. *Am J Public Health.* 2018;108:1220–1222.
12. Lapp NL, Morgan WK, Zaldivar G. Airways obstruction, coal mining, and disability. *Occup Environ Med.* 1994;51:234–238.
13. Kuempel ED, Wheeler MW, Smith RJ, Vallyathan V, Green FHY. Contributions of dust exposure and cigarette smoking to emphysema severity in coal miners in the United States. *Am J Respir Crit Care Med.* 2009;180:257–264.
14. Graber JM, Stayner LT, Cohen RA, Conroy LM, Attfield MD. Respiratory disease mortality among US coal miners; results after 37 years of follow-up. *Occup Environ Med.* 2014;71:30–39.
15. Mossman BT, Churg A. Mechanisms in the pathogenesis of asbestosis and silicosis. *Am J Respir Crit Care Med.* 1998;157:1666–1680.
16. Castranova V, Vallyathan V. Silicosis and coal workers' pneumoconiosis. *Environ Health Perspect.* 2000;108:675–684.
17. Greaves IA. Not-so-simple silicosis: a case for public health action. *Am J Ind Med.* 2000;37:245–251.
18. National Institute for Occupational Safety and Health. *NIOSH Hazard Review—Health Effects of Occupational Exposure to Respirable Crystalline Silica.* DHHS (NIOSH) Publication No. 2002–129. U.S. Department of Health and Human Services, Centers for Disease Control and Prevention, National Institute for Occupational Safety and Health; 2002.
19. Liu Y, Steenland K, Rong Y, et al. Exposure-response analysis and risk assessment for lung cancer in relationship to silica exposure: a 44-year cohort study of 34,018 workers. *Am J Epidemiol.* 2013;178:1424–1433.
20. Finkelstein MM. Silica, silicosis, and lung cancer: a risk assessment. *Am J Ind Med.* 2000;38:8–18.
21. Steenland K, Mannetje A, Boffetta P, et al; International Agency for Research on Cancer. Pooled exposure-response analyses and risk assessment for lung cancer in 10 cohorts of silica-exposed workers: an IARC multicentre study. *Cancer Causes Control.* 2001;12:773–784.

22. Wang D, Yang M, Liu Y, Ma J, Shi T, Chen W. Association of silica dust exposure and cigarette smoking with mortality among mine and pottery workers in China. *JAMA Netw Open.* 2020;3:e202787.
23. Brooks SM, Hammad Y, Richards I, Giovinco-Barbas J, Jenkins K. The spectrum of irritant-induced asthma: sudden and not-so-sudden onset and the role of allergy. *Chest.* 1998;113:42–49.
24. Pronk A, Preller L, Raulf-Heimsoth M, et al. Respiratory symptoms, sensitization, and exposure response relationships in spray painters exposed to isocyanates. *Am J Respir Crit Care Med.* 2007;176:1090–1097.
25. Nicholson PJ, Cullinan P, Taylor AJN, Burge PS, Boyle C. Evidence based guidelines for the prevention, identification, and management of occupational asthma. *Occup Environ Med.* 2005;62:290–299.
26. Brooks S, Weiss MA, Bernstein IL. Reactive airways dysfunction syndrome (RADS): persistent asthma syndrome after high-level irritant exposure. *Chest.* 1985;88:376–384.
27. Tarlo SM, Balmes J, Balkissoon R, et al. Diagnosis and management of work-related asthma: American College of Chest Physicians Consensus Statement. *Chest.* 2008;134:1S–41S.
28. Malo JL, L'archevêque J, Castellanos L, Lavoie K, Ghezzo H, Maghni K. Long-term outcomes of acute irritant-induced asthma. *Am J Respir Crit Care Med.* 2009;179:923–928.
29. Rom WN, Reibman J, Rogers L, et al. Emerging exposures and respiratory health: World Trade Center dust. *Proc Am Thorac Soc.* 2010;7:142–145.
30. Friedman SM, Maslow CB, Reibman J, et al. Case-control study of lung function in World Trade Center Health Registry area residents and workers. *Am J Respir Crit Care Med.* 2011;184:582–589.
31. Banauch GI, Alleyne D, Sanchez R, et al. Persistent hyperreactivity and reactive airway dysfunction in firefighters at the World Trade Center. *Am J Respir Crit Care Med.* 2003;168:54–62.
32. van Rooy FG, Rooyackers JM, Prokop M, Houba R, Smit LAM, Heederik DJJ. Bronchiolitis obliterans syndrome in chemical workers producing diacetyl for food flavorings. *Am J Respir Crit Care Med.* 2007;176:498–504.
33. Boman C, Forsberg B, Sandström T. Shedding new light on wood smoke: a risk factor for respiratory health. *Eur Respir J.* 2006;27:446–447.
34. Raghu G, Remy-Jardin M, Ryerson CJ, et al. Diagnosis of hypersensitivity pneumonitis in adults. An official ATS/JRS/ALAT clinical practice guideline. *Am J Respir Crit Care Med.* 2020;202(3):e36–e69.
35. Fernández Pérez ER, Travis WD, Lynch DA, et al. Diagnosis and evaluation of hypersensitivity pneumonitis: CHEST guideline and expert panel report. *Chest.* 2021;160:e97–e156.
36. Fernández Pérez ER, Swigris JJ, Forssén AV, et al. Identifying an inciting antigen is associated with improved survival in patients with chronic hypersensitivity pneumonitis. *Chest.* 2013;144:1644–1651.
37. Muñoz X, Sánchez-Ortiz M, Torres F, Villar A, Morell F, Cruz MJ. Diagnostic yield of specific inhalation challenge in hypersensitivity pneumonitis. *Eur Respir J.* 2014;44:1658–1665.
38. Adegunsoye A, Ryerson CJ. Diagnostic classification of interstitial lung disease in clinical practice. *Clin Chest Med.* 2021;42:251–261.
39. Wells AU, Flaherty KR, Brown KK, et al; INBUILD trial investigators. Nintedanib in patients with progressive fibrosing interstitial lung diseases-subgroup analyses by interstitial lung disease diagnosis in the INBUILD trial: a randomised, double-blind, placebo-controlled, parallel-group trial. *Lancet Respir Med.* 2020;8:453–460.
40. Van Dyke MV, Martyny JW, Mroz MM, et al. Risk of chronic beryllium disease by HLA-DPB1 E69 genotype and beryllium exposure in nuclear workers. *Am J Respir Crit Care Med.* 2011;183:1680–1688.

Antineoplastic Therapy–Induced Pulmonary Disease

26

Colleen McEvoy

GENERAL PRINCIPLES

- A new era in oncology has ushered in the rapid development of revolutionary drugs and complex multimodality regimens to augment antineoplastic activity.
- However, recent advancements with targeted cell therapy and immunotherapy have also yielded new toxicity profiles.
- Multidrug combinations have led to enhanced toxicity compared to a single agent.
- While most pulmonary toxicities can be controlled, some patients may require discontinuation of anticancer treatment or experience life-threatening respiratory failure.
- Prompt recognition and management is essential as discontinuation of the agent may halt progression.

Classification and Epidemiology

- The incidence of pulmonary toxicity related to antineoplastic agents is difficult to determine as it varies depending on the type of underlying malignancy and the antineoplastic agent.
- Older chemotherapeutics as a cause of pulmonary toxicity have been well described (e.g., bleomycin, busulfan, gemcitabine).[1-3]
- Newer therapies such as tyrosine kinase inhibitors (TKIs), mammalian target of rapamycin (mTOR), antibody–drug conjugates (ADCs), and immune checkpoint inhibitors (ICIs) have led to an increased incidence of drug-induced interstitial lung disease (DILD).[1,2]
- Reports suggest an overall incidence of pulmonary toxicity in approximately 10% of patients treated with antineoplastic agents.[4,5]
- In a large study that evaluated almost 20,000 patients treated with antineoplastic drugs from 2014 to 2018, <1% developed DILD requiring hospitalization, yet those with severe DILD had a high mortality rate of 18%.[6]
- A population-based study found an incidence of respiratory failure attributable to drug-induced lung injury of 6.6 per 100,000 patient-years with 53% of cases associated with chemotherapeutic agents.[3]
- The incidence of DILD is highest in thoracic cancer, followed by hepatobiliary, gastrointestinal cancer, and breast cancer. Thoracic, skin, and hepatobiliary cancer are associated with more severe forms of DILD.[4]
- Among chemotherapeutics, bleomycin and everolimus have the highest incidence of pulmonary toxicity, followed by targeted therapies, and then ICIs. However, with the rising use of ICI and targeted therapies, the frequency will likely continue to increase.
- Agents used in combination may also increase the risk of pulmonary toxicity.
- Radiotherapy is an independent risk factor for pulmonary toxicity. For example, incidence of irinotecan-induced pneumonitis is <2% for monotherapy but increases to 12.5% when combined with paclitaxel and further increases to 56% when given in combination with radiotherapy.[7]
- The combination of programmed cell death protein 1 (PD-1) or programmed cell death ligand 1 (PD-L1) inhibitor with cytotoxic T-lymphocyte associated protein 4 (CTLA-4) inhibitors significantly increases the incidence of pneumonitis.[8,9] DILD caused by a combination of agents is often more severe and has a longer recovery than monotherapy.
- See Table 26-1 for other common examples.

TABLE 26-1 ANTINEOPLASTIC THERAPY–INDUCED PULMONARY DISEASE

Chemotherapy

Bleomycin	Most well-known agent associated with pulmonary toxicity Onset: occurs weeks to months after treatment, Toxicity varies clinically radiographically (diffuse alveolar damage to fibrotic lung disease)
Gemcitabine	Risk of DILD increased when used in combination Predominant radiographic abnormality: diffuse ground glass opacities
Taxanes	Risk 1–5%, most common within 3 wk after administration Predominant radiographic abnormality: hypersensitivity pneumonitis but can vary

Targeted therapy

EGFR inhibitors E.g., gefitinib, erlotinib, afatinib, osimertinib	Improved toxicity profile with third-generation agents Risk increases when given during or after ICI therapy
ALK inhibitors E.g., crizotinib, alectinib, ceritinib, brigatinib	Incidence ~2% in NSCLC Onset time usually within 4 wk of therapy
VEG-F inhibitors E.g., bevacizumab	Improved toxicity profile with third-generation agents, risk increases when given during or after ICI therapy
mTOR inhibitors E.g., everolimus, temsirolimus	Incidence 10% Predominant radiographic abnormality: ground glass opacities with or without diffuse interstitial disease and parenchymal consolidation

Immunotherapy

CTLA-4 E.g., ipilimumab, tremelimumab PD-1 E.g., nivolumab, pembrolizumab PD-L1 E.g., Atezolizumab, durvalumab, avelumab	Pneumonitis varies based on therapy type, tumor type, and ICI regimen Pneumonitis higher in patients with NSCLC or renal cell cancer than melanoma Median time to onset 2.6 months Predominant radiographic abnormalities: OP pattern and ground glass opacities.

ALK, anaplastic lymphoma kinase; CTLA-4, cytotoxic T-lymphocyte associated protein 4; DILD, drug-induced lung disease; EGFR, epidermal growth factor receptor; mTOR, mechanistic target of rapamycin protein; ICI, immune checkpoint inhibitor; NSCLC, non–small-cell lung cancer; OP, organizing pneumonia; PD-1, programmed cell death protein 1; PD-L1, programmed cell death ligand 1, VEG-F, vascular endothelial growth factor.

Pathophysiology
- The pathophysiology of pneumotoxicity is complex, multifactorial and thought to be related to intrinsic action of the drug on the lung and its interaction with malignant cells through direct cytotoxic effects and/or immune-mediated injury.
- Chemotherapeutics cause direct injury to pneumocytes or alveolar capillary endothelium with activation of inflammatory cytokines resulting in endothelial dysfunction, capillary leak syndrome, and noncardiogenic edema.
- Drugs that are metabolized in the lungs may cause oxidative injury from release of free oxygen radicals; bleomycin is a well-described example.
- In immune checkpoint blockade, there is dysregulation of T-cell activation and the immune system leading to pulmonary damage.
- Agents that target epidermal growth factor receptor (EGFR) expressed on type II pneumocytes may impair alveolar repair mechanisms.

Risk Factors
- Although some risk factors are known, most presentations of lung injury are idiosyncratic and unpredictable with some patients being more susceptible than others.
- This increased susceptibility may be related to prior environmental exposures and genetics.
- Other identified risk factors include older age, male sex, smoking history, concurrent/previous interstitial lung disease (ILD), history of thoracic radiotherapy, poor performance states, abnormal baseline lung function, and combinations of cytotoxic agents.[4]
- Cumulative dosing may also affect development and severity of toxicity for some drugs.

DIAGNOSIS
- Pulmonary toxicity related to antineoplastic therapy encompasses a wide, variable, and overlapping spectrum of pulmonary clinical manifestations and severity.
- Any new respiratory symptoms or worsening radiographic changes require a high index of suspicion for the possibility.
- An online resource, www.pneumotox.com, is an invaluable reference for documented complications.[10]
- The severity of pulmonary toxicity is graded according to clinical manifestations by Common Terminology Criteria for Adverse Events (CTCAE v5.0); see Table 26-2.[4]

Clinical Presentation
- Symptoms may be vague including dyspnea and cough or include constitutional symptoms such as fever and malaise. Occasionally, progression to life-threatening respiratory failure requiring mechanical ventilation occurs.
- Up to one-third of patients may be asymptomatic.

History
- It is critical to obtain detailed medication and radiation histories to define the temporal relationship between onset of symptoms and exposure to potentially causative agents.
- Timing of onset varies with some causing damaging effects years later. For example, methotrexate-induced pneumonitis can occur acutely (days to weeks) or be delayed by years.
- Pneumonitis may be triggered or exacerbated by infections. Thus, evaluating and empirically treating for infectious etiologies is often required.

Diagnostic Criteria
- There are no clear criteria for the diagnosis of pulmonary toxicity related to antineoplastic agents. The diagnosis is made based on a history of drug exposure and exclusion of other causes, as well as medical history, clinical, radiographic, and possibly pathologic findings.

TABLE 26-2 COMMON TERMINOLOGY CRITERIA FOR ADVERSE EVENTS GRADING OF DRUG-INDUCED LUNG DISEASE (version 5.0)

Grade	Description
1	Asymptomatic Clinical or diagnostic observations only Intervention not indicated
2	Symptomatic Limiting instrumental ADLs Medical intervention indicated
3	Severe symptoms Limiting self-care ADLs Oxygen indicated
4	Life-threatening respiratory compromise Urgent intervention indicated (e.g., intubation or tracheotomy)
5	Death

ADLs, activities of daily living.

Adapted from Conte P, Ascierto PA, Patelli G, et al. Drug-induced interstitial lung disease during cancer therapies: expert opinion on diagnosis and treatment. *ESMO Open.* 2022;7:100404.

- Clinical improvement after drug discontinuation or clinical worsening with rechallenging of the drug may aid in the diagnosis.

Differential Diagnosis
- Differential diagnosis is broad and includes progression of underlying disease (lymphangitic carcinomatosis, malignant pleural effusion, pulmonary metastases, pulmonary tumor embolism), pulmonary hemorrhage, cardiogenic and noncardiogenic pulmonary edema, radiation pneumonitis, infectious etiologies (viral, bacterial, and fungal), and other causes of ILD.

Imaging
- Radiographic imaging is imperative. High-resolution computed tomography (HRCT) is the imaging modality of choice and should be obtained as early as possible when a patient on antineoplastic therapy presents with respiratory symptoms.
- Typical radiographic features include ground glass opacities. However, a range of findings can be present depending on the drug and the timing of presentation.
- The most common CT pattern observed is hypersensitivity pneumonitis (HP), with diffuse ground glass opacities and centrilobular nodules and air trapping. Other patterns include features of organizing pneumonia (OP) with multifocal bilateral parenchymal consolidations and a peripheral and lower lung distribution, diffuse alveolar damage pattern/acute respiratory distress syndrome (ARDS), nonspecific interstitial pneumonia (NSIP) with ground glass opacities, and progression to pulmonary fibrosis.[11] (See Chapter 24.)
- Pulmonary fibrosis can be observed with bleomycin, methotrexate, or carmustine.
- Cryptogenic OP has been described with trastuzumab, everolimus, and cyclophosphamide.
- Vinblastine, interferon beta, and vemurafenib can cause sarcoid-like reactions in the lung and can mimic metastases.

- Eosinophilic pneumonia, which presents with diffuse pulmonary opacities and bronchoalveolar lavage fluid with eosinophilia, has been associated with bleomycin, lenalidomide, and fludarabine.

Diagnostic Procedures

The role of bronchoscopy and lung biopsy has not been precisely determined. Bronchoscopy is helpful in excluding infectious causes. Transbronchial biopsies are often nonspecific and unable to differentiate the cause of lung injury.

TREATMENT

- The cornerstone of management of toxicity is generally drug withdrawal. However, the need for withdrawal depends on the severity and grade of pulmonary toxicity.
- Withdrawal of the causative agent may result in resolution of signs and symptoms. However, most patients will require treatment.
- Close collaboration with oncology is crucial as cessation of therapy results in withholding of potential lifesaving cancer therapy.
- American Society of Clinical Oncology (ASCO) guidelines are available on the management of immune-related adverse events.[12]

Medications

- Supportive care with oxygen is often required. Supplemental oxygen should be used judiciously in the case of bleomycin and mitomycin toxicity as oxygenation therapy may increase the toxicity.
- Immunosuppressive agents, mainly corticosteroids, are typically first line and may improve symptoms and promote repair of lung injury.
- In ICI-induced pneumonitis, specific guidelines have been developed to help guide treatment. The mainstay of management is discontinuation of ICI and initiation of corticosteroids.[12]
- In severe cases, patients with refractory disease may need additional immunosuppressive agents, such as infliximab, IV immunoglobulin (IVIG), cyclophosphamide, or mycophenolate mofetil.[13]

OUTCOME/PROGNOSIS

- Prognosis is variable depending on the underlying malignancy and degree of lung injury.
- Milder disease and corticosteroid responsiveness portend a better prognosis.
- Unfortunately, only half of the patients respond to corticosteroids, resulting in a high mortality.
- Pneumonitis accounts for 35% of fatalities associated with PD-1/PD-L1 therapy.[12]
- A diffuse alveolar damage (DAD) pattern, concurrent/previous ILD, and lower performance status have been identified as independent risk factors for severe DILD and poor prognosis.

REFERENCES

1. Shroff GS, Sheshadri A, Altan M, Truong MT, Erasmus LT, Vlahos I. Drug-induced lung disease in the oncology patient: from cytotoxic agents to immunotherapy. *Clin Chest Med.* 2024;45:325–337.
2. Long K, Suresh K. Pulmonary toxicity of systemic lung cancer therapy. *Respirology.* 2020;25:72–79.
3. Dhokarh R, Li G, Schmickl CN, et al. Drug-associated acute lung injury: a population-based cohort study. *Chest.* 2012;142:845–850.
4. Conte P, Ascierto PA, Patelli G, et al. Drug-induced interstitial lung disease during cancer therapies: expert opinion on diagnosis and treatment. *ESMO Open.* 2022;7:100404.

5. Raghu G, Nyberg F, Morgan G. The epidemiology of interstitial lung disease and its association with lung cancer. *Br J Cancer.* 2004;91:S3–S10.
6. Kaku S, Horinouchi H, Watanabe H, et al. Incidence and prognostic factors in severe drug-induced interstitial lung disease caused by antineoplastic drug therapy in the real world. *J Cancer Res Clin Oncol.* 2022;148:1737–1746.
7. Charpidou AG, Gkiozos I, Tsimpoukis S, et al. Therapy-induced toxicity of the lungs: an overview. *Anticancer Res.* 2009;29:631–639.
8. Naidoo J, Wang X, Woo KM, et al. Pneumonitis in patients treated with anti-programmed death-1/programmed death ligand 1 therapy. *J Clin Oncol.* 2017;35:709–717.
9. Suresh K, Voong KR, Shankar B, et al. Pneumonitis in non-small cell lung cancer patients receiving immune checkpoint immunotherapy: incidence and risk factors. *J Thorac Oncol.* 2018;13:1930–1939.
10. *Pneumotox.* Accessed October 10, 2024. www.pneumotox.com
11. Johkoh T, Lee KS, Nishino M, et al. Chest CT diagnosis and clinical management of drug-related pneumonitis in patients receiving molecular targeting agents and immune checkpoint inhibitors: a position paper from the Fleischner Society. *Radiology.* 2021;298:550–566.
12. Schneider BJ, Naidoo J, Santomasso BD, et al. Management of immune-related adverse events in patients treated with immune checkpoint inhibitor therapy: ASCO guideline update. *J Clin Oncol.* 2021;39:4073–4126.
13. Gutierrez C, McEvoy C, Munshi L, et al. Critical care management of toxicities associated with targeted agents and immunotherapies for cancer. *Crit Care Med.* 2020;48:10–21.

Solitary Pulmonary Nodule 27

Nathaniel G. Moulton and
Michael Beal

GENERAL PRINCIPLES

- A solitary pulmonary nodule (SPN) is defined as a small, <3 cm, focal, distinct, radiographic density completely surrounded by aerated lung parenchyma without evidence of atelectasis or hilar enlargement.
- Lesions >3 cm are referred to as a mass.
- The primary goal of working up an SPN is to determine as quickly as possible whether the nodule is malignant or benign.
- An SPN can be detected incidentally or by lung cancer screening.
- SPNs can be detected incidentally in up to 30% of all patients undergoing CT scans while abnormal CT scans are found in around 14% of lung cancer screening patients.[1-3]
- Once an SPN is detected, all prior CXR and CT scans should be reviewed.
- Guidelines for follow-up of incidentally and screen-detected nodules based on size, risk factors, and nodule type are published and should be referenced.[4,5]
- SPNs can further be described as solid, part solid, or pure ground glass (Figure 27-1):
  - Ground glass refers to a nodule with a density in which the lung architecture is not obscured by the nodule.
  - Part solid refers to a nodule that has both ground-glass and solid components.
  - While subsolid nodules may also be secondary to benign or malignant etiologies, malignant subsolid nodules grow at a slower pace than malignant solid nodules. Malignant subsolid nodules typically represent adenocarcinoma-spectrum lesions such as adenocarcinoma in situ (AIS) or minimally invasive adenocarcinoma (MIA).
- Once imaging and history have been reviewed, the risk for malignancy should be determined. In general:
  - For nodules with low malignancy likelihood, serial imaging is recommended.
  - An intermediate risk of malignancy requires additional diagnostic workup.
  - Nodules with high likelihood of malignancy should be referred for definitive management, such as surgical resection or radiation therapy (Figure 27-2).
- Solid nodules which have been stable without growth for more than 2 years are likely benign, while subsolid nodules should be monitored for up to 5 years prior to cessation of follow-up.[1,6,7]

DIAGNOSIS

Clinical Presentation

History
- The most important aspect of the history in a patient with an SPN is the reviewing of prior imaging.

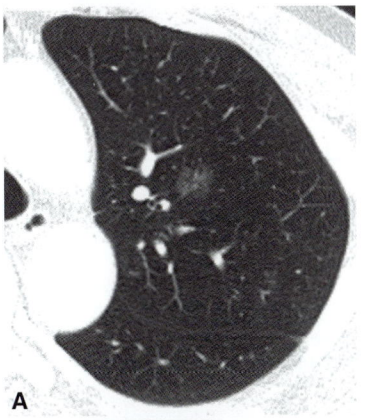
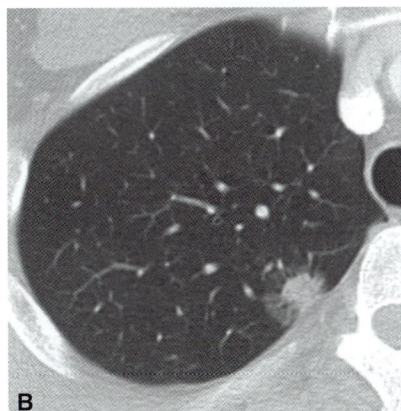
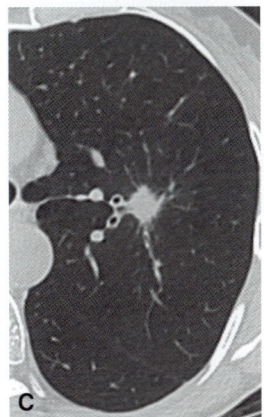

Figure 27-1 Nodule types: **A.** Pure Ground-glass nodule. **B.** Part-solid nodule. **C.** Solid spiculated nodule.

- Additionally, while SPN is a radiographic diagnosis, one should obtain a complete history with an emphasis on risk factors for malignancy, infection, autoimmune, or inflammatory disease.[1,7]
  - A detailed smoking history is essential because tobacco is the leading risk factor for primary lung cancer.
  - Age is also important, with increased odds of malignancy for every 10 years above 50 years old.
  - Other risk factors for malignancy include exposures to asbestos, second-hand smoke, radon, arsenic, radiation, haloethers, nickel, and polycyclic aromatic hydrocarbons.
  - History of chronic obstructive pulmonary disease (COPD) and evidence of emphysema on CT imaging may indicate past or current smoking history and increases the risk for malignancy.

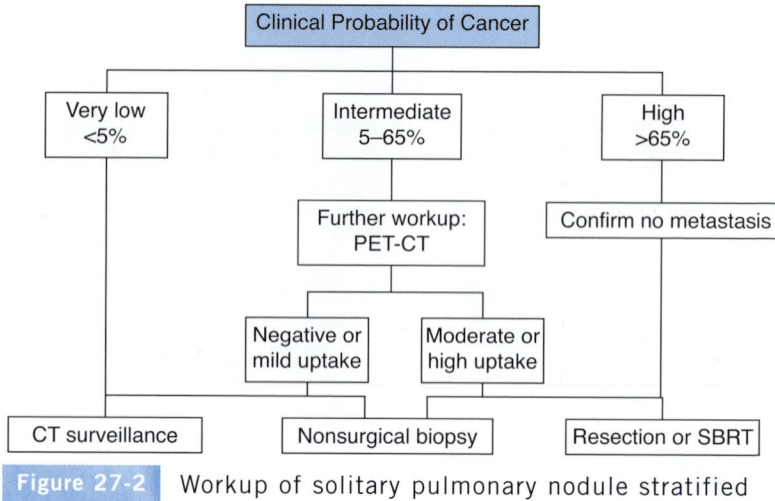

Figure 27-2 Workup of solitary pulmonary nodule stratified by risk assessment. (Adapted from 2013 ACCP Guidelines.)

- History of any malignancy, but especially cancers that metastasize to the lung (e.g., lung cancer, malignant melanoma, sarcomas, and colon, breast, renal, germ cell, and bladder cancers), raises suspicion of a metastatic lung nodule.
- Any immunosuppressed state including HIV, chronic corticosteroids or other immune-modulating medications, or posttransplantation status broadens the differential diagnosis for infection as well as malignancy.

Clinical Manifestations and Symptoms

SPNs, as a function of their small size, are usually asymptomatic. If symptoms are present they may or may not be related to the same process as the SPN. Clinical correlation is advised, but the following should be kept in mind:

- Chest pain, especially pleuritic, may indicate pleural, mediastinal, or pericardial involvement.
- New diffuse pain or bone pain may indicate metastatic disease or hypertrophic osteoarthropathy.
- Weight loss is nonspecific, but if present with malignancy is a poor prognostic factor.
- Cough may or may not be present and is nonspecific.
- Hemoptysis with an SPN can suggest malignancy such as a squamous cell carcinoma, a proximal lesion, or infectious or inflammatory etiologies.
- Hoarseness may be present from compression or invasion of the left recurrent laryngeal nerve.

Physical Examination

While the physical exam is typically normal in the workup of SPNs, a thorough examination can yield clues to complications of direct involvement of the SPN, metastatic disease, paraneoplastic disease, or evidence of infection. Signs to look for include clubbing and long bone swelling (hypertrophic osteoarthropathy), hepatomegaly, bone tenderness (metastases), plethoric face, engorged neck, and superficial veins (superior vena cava syndrome), wasting, lymphadenopathy, and focal neurologic deficits.

Differential Diagnosis
- The differential diagnosis can be divided into malignant and nonmalignant causes; see Table 27-1.
- Malignant causes include primary lung cancers (adenocarcinoma, squamous cell carcinoma, large-cell carcinoma, small-cell carcinoma, adenocarcinoma in situ [formerly referred to as bronchoalveolar cell carcinoma]), metastatic cancers, and carcinoid tumors.
- Nonmalignant causes include benign neoplasms, vascular malformations, developmental abnormalities, inflammatory nodules, and infections (granulomatous and nongranulomatous).

Diagnostic Testing
Laboratory Evaluation
- Laboratory evaluation does not have a routine role in the workup of SPNs.
- Basic laboratory evaluation may be desired based on the history, imaging, and physical exam findings to detect suspected blood count abnormalities or metabolic derangements.
- Hypercalcemia may be due to bony metastases or release of parathyroid hormone (PTH)-related peptide from a squamous cell carcinoma as well as sarcoidosis.
- Hyponatremia may be due to the syndrome of inappropriate antidiuretic hormone secretion (SIADH), which can be seen in small-cell carcinoma or significant pulmonary or neurologic disease.
- Liver abnormalities may suggest liver metastases.
- If the history includes risk factors for endemic fungi or tuberculosis (TB), additional focused laboratory testing should be obtained with fungal antibody titers, interferon-gamma release assay (IGRA) for TB, or serum aspergillus galactomannan antigen.
- Rheumatologic serologies should be obtained if there is suspicion for an autoimmune etiology.

Imaging
Characteristics on CT imaging can be suggestive of malignant or benign etiologies[1,4,7]:

- Size: Increasing size increases the risk of malignancy.
  - SPNs less than 10 mm in size are less likely to be malignant.
  - As an independent risk factor, nodules 4–6 mm in size have been shown to have a 0.5% probability of malignancy, while nodules 7–10 mm having a 1.7% probability.
  - SPNs >2 cm in size have a 60–80% risk of malignancy.
- Location: Nodules located in the upper lobes are more likely to be malignant.
- Calcification patterns
  - Diffuse, central, popcorn, or laminated calcifications are suggestive of benign disease processes such as infectious granuloma or hamartomas.

TABLE 27-1 DIFFERENTIAL DIAGNOSIS OF THE SOLITARY PULMONARY NODULE

Malignant
  Primary lung cancer (adenocarcinoma, squamous cell carcinoma, large cell carcinoma, small cell carcinoma, adenocarcinoma in situ)
  Lymphoma
  Carcinoid
  Metastasis (breast, kidney, thyroid, lung, melanoma, sarcoma, bladder, colon, kidney, testicle)

Benign
  Infectious granuloma
    Histoplasmosis
    Coccidioidomycosis
    TB
    Atypical mycobacteria
    Cryptococcosis
    Blastomycosis
  Other infections
    Bacterial abscess
    Dirofilaria immitis
    Echinococcal cyst
    Ascariasis
    Pneumocystis carinii
    Aspergilloma
  Benign neoplasms
    Hamartoma
    Lipoma
    Fibroma
  Vascular
    Arteriovenous malformation
    Pulmonary varix
  Developmental
    Bronchogenic cyst
  Inflammatory
    Amyloidoma
    ANCA-positive vasculitis
    Foreign body
    Posttransplant lymphoproliferative disorder
    Rheumatoid nodule
    Rounded atelectasis
    Sarcoidosis

ANCA, antineutrophil cytoplasmic antibody.

- Stippled or eccentric calcifications can occur in malignant disease and should raise suspicion.
- Doubling time:
  - Refers to the amount of time it takes for an SPN to double in volume.
  - One doubling time corresponds to 25% increase in diameter on CT imaging.
  - The doubling time of malignant tumors ranges from 100 to 400 days, while benign lesions may be shorter or longer in their doubling time.
- Border
  - Smooth or well-rounded nodules suggest a benign process.
  - A scalloped or spiculated (corona radiata) appearance suggests a malignant SPN.
  - Rounded atelectasis is thought to be due to inflammatory process.
  - A halo sign can indicate fungal infection.
- Density: subsolid nodules with large or growing solid components are suggestive of malignancy.
- Cavitation:
  - Cavity wall thickness <5 mm are most likely benign.
  - Cavity wall thickness >15 mm are malignant 95% of the time.
- Pleural retraction or dilated bronchus near an SPN suggests malignancy.
- Attenuation
  - Fat attenuation (–400 to –120 HU) is strongly suggestive of a hamartoma or lipoma.
  - Some metastatic malignancies (e.g., liposarcoma or renal cell carcinoma) may occasionally contain fat.
- Vascular structures: contrast can identify a feeding artery and draining vein as can be seen in arteriovenous malformations.
- Positron emission tomography (PET) with 18-fluorodeoxyglucose (FDG) identifies metabolically active lesions.
  - PET can discriminate between malignant and nonmalignant nodules with sensitivity of 95% and specificity of 82%.[8]
  - Specificity will vary depending on area and likelihood of granulomatous disease.
  - False positives can occur with infectious or inflammatory lesions.
  - False negatives may occur with slow-growing or subsolid tumors such as carcinoid or adenocarcinoma in situ.
  - This modality is of limited use in very small nodules <8 mm in size due to lower resolution.
  - PET scanning is not indicated for low-risk or high-risk lesions but can provide guidance in the management of nodules at intermediate risk of malignancy.

Further Evaluation of the SPN
Follow-Up Interval and Next Steps in Management
- Radiologic societal guidelines are helpful in determining the next steps in the evaluation of SPNs.
- The Fleischner Society Guidelines provide recommendations for next steps in management for incidentally detected lung nodules. Recommendations are based on size, risk factors for malignancy, and type of nodule (solid, subsolid, or ground glass). See Tables 27-2 and 27-3.[4] Notably, these guidelines are not applicable for patients with a history of malignancy, <35 years old, or immunosuppressed patients.

TABLE 27-2. GUIDELINES FOR INCIDENTAL SOLID SOLITARY PULMONARY NODULES

Nodule Size	Low Risk	High Risk
<6 mm	No follow-up	Optional CT at 12 mo
6–8 mm	CT at 6–12 mo, then consider CT at 18–24 mo	CT at 6–12 mo, then at 18–24 mo
>8 mm	CT at 3 mo, PET-CT, or tissue sampling	CT at 3 mo, PET-CT, or tissue sampling

PET, positron emission tomography.
Adapted from MacMahon H, Naidich DP, Goo JM, et al. Guidelines for management of incidental pulmonary nodules detected on CT images: From the Fleischner Society 2017. *Radiology*. 2017;284(1):228–243.

- Lung Imaging Reporting and Data System (Lung-RADS) provides recommendations for the further evaluation of nodules detected as part of lung cancer screening. See Table 27-4.[5] Guidelines for Incidental Subsolid Solitary Pulmonary Nodules[9]:
  - Age 50–80
  - >20 pack-year history of smoking
  - Current smoker or have quit smoking within the past 15 years

Risk Stratification
- After review of the history, imaging, physical exam, and laboratory evaluation, the pretest probability of malignancy should be calculated by either expert clinical judgment or quantitatively by using a validated model, such as the Brock, Mayo, Herder, or VA model.[10] Expert clinicians may still have better accuracy for malignancy than risk models.[11]
- The American College of Chest Physicians (ACCP) guidelines recommend further evaluation of SPNs based on risk of malignancy.[7] SPNs are typically

TABLE 27-3. GUIDELINES FOR INCIDENTAL SUBSOLID SOLITARY PULMONARY NODULES

Nodule Type	<6 mm	≥6 mm
Ground glass	No routine follow-up	CT at 6–12 mo, then CT every 2 y until 5 y
Part solid	No routine follow-up	CT at 3–6 m; if unchanged and solid component remains <6 mm, annual CT until 5 y

Adapted from MacMahon H, Naidich DP, Goo JM, et al. Guidelines for management of incidental pulmonary nodules detected on CT images: From the Fleischner Society 2017. *Radiology*. 2017;284(1):228–243.

TABLE 27-4 GUIDELINES FOR NODULE MANAGEMENT IN LUNG CANCER SCREENING

Lung-RADS Score	Category Description	Management
0	Incomplete	Additional images needed
1	Negative	Annual low-dose CT
2	Benign	Annual low-dose CT
3	Probably benign	6-month low-dose CT
4A	Suspicious	3-month low-dose CT or PET-CT
4B, 4X	Very suspicious	Diagnostic chest CT, PET-CT, tissue sampling, or referral for clinical management

PET, positron emission tomography.
Adapted from Martin MD, Kanne JP, Broderick LS, et al. *RadioGraphics* update: Lung-RADS 2022. *Radiographics*. 2023;43(11):e230037.

---

grouped as low risk (<5%), intermediate risk (5–65%), and high risk of malignancy (>65%).
- Low-risk nodules (<5%) should be followed with serial imaging based on the appropriate societal guidelines.
- Intermediate-risk nodules (5–65%) warrant further characterization with either close follow-up imaging, functional imaging such as PET, biomarker evaluation, or biopsy.
- High-risk nodules (>65%), nodules with evidence of malignant growth on serial CT scans, and nodules hypermetabolic on PET scan should be considered for biopsy or definitive management unless contraindicated.
- For nodules with discordant test results, patients with high-risk nodules who do not desire surgery, or patients not suitable for surgery, nonsurgical biopsy should be considered.

Biomarker Evaluation
- Research on biomarkers is ongoing and aims at providing another tool for the risk stratification of SPNs.[12]
- One commercially available classifier, Nodify XL2, uses two proteins in conjunction with clinical and imaging features and has been clinically validated to improve accuracy in assessing probability of cancer risk for SPNs and have been shown to reduce invasive procedures in patients with benign nodules.[13]
- Additional research is ongoing for additional biomarker such as blood protein–based biomarkers, exhaled volatile organic compounds, bronchial or nasal epithelium genomic classifiers, and quantitative imaging analysis.

Biopsy
- Biopsy is recommended for SPNs in patients when:
  - The clinical likelihood of malignancy and results of imaging studies are not in agreement (e.g., high clinical suspicion but a negative fluorodeoxyglucose positron emission tomography scan [FDG PET scan]).

- When the probability of malignancy is intermediate (5–65%) after further image characterization or biomarker evaluation.
- A specific treatment is available for a benign diagnosis (e.g., fungal infection).
- The patient wants biopsy confirmation prior to committing to surgery or radiation (this may be most useful when the risks of surgery are high).
• Options for biopsy include transthoracic ultrasound-guided or CT-guided biopsy, bronchoscopic biopsy, or surgical biopsy.
  - US- or CT-guided transthoracic needle aspiration may be performed for peripheral nodules when there is no indication for pathologic staging of the mediastinum or hila, such as in cases of small, peripheral pulmonary lesions.
    - The pooled diagnostic yield of CT-guided biopsy can be over 90%, but is dependent on multiple factors including lesion size, expertise of the radiologist, availability of an onsite cytopathologic examination, needle size, and number of needle passes.[14]
    - Despite the high diagnostic yield, complications of CT-guided biopsy can be as high as 25% and include pulmonary hemorrhage, pneumothorax, and air embolism.[14]
  - Bronchoscopic biopsy utilizes a flexible bronchoscope in addition to radial-probe endobronchial ultrasound and fluoroscopy to biopsy nodules from within the airways.
    - Pooled diagnostic yield for SPNs is ~70% and is largely dependent on nodule size, location, and a visible airway leading to the nodule.[15]
    - Newer technology utilizing virtual bronchoscopic guidance with electromagnetic navigation and robotic assistance in addition to intraprocedural CT imaging aims to improve diagnostic yield and is becoming routine in the workup of SPNs.[16,17]
• Surgical evaluation of SPN can be performed in nodules which are difficult to biopsy via CT-guided or bronchoscopic approaches, or in nodules with a high suspicion for malignancy undergoing definitive management.[7] Surgery can be performed with robotic-assisted minimally invasive surgery, video-assisted thoracoscopic surgery, or open thoracotomy to obtain a wedge biopsy of the SPN. If frozen sectioning indicates malignancy, additional resection, and staging can be performed based on surgical margins and guidelines.

TREATMENT

• Many benign nodules such as AVMs, granulomas, or hamartomas do not need further treatment following appropriate diagnosis and follow-up.
• Infectious and inflammatory etiologies of SPNs may warrant further treatment depending on patient and disease-specific factors.
• When malignant, SPNs often represent early, stage I non–small-cell lung cancer (NSCLC). Definitive treatment options for stage I NSCLC include surgical resection or stereotactic body radiation therapy (SBRT), which is a nonsurgical approach using highly focused radiation.

REFERENCES

1. Mazzone PJ, Lam L. Evaluating the patient with a pulmonary nodule: a review. *JAMA.* 2022;327:264–273.
2. Gould MK, Tang T, Liu I-LA, et al. Recent trends in the identification of incidental pulmonary nodules. *Am J Respir Crit Care Med.* 2015;192:1208–1214.
3. Pinsky PF, Gierada DS, Black W, et al. Performance of Lung-RADS in the National Lung Screening Trial: a retrospective assessment. *Ann Intern Med.* 2015;162:485–491.
4. MacMahon H, Naidich DP, Goo JM, et al. Guidelines for management of incidental pulmonary nodules detected on CT images: from the Fleischner Society 2017. *Radiology.* 2017;284:228–243.
5. Martin MD, Kanne JP, Broderick LS, Kazerooni EA, Meyer CA. *RadioGraphics* Update: Lung-RADS 2022. *Radiographics.* 2023;43:e230037.
6. Shin KE, Lee KS, Yi CA, Chung MJ, Shin MH, Choi YH. Subcentimeter lung nodules stable for 2 years at LDCT: long-term follow-up using volumetry. *Respirology.* 2014;19: 921–928.
7. Gould MK, Donington J, Lynch WR, et al. Evaluation of individuals with pulmonary nodules: when is it lung cancer? Diagnosis and management of lung cancer, 3rd ed: American College of Chest Physicians evidence-based clinical practice guidelines. *Chest.* 2013;143:e93S–e120S.
8. Groheux D, Quere G, Blanc E, et al. FDG PET-CT for solitary pulmonary nodule and lung cancer: literature review. *Diagn Interv Imaging.* 2016;97:1003–1017.
9. Jonas DE, Reuland DS, Reddy SM, et al. Screening for lung cancer with low-dose computed tomography: updated evidence report and systematic review for the US Preventive Services Task Force. *JAMA.* 2021;325:971–987.
10. Choi HK, Ghobrial M, Mazzone PJ. Models to estimate the probability of malignancy in patients with pulmonary nodules. *Ann Am Thorac Soc.* 2018;15:1117–1126.
11. Tanner NT, Porter A, Gould MK, Li X-J, Vachani A, Silvestri GA. Physician assessment of pretest probability of malignancy and adherence with guidelines for pulmonary nodule evaluation. *Chest.* 2017;152:263–270.
12. Paez R, Kammer MN, Tanner NT, et al. Update on biomarkers for the stratification of indeterminate pulmonary nodules. *Chest.* 2023;164:1028–1041.
13. Pritchett MA, Sigal B, Bowling MR, Kurman JS, Pitcher T, Springmeyer SC; ORACLE Study Investigators. Assessing a biomarker's ability to reduce invasive procedures in patients with benign lung nodules: Results from the ORACLE study. *PLoS One.* 2023;18: e0287409.
14. Han Y, Kim HJ, Kong KA, et al. Diagnosis of small pulmonary lesions by transbronchial lung biopsy with radial endobronchial ultrasound and virtual bronchoscopic navigation versus CT-guided transthoracic needle biopsy: a systematic review and meta-analysis. *PLoS One.* 2018;13:e0191590.
15. Ali MS, Trick W, Mba BI, Mohananey D, Sethi J, Musani AI. Radial endobronchial ultrasound for the diagnosis of peripheral pulmonary lesions: a systematic review and meta-analysis. *Respirology.* 2017;22:443–453.
16. Diddams MJ, Lee HJ. Robotic bronchoscopy: review of three systems. *Life (Basel).* 2023;13:354.
17. Reisenauer J, Duke JD, Kern R, Fernandez-Bussy S, Edell E. Combining shape-sensing robotic bronchoscopy with mobile three-dimensional imaging to verify tool-in-lesion and overcome divergence: a pilot study. *Mayo Clin Proc Innov Qual Outcomes.* 2022; 6:177–185.

Lung Transplantation

28

**Laura Halverson and
James McMenimen**

GENERAL PRINCIPLES

- This chapter touches on the logistical background of lung transplantation, common terminology, candidate selection, as well as postoperative management of adult lung transplant patients, including a comprehensive review of immunosuppressive agents.
- There are three general arms to the organ transplantation system in the US:
  - United network for organ sharing (UNOS) operates the organ procurement and transplantation network (OPTN) and maintains a national registry for organ matching.
  - Organ procurement organizations (OPOs) are nongovernmental organizations that recover organs in their respective service areas and allocate them based on UNOS policies.
  - Transplant centers: as of November 2023, there are 74 transplant centers in the United States performing adult lung transplantation.
- The most common underlying lung diseases leading to transplantation are pulmonary fibrosis (both idiopathic and interstitial lung diseases [ILDs] with known etiologies), chronic obstructive pulmonary disease (COPD)/emphysema (including α1-antitrypsin deficiency), cystic fibrosis (CF), sarcoidosis, and idiopathic pulmonary arterial hypertension (IPAH). Transplant for the indication of CF is decreasing in the CFTR modulator era.
- Dual-organ lung transplantation is relatively rare. Heart–lung transplantation is generally reserved for patients with Eisenmenger syndrome and an uncorrectable congenital heart defect. Liver–lung transplantation is indicated in the setting of CF with CF-related cirrhosis, hepatopulmonary syndrome, pulmonary hypertension secondary to liver disease, and alpha-1 antitrypsin deficiency with subsequent emphysema and cirrhosis.
- The majority of lung transplant recipients are between 18 and 64 years of age, though the percentage of recipients >65 years has increased in recent years commensurate with increased transplantation of patients with idiopathic pulmonary fibrosis (IPF).[1]
- When referring a patient for transplantation, both absolute and relative contraindications must be considered, in addition to their age and significant comorbidities (Table 28-1).[2-4]

DONOR AND CANDIDATE SELECTION

Indications and Timing of Referral by Diagnosis

- In general, a transplant evaluation should occur if a patient meets three basic criteria: (1) they are experiencing progressive disease despite maximal therapy,

TABLE 28-1 CONTRAINDICATIONS TO LUNG TRANSPLANTATION

Absolute

Significant dysfunction of major nonpulmonary organs, e.g., renal dysfunction (which can worsen with immunosuppression), low ejection fraction, cirrhosis

CVA history or serious musculoskeletal disease (active myositis) preventing rehabilitation both pre- and posttransplant

Acute medical instability (critical illness)

Active infection with *Mycobacterium abscessus* or *Burkholderia cenocepacia*

Active substance use and dependence; most commonly tobacco, alcohol, and narcotics (a minimum of 6-mo cessation of alcohol, tobacco, and illicit drugs is needed in addition to participation in substance use counseling or support groups)

Active malignancy (other than basal or squamous cell carcinoma of the skin); in general, previous cancer should be in continuous remission for 5 y before transplantation

Poor rehabilitation potential (severe prolonged frailty or critical illness myopathy)

Active extrapulmonary infection

Relative

Mild to moderate coronary artery disease

Frailty, deconditioning, and decreased functional status

Symptomatic osteoporosis (disease must be treated before transplantation)

Ideal body weight <70% or >130%, BMI >30

Substance abuse

Cognitive impairment or severe uncontrolled psychiatric disease

Lack of social support, specifically inadequate posttransplant caregiver options

Longstanding documented medical nonadherence

Mechanical ventilation

BMI, body mass index; CVA, cerebrovascular accident.

---

(2) they are deemed to be at high risk of death from their lung disease within 2 years, and (3) they have a high likelihood of survival at 5 years from a general medical perspective provided there is adequate graft function.
- Different disease processes have benchmarks that are used to determine appropriate timing for both referral to a transplant center for evaluation and to help to guide timing of waitlist placement.

COPD/Emphysema
- Referral should take place when a patient has a BODE score of 5–6, a forced expiratory volume at 1 second (FEV1) <25% predicted, is experiencing increased

frequency of exacerbations or hospitalizations, and has developed elevated $PaCO_2$ or resting hypoxemia.
- Listing for transplant is reasonable when FEV1 is <15–20% predicted, BODE score is 7 or greater, the patient has developed group 3 pulmonary hypertension, or if their quality of life has declined significantly.
- Lung transplant for COPD/emphysema offers improvement in quality of life but no survival benefit, so meeting the above criteria prior to listing is paramount.

Pulmonary Fibrosis/Interstitial Lung Disease
- Referral should take place when a patient increasing oxygen requirements and progressive decline in FVC despite appropriate therapies. It is appropriate to refer a patient for transplant evaluation at the time of diagnosis of IPF (depending on their age and comorbidities) given the unpredictable and at times rapid progression of the disease.
- Listing for transplant is reasonable when there is a more precipitous decline in pulmonary function tests (PFTs) or oxygenation over the prior 6 months, development of group 3 pulmonary hypertension or increasing exacerbations and hospitalizations.

Cystic Fibrosis
- Referral should take place when FEV1 is <30% predicted, the patient experiences more frequent exacerbations with poor recovery, episodes of significant hemoptysis and/or worsening nutritional status.
- Listing for transplant is reasonable when there is chronic resting hypoxemia, chronic hypercapnic respiratory failure requiring the use of noninvasive positive pressure ventilation (NIPPV), development of group 3 pulmonary hypertension, or more frequent hospitalizations.

Pulmonary Arterial Hypertension
- Referral should take place when a patient has a New York Heart Association (NYHA) functional class III or IV symptoms despite escalating (parenteral) therapy, or known pulmonary veno-occlusive disease.
- Listing for transplant is reasonable when there is evidence of worsening right heart failure, development of significant pericardial effusion, decreased cardiac index (<2), and/or decreasing 6-minute walk test (6MWT) (<350 m).

Recipient Selection and Organ Allocation
- Each transplant center has specific evaluation requirements. Generally, patients undergo a thorough battery of laboratory tests (infectious disease serologies, drug screen, HLA typing, in addition to complete blood count [CBC], complete metabolic panel [CMP] and autoimmune disease screening), pulmonary function testing including 6MWT, imaging tests including high-resolution CT of the chest, V/Q scan for surgical planning and a cardiac catheterization to assess for coronary disease and pulmonary hypertension. Additional vital organ functions are evaluated as needed based on the results of screening tests, and often include liver ultrasound, esophageal pH probe and motility studies, 24-hour urine for creatinine clearance, or carotid dopplers.

- Following this evaluation, the suitability for transplantation and appropriate timing for listing are decided by a multidisciplinary committee of individuals which includes pulmonary physicians, thoracic surgeons, dieticians, social workers, financial/insurance experts, and psychologists.
- Relative contraindications are common and underscore the importance of early referral to a transplant center so that the potential candidate has time to improve modifiable factors in order to optimize their chance at a successful transplant. Common modifiable relative contraindications include obesity or protein calorie malnutrition, deconditioning, reliance on chronic opioids or benzodiazepines, and lack of social support or adequate financial resources.
- The donor and the recipient are matched for ABO blood groups, height, and the absence of circulating anti–donor-specific HLA antibodies (discussed further in the section on Rejection).
- Prior to 2005, priority for lung organ allocation was determined primarily by waiting time. In 2005, the Lung Allocation System (LAS) was developed with the goal to allocate organs based primarily on medical urgency and expected outcome (i.e., success) after transplantation.[5] In 2023, the Lung Composite Allocation Score (CAS) was released, which was developed to further account for biologic disadvantages (rarer blood types, high-level allosensitization, extremes of height) in addition to accounting for predicted waitlist and post-transplant survival.[6]
- We do not yet have adequate longitudinal data to determine the impact of this current system.

Donor Selection
- Donor organs remain in short supply.
- Given the limitation in the organ pool, donor criteria have become increasingly liberalized. Standard criteria for acceptance are listed in Table 28-2.[5]
- Efforts to broaden the donor pool include acceptance of marginal donors, acceptance of Hepatitis C Virus (HCV)-positive donors, donation after cardiac death (so-called DCD donor), and development of ex vivo organ reconditioning protocols.

TABLE 28-2 STANDARD LUNG TRANSPLANT DONOR CRITERIA

Age <55 y
ABO compatibility
Clear CXR
PaO_2 ≥300 mm Hg, ventilated with a fraction of inspired oxygen = 1, and positive end-expiratory pressure = 5 cm H_2O
≤20 pack-year smoking history
Satisfactory bronchoscopic examination and gross inspection (before harvest)

Adapted from Snell GI, Westall GP. Selection and management of the lung donor. *Clin Chest Med.* 2011;32:223–232.

- Potential organ donors are screened for past medical history (particularly respiratory and oncologic disease), social history (tobacco use, vaping/marijuana use frequency, intravenous drug abuse [IVDA]), pertinent physical examination findings (e.g., chest trauma), cause of death, vital signs, bronchoscopic findings, sputum cultures, viral swab results, and CT imaging of the chest.
- Donors are also tested for HIV, hepatitis B and C, human T-cell leukemia virus type 1 (HTLV-1), syphilis, and cytomegalovirus (CMV, pretransfusion preferred). Organs that are positive for HIV or HTLV-1 are excluded from transplantation.
- Malignancy usually prevents transplantation, except for localized skin cancers, cervical cancer, or neurologic tumors that rarely metastasize.

Surgical Considerations
- Single lung transplantation (SLT) and bilateral lung transplantation (BLT) are possible for COPD, α1-antitrypsin–deficiency emphysema, IPF, IPAH, and some cases of Eisenmenger syndrome.
- BLT is mandatory for diffuse bronchiectasis associated with CF or other diseases, or for patients with pretransplantation history of colonization with pseudomonas, aspergillus or mycobacterial disease regardless of underlying lung disease.
- Heart–lung transplantation is usually reserved for complex congenital heart diseases with pulmonary hypertension.
- BLT is the most common procedure performed currently.

TREATMENT

Immunosuppressive Therapy
- Randomized controlled trials are very sparse in lung transplantation; a majority of protocols are derived from renal transplantation or are the result of historical practice patterns. As such, the regimen varies from center to center.
- Induction: High-dose immunosuppression is initiated in the operating room and continued in the initial posttransplant hospitalization. Treatment options have included interleukin (IL-2) receptor antagonists, antilymphocyte antibody preparations, or alemtuzumab (anti-CD52).[7]
- Maintenance: Immunosuppression strategies vary among transplant centers but most use a triple-drug maintenance regimen consisting of a corticosteroid (methylprednisolone perioperatively, followed by prednisone), an antimetabolite (azathioprine or mycophenolate mofetil [MMF]), and a calcineurin inhibitor (cyclosporine [CsA] or tacrolimus).[7]

Specific Agents
Corticosteroids
- Steroids have anti-inflammatory effects in both the innate and adaptive arms of the immune system. Dosing is variable.
- Metabolism and excretion: Hepatic metabolism, including cytochrome P450-3A4 isoform (CYP3A4), and urinary excretion.
- Interactions: Barbiturates, phenytoin, rifampin, and St. John's wort decrease corticosteroid effectiveness by inducing CYP3A4. Conversely, inhibitors of

CYP3A4, such as azole antifungals and macrolides, may increase steroid levels. Steroids may also increase CsA levels and potentiate aspirin or NSAID-induced gastritis.
- Adverse drug reactions: Chronic steroid use contributes to multiple complications including skin thinning, impaired wound healing, fat redistribution, hypertension, hypokalemia, hyperglycemia, adrenal insufficiency, osteoporosis, and mental status changes (ranging from restlessness and poor sleep to agitation and steroid psychosis). Corticosteroids may also increase or decrease the prothrombotic effect of warfarin.

Azathioprine
- Azathioprine is a purine analog that inhibits DNA and RNA synthesis, ultimately blocking proliferation of activated lymphocytes.
- Initial dosing is 1–3 mg/kg PO/IV daily.
- Bioavailability: Azathioprine is well absorbed after oral administration. Azathioprine and its metabolite 6-mercaptopurine are 30% bound to plasma proteins.
- Metabolism and excretion: Hepatic metabolism and urinary excretion.
- Interactions: Allopurinol may reduce metabolism and increase azathioprine levels. Drugs with bone marrow toxicity should be avoided, as the effects can be additive. Warfarin levels may increase via unknown mechanisms.
- Adverse drug reactions: Bone marrow toxicity (thrombocytopenia, anemia, and leukopenia). Leukopenia is common in patients with mutations in thiopurine S-methyltransferase, which can be screened with genetic testing if needed. Gastrointestinal (GI) side effects include hepatitis, cholestatic jaundice, and pancreatitis.

Mycophenolate Mofetil
- MMF was initially developed as an antibiotic/antineoplastic/antipsoriatic agent. It is a selective, noncompetitive, and reversible inhibitor of inosine monophosphate dehydrogenase, blocking de novo purine synthesis. As B and T cells lack the salvage pathway of purine synthesis, they are selectively inhibited.
- Initial dosing is 1–1.5 g PO/IV bid.
- Bioavailability: MMF is given as an ester derivative owing to poor absorption. In this form, it is rapidly absorbed orally. It is 97% albumin bound in plasma.
- Metabolism and excretion: MMF is rapidly hydrolyzed to an active metabolite mycophenolic acid (MPA) in the liver. Also, it is later inactivated in the liver by glucuronidation. MPA is eliminated primarily in the urine as MPA glucuronide. In renal failure, accumulated MPA glucuronide may be converted to MPA, causing toxicity.
- Interactions: Relatively few drug interactions occur. Antacids may reduce absorption. Cholestyramine and antibiotics that alter gut flora can decrease levels by reducing enterohepatic circulation. Drugs that interfere (e.g., probenecid) or compete for renal tubular secretion may increase MPA glucuronide levels. High doses of salicylates may increase free MPA levels.
- Adverse drug reactions: MMF is generally well tolerated. GI side effects are most common (abdominal pain, nausea, vomiting, dyspepsia, diarrhea). These can be overcome by splitting doses or administering the drug with small amounts of food. Bone marrow toxicity (anemia, leukopenia, and thrombocytopenia) is another clinically significant side effect.

- Monitoring: Therapeutic monitoring is not routinely performed. Concentrations may be monitored in renal failure or coadministration with CsA.

Cyclosporine
- CsA is a fat-soluble fungal polypeptide that inhibits production of IL-2 from CD4+ cells. It binds cyclophilin in lymphocytes, and the complex then binds calcineurin, inhibiting cytokine gene transcription and lymphocyte proliferation.
- Initial dosing is 5–10 mg/kg/d split into two doses.
- Bioavailability: Oral bioavailability is variable and dependent on the drug formulation (sandimmune 10–90%, neoral 30–45%). It is also bile dependent and can be influenced by fat intake, diarrhea, and GI motility. CsA is mostly distributed outside of the blood volume and the fraction in plasma is 90% lipoprotein bound.
- Metabolism and excretion: CsA is extensively metabolized in liver and intestine (CYP3A4). Elimination is primarily by excretion of metabolites in the bile. Only a small fraction is excreted unchanged via GI and genitourinary tracts.
- Interactions: Drug interactions are very common because of CYP3A4 induction or inhibition. Drugs that decrease CsA levels include rifampin, phenytoin, carbamazepine, phenytoin, St. John's wort, and hydroxymethylglutaryl (HMG) coenzyme A reductase inhibitors. Increased levels are seen with azole antifungals, macrolides, calcium channel blockers (verapamil and diltiazem; nifedipine has less effect), and grapefruit juice. Many nephrotoxic drugs have synergistic toxicity with CsA. Potassium-sparing diuretics should be avoided owing to the potential for hyperkalemia. Concomitant use of HMG coenzyme A reductase inhibitor therapy increases the risk of myopathy and rhabdomyolysis.
- Adverse drug reactions: Renal side effects are common (hyperkalemia, hypomagnesemia, hypertension). Metabolic side effects include hyperlipidemia, gout, osteoporosis, hirsutism, and hyperglycemia. Neurologic effects include tremors, peripheral neuropathy, headaches, mental status changes, and, in rare instances, reversible posterior leukoencephalopathy syndrome. Gingival hypertrophy (especially in conjunction with nifedipine), a thrombotic thrombocytopenic purpura–like syndrome, and hepatotoxicity can be seen as well.
- Monitoring: Therapeutic monitoring is performed due to intra- and interpatient variability of absorption, metabolism, and excretion, as well as the considerable side effect profile. Levels measured include trough, area under the curve, and C2 pseudopeak levels. Target levels vary with time interval after transplant, organ type, and rejection history.

Tacrolimus
- Tacrolimus is a fungal-derived macrolide that inhibits IL-2 production. It binds to immunophilin FKBP12, and blocks calcineurin activity in a fashion similar to CsA.
- Initial dosing range is about 0.1 mg/kg/d PO divided into two doses.
- Bioavailability: Oral bioavailability is poor (20–25%) but not bile acid dependent. It is fat soluble, and ~80% of serum drug is red blood cell (RBC) membrane bound.
- Metabolism and excretion: Tacrolimus is metabolized in the liver and intestine (CYP3A4). Tacrolimus is excreted unchanged in bile, thus there is no need for adjustment in renal failure or hepatic disease.

- Interactions: Similar to those with CsA.
- Adverse drug reactions: Similar to those with CsA.
- Monitoring: Trough levels are routinely used (and correlate with area under the curve measurements).

Sirolimus
- Sirolimus is a fungal-derived macrolide, also known as rapamycin. Unlike the calcineurin inhibitors tacrolimus and CsA, the sirolimus–immunophilin complex inhibits the mammalian target of rapamycin (mTOR) and blocks cytokine-mediated cell cycling and B- and T-cell function.
- Initial dosing is 2 mg/d. It is diluted with water or juice (except grapefruit juice). A long half-life allows for once-daily dosing.
- Bioavailability: Sirolimus is rapidly absorbed after oral administration but has poor bioavailability (about 14% with the oral solution but higher with tablets). It is 92% bound to plasma proteins.
- Metabolism and excretion: It is metabolized in the liver and intestine (CYP3A4). More than 90% is eliminated via the gut.
- Interactions: Similar to those with CsA. There is marked interaction with CsA itself, increasing the levels of CsA by >300%. CsA can be dosed 4 hours before sirolimus (but this complicates monitoring of blood levels).
- Adverse drug reactions: Side effects include hypertension, hypercholesterolemia, and hypertriglyceridemia. Bone marrow toxicity (thrombocytopenia and anemia) may occur. Other effects include interstitial pneumonitis and hepatotoxicity. Sirolimus has a boxed warning regarding immediate use after lung transplant, as it has been associated with bronchial anastomotic dehiscence. It can be safely used later (after anastomotic healing), but caution is warranted if additional operations are required.
- Monitoring: Monitoring is essential as target levels also depend on whether CsA or tacrolimus is used.

Interleukin-2 Receptor Antagonists
- IL-2 receptor antagonists are chimeric murine–human monoclonal antibodies. They bind the IL-2 receptor on the surface of activated T lymphocytes and inhibit proliferation and differentiation of T cells. Basiliximab is a true chimeric antibody (25% mouse) used for induction immunosuppression. Daclizumab is a humanized antibody (10% mouse) that is no longer available.
- Basiliximab has a half-life of about 14 days. It is given as a 20-mg IV infusion once before transplant and then again on the fourth day posttransplant.
- Adverse effects: Basiliximab is well tolerated, much better than predecessors OKT3 and muromonab-CD3. Side effects are generally similar to placebo but there remains a theoretical risk for infection and posttransplant lymphoproliferative disorder (PTLD). A severe, acute hypersensitivity syndrome (including a pulmonary edema/acute respiratory distress [ARDS]-like picture) can occur with basiliximab and is a contraindication to continued use.

Antithymocyte Globulin
- Antithymocyte globulin (ATG) is a polyclonal antilymphocyte globulin commonly used for both treatments of rejection and as an induction immunosuppression agent. Atgam is derived from horses, whereas thymoglobulin is of

rabbit origin. There is profound B- and T-cell depletion after administration owing to complement-mediated cytolysis of antibody-coated cells.
- Dosing: Atgam: 10–20 mg/kg IV infusion. Thymoglobulin: 1–1.5 mg/kg IV infusion. Atgam has a half-life of 6 days, whereas thymoglobulin has a half-life of 30 days. Thymoglobulin is about 10 times more potent than atgam.
- Adverse drug reactions: There are numerous reactions, including flulike symptoms secondary to cytokine release syndrome (IL-1, IL-6, tumor necrosis factor-α). These symptoms can be attenuated with premedication (using a combination of prednisone, acetaminophen, diphenhydramine, and IV fluids). There is a potential risk of infection and PTLD, but the data in lung transplantation are variable. Leukopenia is the most serious complication of therapy. Thrombocytopenia may complicate therapy and anaphylaxis is documented but rare.
- Monitoring: Some centers monitor CD3+ levels to gauge adequacy of therapy.

Other Agents
- Alemtuzumab (anti-CD52) has been used by a few centers for induction immunosuppression or for treatment of rejection. However, this drug is no longer widely available and is used under a special distribution program.
- Azithromycin is a macrolide antibiotic that has demonstrated efficacy to delay the development of bronchiolitis obliterans syndrome (BOS) and chronic rejection in several studies. Dosing schedules are usually three times per week.
- Leflunomide is an antimetabolite that blocks pyrimidine synthesis and lymphocyte proliferation, similar to purine synthesis inhibitors.
- Rituximab (anti-CD20) is a chimeric monoclonal antibody that destroys B cells and commonly used for connective tissue diseases, such as lupus. It is also used in the treatment of antibody-mediated rejection (AMR) in some centers.
- Bortezomib is a proteasome inhibitor used in the treatment of multiple myeloma. Given the effect on plasma cells, some centers have used bortezomib in patients with severe AMR.

COMPLICATIONS

Hyperacute Rejection
- Immediate response due to preformed circulating antibodies to donor antigens (HLA, ABO, and other antigens) that bind the vascular endothelium and initiate the host immunologic response and lead to thrombus formation, inflammatory cell infiltrates, and fibrinoid necrosis of the vessels.[8]
- Clinically, this results in fulminant allograft failure, although there have been reported cases of successful management with intensive immunosuppression and plasma exchange.
- This complication has become exceedingly rare in recent years because of sensitive screening methods to avoid donors with reactivity to preformed anti-HLA antibodies in potential transplant recipients.

Acute Rejection
- Despite standard three-drug immunosuppressive therapy, many lung transplant patients still experience one or more episodes of acute rejection, especially in

the first 6 months after transplantation. Recurrent episodes of rejection, particularly grade A2 or higher, are associated with an increased risk of chronic lung allograft dysfunction (CLAD) development.[8]
- Acute rejection is primarily a cell-mediated immune response triggered by recognition of major histocompatibility complex antigens. Pathologic findings include perivascular and/or peribronchiolar lymphocytic infiltrate, with the extent of the inflammation into the surrounding tissue determining the grade of rejection.[9]
- Most cases of mild acute rejection are asymptomatic and discovered only with surveillance bronchoscopy during the first year following transplantation. Rarely, more severe cases may present with shortness of breath, nonproductive cough, low-grade fever, and decline in exercise oximetry and spirometry (FEV1 decrease by >10%).[9]
- Pathologic findings in transbronchial biopsies are the gold standard. Since early stages of acute rejection may be asymptomatic, surveillance bronchoscopies can improve early detection and are used by some centers during the first year after transplantation. However, while the performance of surveillance biopsies is a common standard of practice, it does not necessarily improve survival nor decrease the incidence of chronic rejection.[9]
- Noninvasive techniques to assist in the diagnosis of acute rejection have been developed in the form of cell-free DNA (cfDNA), measuring the amount of free donor DNA circulating in the peripheral blood. These are in the early phases of clinical use, but serve as another tool to allow for earlier detection of acute rejection with elevated levels of cfDNA circulating prior to decline in spirometry. The primary disadvantage is lack of specificity, as any source of pulmonary inflammation (infection, edema, rejection) can result in an increased laboratory result of cfDNA.[10,11]
- The International Society for Heart and Lung Transplantation (ISHLT) criteria for acute rejection are listed in Table 28-3 and are based on severity and location.[12] Most centers treat detectable acute rejection grades A1 and higher, given their correlation with development of CLAD, but practices vary for grade A1 depending on clinical parameters such as lung function or history of prior episodes of acute rejection.
- Initial treatment includes high-dose IV corticosteroids (methylprednisolone, 0.5–1 g IV daily for 3 days). An oral prednisone taper starting at 0.5–1 mg/kg/d over a few weeks may also be used.[8,9]
- Refractory cases of acute cellular rejection may be treated with repeat courses of steroids, by alteration of maintenance immunosuppression, and/or with antilymphocyte antibody therapy.[8]

Antibody-Mediated Rejection
- Development of donor-specific antibody (DSA) to mismatched HLA is common following lung transplantation and is associated with increased CLAD and worse clinical outcomes. A prospective, multicenter study observed development of DSA in 36% of lung transplant recipients within 4-months of transplant.[13] Given this, many transplant centers have developed routine DSA screening protocols.
- AMR occurs with the development of antibodies against non-self HLA expressed on the donor lung, leading to endothelial cell injury and graft dysfunction.

TABLE 28-3	CLASSIFICATION AND GRADING OF LUNG ALLOGRAFT REJECTION

A. Acute vascular rejection (vascular rejection of any grade may occur with or without acute airway rejection)
A0: none
A1: minimal
A2: mild
A3: moderate
A4: severe
B. Lymphocytic bronchiolitis
B0: none
B1R: mild
B2R: severe
C. Chronic airway rejection
C1: bronchiolitis obliterans
D. Chronic vascular rejection
Accelerated graft vascular sclerosis

Adapted from Stewart S, Fishbein MC, Snell GI, et al. Revision of the 1996 working formulation for the standardization of nomenclature in the diagnosis of lung rejection. *J Heart Lung Transplant.* 2007;26:1229–1242.

More specifically, AMR involves activation of allospecific B cells and plasma cells leading to the formation of DSA, usually against either class I or class II HLAs.[8,9]
- There is also evidence that the development of antibodies to lung-restricted self-antigens (SAgs) also plays an important role in the development of AMR and CLAD. This autoimmunity occurs when tissue allograft injury leads to exposure of normally sequestered SAgs and the development of non-HLA antibodies. Collagen V, an extracellular matrix protein, and K-alpha-1 tubulin, a gap junction protein, are both expressed on airway epithelial cells and are the best-studied examples of SAgs.
- A complex formal algorithm for the diagnosis of AMR has been developed, with distinctions between probable and possible AMR. However, the detection of new donor-specific anti-HLA antibodies with allograft dysfunction, pulmonary infiltrates, and evidence of C4d complement deposition and associated pathologic changes in transbronchial lung biopsies help to confirm the diagnosis.[9,14] These are displayed in Table 28-4.
- Treatment may include a combination of high-dose steroids, intravenous immunoglobulin (IVIG), carfilzomib, tocilizumab, rituximab, and plasma exchange. Treatment regimens are chosen largely by patient factors (severity of symptoms, current infectious or hematologic comorbidities) as no head-to-head clinical trials comparing regimens exist currently.
- There is emerging evidence suggesting use of tocilizumab, an IL-6 inhibitor, may be a useful treatment for AMR. A single-center study demonstrated increased

TABLE 28-4 ISHLT CONSENSUS CRITERIA FOR THE DIAGNOSIS OF AMR

Diagnostic Criteria	Definite AMR	Probable AMR (dysfunction plus any four criteria met)	Possible AMR (dysfunction plus any three criteria met)
Allograft dysfunction	+	+	+
Circulating DSA	+	±	±
C4d Deposition	+	±	±
Lung injury histopathology	+	±	±
Exclusion of other causes	+	±	±

AMR, antibody-mediated rejection; DSA, donor-specific antibody; ISHLT, International Society of Heart and Lung Transplantation.

- clearance of DSA and less recurrence or development of new DSA with use of tocilizumab. There was also decreased graft failure compared to AMR treatment regimens that did not include tocilizumab.[15]
- The diagnosis of AMR remains associated with poor short- and long-term prognosis. There is both increased mortality and incidence of CLAD among survivors, with retrospective studies demonstrating between 38% and 47% 1-year mortality, and for those who survived past 1 year, a >90% risk of developing CLAD.[16]

Chronic Rejection

- Chronic rejection can be summarized broadly as lung allograft dysfunction over time not due to another identifiable underlying cause, most commonly infection, weight gain, severe gastroesophageal reflux disease (GERD)/reflux, pulmonary edema due to renal or liver disease, or airway stenosis. Previously referred to as BOS based on progressive obstructive ventilatory defects over time, chronic lung allograft syndrome, or CLAD, is now understood to have three possible phenotypes: obstructive, restrictive, and mixed.
- Histologic confirmation of CLAD is difficult and not necessary for the definition.
- The prevalence of CLAD approaches 50% within 3–5 years after lung transplantation.
- CLAD is the end result of multifactorial insults to the transplanted tissue. Table 28-5 lists the risk factors linked to chronic rejection.[17-23] The BOS phenotype of CLAD is a fibroproliferative process that begins with lymphocytic infiltration of the submucosa. As the infiltrate migrates into the epithelium, destruction and loss of bronchiolar mucosa follow. Fibroblasts and myofibroblasts are stimulated by this reaction, and subsequently lay down intraluminal granulation tissue. Some airways may remain patent, whereas others are obliterated.

TABLE 28-5	MECHANISMS OF CHRONIC LUNG ALLOGRAFT REJECTION

Immune Mechanisms
Acute rejection: The risk of CLAD has been correlated with higher grades of histologic rejection, persistent rejection, or recurrent rejection after treatment; in particular patients with more than three episodes of acute rejection were noted to be at increased risk of developing subsequent CLAD. There is some suggestion that in certain cases, severe acute rejection may lead directly to airway fibrosis
HLA mismatching: Lung transplants are not HLA matched with recipients; however, although the significance of HLA mismatch remains controversial, the development of donor-specific HLA antibodies after transplantation is strongly linked to CLAD

Nonimmune Mechanisms
Primary Graft Dysfunction has been identified as an independent risk factor for CLAD
CMV infection: CMV pneumonitis is a risk factor for developing CLAD; prophylaxis may attenuate this risk
Hemodynamic factors: Donor cold ischemic time at the time of transplantation (between procurement and surgery) increases the risk of CLAD; reperfusion injury, after vascular anastomosis, may cause oxidative damage to the allograft tissue; this disruption of the bronchial circulation in the transplanted lung may be a contributing factor
Community-acquired respiratory tract infection (especially viral illness such as RSV, Parainfluenza, Influenza, and COVID-19)
Pseudomonas colonization in the allograft
Gastroesophageal reflux disease
Recurrent aspiration events, usually in setting of esophageal dysfunction

CLAD, chronic lung allograft dysfunction; COVID-19, coronavirus disease 2019; CMV, cytomegalovirus; RSV, respiratory syncytial virus.

- Chronic rejection manifests as progressive decline in spirometric lung function. Depending on their reference FEV1 and overall functional status, patients may be relatively asymptomatic or present with worsening dyspnea, cough, wheezing, and decreased exercise tolerance.
- Several approaches to treatment include[8,24]:
  - Alteration of maintenance immunosuppression regimen by transitioning from CsA to tacrolimus and/or transition from azathioprine to MMF. There is limited case-series evidence for mitigation of lung function decline or reversal with substitution of tacrolimus for CsA. There may be an increase in hyperglycemia or nephrotoxicity following transition.[24]
  - Azithromycin administered 250 mg daily for 5 days, then continued three times weekly should be considered in patients with chronic rejection. There may be complete reversal of FEV1 decline and increased response may be seen

in patients with bronchoalveolar lavage (BAL) neutrophilia. Trial of azithromycin should be continued for a minimum of 3 months.
- ○ ATG therapy can be considered and has previously been evaluated in patients with BOS phenotype and has been shown to temporarily slow the rate of decline of FEV1.
- ○ Extracorporeal photopheresis (ECP) involves collection of peripheral blood lymphocytes by apheresis which are treated with 8-methoxypsoralen and then exposed to ultraviolet A light and then reinfused to the patient. This is thought to induce lymphocyte apoptosis and induction of T regulatory cells. A single-center randomized clinical trial demonstrated that 61% of patients with BOS who were treated with ECP had their FEV1 stabilize over the following 6 months.[25]
- ○ Repeat lung transplantation can be considered in carefully selected patients. The most common reasons for retransplantation are early graft failure, airway complications, and CLAD. Outcomes are worse with retransplant compared to primary lung transplant. In general, retransplant should only be considered in younger, ambulatory patients who would meet all requirements to have primary lung transplant.
- ○ Prevention of chronic rejection with empiric three-drug immunosuppression, early and aggressive treatment of respiratory infections, management of GERD, and regular spirometric testing are important aspects of prevention and management.

Infection in the Lung Transplant Patient
- Infections confer a risk of increased morbidity and mortality in the transplant population. The combination of immunosuppression, denervated lung, impaired lymphatic drainage, abnormal mucociliary clearance, and suboptimal cough reflex all increase the susceptibility to infection in lung transplant recipients disproportionate to other solid organ transplant recipients.
- Empiric broad-spectrum antibiotics at the time of transplantation help to prevent early postoperative pneumonia after transplantation. Vancomycin and cefepime or meropenem are reasonable choices while awaiting culture results.

Bacterial Pneumonia
- Bacterial infections account for >50% of infection-related transplant deaths.
- Most of these infections occur within the first 2 weeks after transplantation but can re-emerge in the setting of BOS or with chronic airway colonization (e.g., CF).
- Gram-negative pneumonia: Gram-negative rods are consistently the most common bacterial organisms involved.[26,27]
- Multidrug-resistant Pseudomonas and related species are a considerable problem in transplant recipients colonized with these organisms before transplant. The presence of Pseudomonas in respiratory specimens has been associated with the development of DSA.[28]
- There is no consensus regarding management of these multidrug-resistant infections in the perioperative period, and institutions vary their prophylaxis based on individual culture data and sensitivities.
- Lung transplant patients are more prone to Legionella infection, but the rates of infection are widely variable among institutions.

- Gram-positive pneumonia: *Staphylococcus aureus* (including methicillin-sensitive and resistant strains) is the most common gram-positive bacterial airway infection in lung transplant recipients. This often occurs in the early posttransplant or perioperative setting and can be transferred from the donor.[29]
- Atypical pneumonia: Listeria and Nocardia infections are uncommon perhaps because they are susceptible to trimethoprim-sulfamethoxazole (TMP-SMX), used as *Pneumocystis jirovecii* prophylaxis (PJP). TB is an uncommon infection in lung transplant recipients. However, antimycobacterial treatment can be problematic owing to frequent interactions between these agents and immunosuppressive medications. Patients undergoing transplantation should receive a tuberculin skin test and receive appropriate therapy before surgery.

Viral Pneumonias
- CMV is the second most frequent infection in lung transplant patients.
- CMV can be acquired via the allograft from a seropositive donor, transfusion of seropositive blood products, or activation of latent disease in a seropositive recipient.
- Pneumonitis is the most common manifestation, but patients may also present with colitis, gastroenteritis, and hepatitis. CMV pneumonia may be confused with acute rejection but usually does not develop until 7–8 weeks after transplantation.
- Risk of reactivation is linked to the serologic status of donor and recipient[30,31]:
  - Donor CMV Ig–/recipient CMV Ig–: low risk
  - Donor CMV Ig–/recipient CMV Ig+: moderate risk
  - Donor CMV Ig+/recipient CMV Ig+: moderate risk
  - Donor CMV Ig+/recipient CMV Ig–: highest risk
- Symptoms include low-grade fever, cough, and shortness of breath.
- Decreased spirometric function may occur and CXRs may demonstrate perihilar infiltrates, interstitial edema, or pleural effusions.
- Quantitative polymerase chain reaction (PCR) is now widely used but there is no standardized assay. Hence, threshold levels vary from assay to assay and between centers.[26,30]
- Shell vial cultures of BAL fluid (or blood or urine) can rapidly determine active infection in 24–48 hours via fluorescent antibodies to CMV antigen.
- Bronchoscopy for culture of airway secretions and transbronchial lung biopsies may be done. Viral cytopathic effect on transbronchial biopsy is the gold standard for diagnosis of CMV pneumonitis. Some centers also use immunohistochemical stains to aid in diagnosis.
- Prevention: The most common method of prophylaxis is antiviral therapy, that is, valganciclovir or human CMV immunoglobulin (cytogam). Centers differ on approach and duration of prophylactic therapy.[26,30] Our center uses the following approach:
  - Prophylactic strategy for high-risk patients: valganciclovir, 450–900 mg/d, for 6 months after transplantation. Some centers may extend prophylaxis to 12 months.
  - Preemptive strategy for medium- and low-risk patients: serum CMV PCR is monitored once a week for the first 3 months.
- Treatment[26,30]:
  - Acyclovir has no role in the treatment of CMV.
  - Valganciclovir PO or ganciclovir IV for 2–3 weeks is the therapy of choice. The major side effect is leukopenia. Relapses are frequent after therapy and

can be attenuated by maintenance therapy for 3–6 weeks after treatment. Ganciclovir resistance must be considered in patients who do not respond to therapy.
  - Other therapies may include cytogam, foscarnet, or cidofovir.
- Other herpesviruses: Epstein–Barr virus (EBV) is implicated in development of posttransplant lymphoproliferative disease (PTLD). Varicella zoster virus (VZV) manifests as chickenpox with primary exposure and as zoster with reactivation. The American Society of Transplantation recommends seronegative transplant patients be vaccinated against VZV before transplantation.[26] Immunocompromised patients with acute exposure may receive VZV immune globulin or acyclovir prophylaxis to protect against or attenuate infection.
- Community-acquired respiratory viruses (e.g., respiratory syncytial virus [RSV], influenza virus, parainfluenza virus, adenovirus, rhinovirus, and metapneumovirus) have been implicated in the development of BOS. Ribavirin may be used for RSV and even parainfluenza virus, although the evidence to support these therapies is limited.[26,32] Neuraminidase inhibitors are recommended for immunosuppressed patients infected with influenza viruses.[26,32]

Fungal Infections
- The most common fungal infections are Candida and Aspergillus following transplantation.
- Candidal infections of relevance to lung transplant recipients include candidal tracheobronchitis (common but candidal pneumonitis/pneumonia is rare), thrush (increased with higher doses of steroids and/or concurrent treatment with broad-spectrum antibiotics), wound infections/cellulitis (cross-sectional imaging can help to determine the extent of disease) and disseminated disease (patients with indwelling catheters are at higher risk).
- Candidal infections were once associated with a high mortality but now they are easier to control with newer and more effective therapies. Treatment options include azoles, echinocandins, and liposomal amphotericin B (decreases kidney toxicity).[33]
- Azoles increase the levels of calcineurin inhibitors, so therapeutic monitoring and dose adjustments are necessary.
- Resistance is also an increasing problem, notably with non-albicans candida species: *C. glabrata* and *C. tropicalis* (high minimum inhibitory concentration [MIC] to fluconazole), *C. krusei* (resistant to fluconazole); *C. lusitaniae* (resistant to amphotericin B), and *C. guilliermondii* (resistant to amphotericin B and caspofungin).
- Aspergillus is contracted via inhalation of spores. Common species include *A. fumigatus* (most common), *A. flavus, A. terreus.*
- Disease manifestations include tracheobronchial aspergillosis (occurs within 3 months following transplantation, early colonization increases the risk of developing more invasive disease), pulmonary aspergillosis (develops after tracheobronchial aspergillosis), and disseminated aspergillosis (can be devastating, central nervous system [CNS] involvement should be identified).[26]
- Infection can be detected clinically by screening sputum or BAL fluid for hyphae but invasive pneumonia is confirmed only by biopsy (transbronchial or surgical). Serum galactomannan may aid in diagnosis.[34]
- Treatment: Bronchitis can be treated with itraconazole, voriconazole, or inhaled amphotericin B.[26,34] Disseminated disease is usually treated with liposomal

amphotericin B but nephrotoxicity is a major source of morbidity, especially with calcineurin inhibitors. Voriconazole is superior to amphotericin B in invasive disease. Echinocandins may prove to be a less toxic option.
- *Pneumocystis jirovecii* pneumonia:
  - Infection with *P. jirovecii* is uncommon as the result of widespread routine prophylaxis with TMP-SMX.[26,35]
  - Prophylaxis is accomplished with one double-strength tablet three times a week. Alternatives include dapsone, atovaquone, and monthly inhaled pentamidine.
  - Treatment for Pneumocystis pneumonia is TMP-SMX, 15–20 mg of the TMP component/kg/d PO/IV in 3–4 divided doses daily. IV pentamidine can also be used for treatment.

Posttransplant Lymphoproliferative Disorder

- PTLD falls in the spectrum of non-Hodgkin lymphoma and is predominantly of B-cell lineage.[36,37]
- PTLD is often, although not always, associated with EBV infection. B lymphocytes are transformed by EBV and undergo uncontrolled clonal expansion in the setting of drug-induced T-lymphocyte suppression.
- Intrathoracic PTLD, with or without involvement of the allograft, typically occurs within the first year after transplant. Intrathoracic PTLD presents as a pulmonary nodule, pulmonary infiltrate, or lymphadenopathy on routine CXR.
- Extrathoracic PTLD, especially the GI tract, is more common after the first posttransplant year. It can present as nonhealing ulcers, bowel perforations, GI bleeding, and masses.
- De-escalation of immunosuppression is the first step in management.
- Other approaches include a combination of rituximab, chemotherapy, and surgical excision.
- A retrospective analysis demonstrated no difference in survival based on time of PTLD diagnosis (early vs. late), but disease involving the allograft had a better prognosis than PTLD without allograft involvement (median survival postdiagnosis 2.6 vs. 0.2 years).[38]

Other Complications

- Primary graft dysfunction (PGD) (so-called reperfusion edema or primary graft failure) is a form of acute lung injury (ALI) that occurs in the immediate postoperative period (72 hours). Up to 25% of patients develop PGD following lung transplantation. PGD severity is graded (0–3) based on PaO_2/FiO_2 ratio and radiographic infiltrates, analogous to ALI/ARDS. PGD 3 is associated with significant posttransplant morbidity and mortality, as well as increased risk for the development of BOS.
- Lung transplant recipients have a higher risk of malignancy than individuals in the general population. Squamous cell carcinoma of the skin is more common, as are cancers of the cervix, anogenital region, and the hepatobiliary system. Routine cancer screening and prevention are therefore essential.
- Lung transplant recipients are at a higher risk for venous thromboembolism and hypercoagulability. Initial treatment with low–molecular-weight heparin

(LMWH) should be initially dosed at 0.8 mg/kg q12h, instead of standard 1 mg/kg q12h regimens. Monitoring of anti-factor Xa levels is encouraged to avoid over-anticoagulation.
- GI complications: Lung transplant recipients are at an increased risk for chronic gastritis, peptic ulcer disease, and gastroparesis. GERD is a risk factor for the development of CLAD and medication-refractory cases are often treated with fundoplication. Secondary malnutrition can lead to several other systemic problems.
- Recurrent primary disease has been reported in sarcoidosis, bronchoalveolar carcinoma, lymphangioleiomyomatosis, Langerhans cell histiocytosis, pulmonary alveolar proteinosis, diffuse panbronchiolitis, and giant cell pneumonitis.

OUTCOMES

- Survival after transplant is a complicated issue.
- Based on data from the ISHLT registry, the unadjusted median time to survival was 5.7 years for all adult lung transplants between 1994 and 2012.[39] Rates of long-term survival improve for those who survive to year 1. Thus, the conditional median survival for recipients who are alive at 1 year is 7.9 years.[39]
- Initial differences in 1-month survival usually reflect perioperative mortality associated with the complexity and severity of the surgery for each disease type (e.g., lung transplantation for IPAH has higher perioperative mortality than for COPD). These outcomes must be considered in light of the fact that these patients would probably have a higher mortality without transplantation when compared to a patient with COPD.
- A number of risk factors have been associated with an increased risk of death at 1 and 5 years posttransplantation.[39]
  - Severity of disease process: CLAD (retransplantation) > IPAH > bronchiectasis (including CF) > IPF > COPD
  - Renal failure, requiring hemodialysis
  - Diabetes mellitus
  - Hospitalization (requiring IV inotropes, respiratory failure)
  - Pulmonary embolism
  - CMV mismatch (donor positive, recipient negative)

REFERENCES

1. Patterson GA. Indications: unilateral, bilateral, heart–lung, and lobar transplant procedures. *Clin Chest Med.* 1997;18:225–230.
2. The American Society for Transplant Physicians; American Thoracic Society; European Respiratory Society; International Society for Heart and Lung Transplantation. ATS guidelines: lung transplantation: report of the ATS workshop on lung transplantation. *Am Rev Respir Dis.* 1993;147:772–776.
3. The American Society for Transplant Physicians; American Thoracic Society; European Respiratory Society; International Society for Heart and Lung Transplantation. ATS guidelines: international guidelines for the selection of lung transplant candidates. *Am J Respir Crit Care Med.* 1998;158:335–339.
4. Orens JB, Estenne M, Arcasoy S, et al; Pulmonary Scientific Council of the International Society for Heart and Lung Transplantation. International guidelines for the selection of lung transplant candidates: 2006 update—a consensus report from the Pulmonary

Scientific Council of the International Society for Heart and Lung Transplantation. *J Heart Lung Transplant.* 2006;25:745–755.
5. Snell GI, Westfall GP. Selection and management of the lung donor. *Clin Chest Med.* 2011;32:223–232.
6. OPTN Lung Transplantation Committee. Establish continuous distribution of lungs. Accessed December 25, 2023. https://optn.transplant.hrsa.gov/media/esjb4ztn/20211206-bp-lung-establish-cont-dist-lungs.pdf()
7. Floreth T, Bhorade SM, Ahya VN. Conventional and novel approaches to immunosuppression. *Clin Chest Med.* 2011;32:265–277.
8. Hachem RR. Lung allograft rejection: diagnosis and management. *Curr Opin Organ Transplant.* 2009;14:477–482.
9. Martinu T, Pavlisko EN, Chen DF, Palmer SM. Acute allograft rejection: cellular and humoral processes. *Clin Chest Med.* 2011;32:295–310.
10. Agbor-Enoh S, Jackson AM, Tunc I, et al. Late manifestation of alloantibody-associated injury and clinical pulmonary antibody-mediated rejection: evidence from cell-free DNA analysis. *J Heart Lung Transplant.* 2018;37:925–932.
11. Agbor-Enoh S, Wang Y, Tunc I, et al. Donor-derived cell-free DNA predicts allograft failure and mortality after lung transplantation. *EBioMedicine.* 2019;40:541–553.
12. Stewart S, Fishbein MC, Snell GI, et al. Revision of the 1996 working formulation for the standardization of nomenclature in the diagnosis of lung rejection. *J Heart Lung Transplant.* 2007;26:1229–1242.
13. Hachem RR, Kamoun M, Budev MM, et al. Human leukocyte antigens antibodies after lung transplantation: primary results of the halt study. *Am J Transplant.* 2018;18:2285–2294.
14. Levine DJ, Glanville AR, Aboyoun C, et al. Antibody-mediated rejection of the lung: a consensus report of the international society for heart and lung transplantation. *J Heart Lung Transplant.* 2016;35:397–406.
15. January SE, Fester KA, Halverson LP, et al. Tocilizumab for antibody-mediated rejection treatment in lung transplantation. *J Heart Lung Transplant.* 2023;42:1353–1357.
16. Witt CA, Gaut JP, Yusen RD, et al. Acute antibody-mediated rejection after lung transplantation. *J Heart Lung Transplant.* 2013;32:1034–1040.
17. Husain AN, Siddiqui MT, Holmes EW, et al. Analysis of risk factors for the development of bronchiolitis obliterans syndrome. *Am J Respir Crit Care Med.* 1999;159:829–833.
18. Jaramillo A, Smith MA, Phelan D, et al. Development of ELISA-detected anti-HLA antibodies precedes the development of bronchiolitis obliterans syndrome and correlates with progressive decline in pulmonary function after lung transplantation. *Transplantation.* 1999;67:1155–1161.
19. Schulman LL, Weinberg AD, McGregor CC, Suciu-Foca NM, Itescu S. Influence of donor and recipient HLA locus mismatching on development of obliterative bronchiolitis after lung transplantation. *Am J Respir Crit Care Med.* 2001;163:437–442.
20. Estenne M, Hertz MI. Bronchiolitis obliterans after human lung transplantation. *Am J Respir Crit Care Med.* 2002;166:440–444.
21. Palmer SM, Davis RD, Hadjilladis D, et al. Development of an antibody specific to major histocompatibility antigens detectable by flow cytometry after lung transplant is associated with bronchiolitis obliterans syndrome. *Transplantation.* 2002;74:799–804.
22. Daud SA, Yusen RD, Meyers BF, et al. Impact of immediate primary lung allograft dysfunction on bronchiolitis obliterans syndrome. *Am J Respir Crit Care Med.* 2007;175:507–513.
23. Knoop C, Estenne M. Chronic allograft dysfunction. *Clin Chest Med.* 2011;32:311–326.
24. Meyer KC, Raghu G, Verleden GM, et al; ISHLT/ATS/ERS BOS Task Force Committee; ISHLT/ATS/ERS BOS Task Force Committee. An international ISHLT/ATS/ERS clinical practice guideline: diagnosis and management of bronchiolitis obliterans syndrome. *Eur Respir J.* 2014;44:1479–1503.

25. Jaksch P, Scheed A, Keplinger M, et al. A prospective interventional study on the use of extracorporeal photopheresis in patients with bronchiolitis obliterans syndrome after lung transplantation. *J Heart Lung Transplant.* 2012;31:950–957.
26. Sims KD, Blumberg EA. Common infections in the lung transplant recipient. *Clin Chest Med.* 2011;32:327–341.
27. van Delden C, Blumberg EA; AST Infectious Diseases Community of Practice. Multidrug resistant gram-negative bacteria in solid organ transplant recipients. *Am J Transplant.* 2009;9:S27–S34.
28. Kulkarni HS, Tsui K, Sunder S, et al. Pseudomonas aeruginosa and acute rejection independently increase the risk of donor-specific antibodies after lung transplantation. *Am J Transplant.* 2020;20:1028–1038.
29. AST Infectious Diseases Community of Practice; Garzoni C. Multiply resistant gram-positive bacteria, methicillin-resistant, vancomycin-intermediate and vancomycin-resistant Staphylococcus aureus (MRSA, VISA, VRSA) in solid organ transplant recipients. *Am J Transplant.* 2009;9:S41–S49.
30. AST Infectious Diseases Community of Practice; Humar A, Snydman D. Cytomegalovirus in solid organ transplant recipients. *Am J Transplant.* 2009;9:S78–S86.
31. Ettinger NA, Bailey TC, Trulock EP, et al. Cytomegalovirus infection and pneumonitis. Impact after isolated lung transplantation. Washington University Lung Transplant Group. *Am Rev Respir Dis.* 1993;147:1017–1023.
32. AST Infectious Diseases Community of Practice; Ison MG, Michaels MG. RNA respiratory viral infections in solid organ transplant recipients. *Am J Transplant.* 2009;9: S166–S172.
33. AST Infectious Diseases Community of Practice; Pappas PG, Silveira FP. Candida in solid organ transplant recipients. *Am J Transplant.* 2009;9:S173–S179.
34. AST Infectious Diseases Community of Practice; Singh N, Husain S. Invasive aspergillosis in solid organ transplant recipients. *Am J Transplant.* 2009;9:S180–S191.
35. AST Infectious Diseases Community of Practice; Martin SI, Fishman JA. Pneumocystis pneumonia in solid organ transplant recipients. *Am J Transplant.* 2009;9:S227–S233.
36. Straathof KC, Savoldo B, Heslop HE, Rooney CM. Immunotherapy for post-transplant lymphoproliferative disease. *Br J Haematol.* 2002;118:728–740.
37. Robbins HY, Arcasoy SM. Malignancies following lung transplantation. *Clin Chest Med.* 2011;32:343–355.
38. Paranjothi S, Yusen RD, Kraus MD, Lynch JP, Patterson GA, Trulock EP. Lymphoproliferative disease after lung transplantation: comparison of presentation and outcome of early and late cases. *J Heart Lung Transplant.* 2001;20:1054–1063.
39. Yusen RD, Edwards LB, Kucheryavaya AY, et al; International Society for Heart and Lung Transplantation. The registry of the International Society for Heart and Lung Transplantation: thirty-first adult lung and heart–lung transplant report—2014; focus theme: retransplantation. *J Heart Lung Transplant.* 2014;33:1009–1024.

Index

Page numbers followed by f refer to figures; page numbers followed by t refer to tables.

A

A1ATD. *See* Alpha1 (α1)-antitrypsin deficiency (A1ATD)
Abatacept, 173
ABPA. *See* Allergic bronchopulmonary aspergillosis (ABPA)
ABRS. *See* Acute bacterial rhinosinusitis (ABRS)
Accelerated silicosis, 300
Acetaminophen, 176
Acinetobacter species, 116
Active pulmonary TB/tuberculosis disease, 125
   diagnosis of, 127
   special considerations, 127–128
   treatment, 128
Active TB, 125
Acute asthma exacerbations, 77–80. *See also under* Asthma
Acute bacterial rhinosinusitis (ABRS), 157, 160
Acute bronchitis, 161
Acute cough, 61
Acute exacerbations of chronic obstructive pulmonary disease (AECOPD), 55
Acute hypoxemic respiratory failure trauma, 56
Acute respiratory disease (ARD), 169–170
Acute silicosis, 300
Acute viral rhinosinusitis (AVRS)
   management, 160
   symptoms of, 157
Acyclovir, for CMV, 338
Adaptive/auto-servo ventilation (ASV), 274
ADCs. *See* Antibody–drug conjugates (ADCs)
Adenocarcinoma in situ (AIS), 314
Adenovirus, 167, 169–170
   clinical presentation, 170
   diagnosis, 170
   epidemiology, 169–170
   treatment, 170
   virology, 167
AECOPD. *See* Acute exacerbations of chronic obstructive pulmonary disease (AECOPD)

AHI. *See* Apnea-hypopnea index (AHI)
Air bronchogram sign, 8
Air trapping, 26
AIS. *See* Adenocarcinoma in situ (AIS)
Albuterol, 91
Alemtuzumab, in lung transplantation, 332
Allergic bronchopulmonary aspergillosis (ABPA), 134
   diagnosis of, 139–140, 140f
   diagnostic testing for, 140–141
   overview, 139
   treatment of, 141
Allergic phenotype, 73, 75
Allergic rhinitis, 62, 76
All-night polysomnogram (ANPSG), 273–274
Alpha1 (α1)-antitrypsin deficiency (A1ATD), 85
Ambrisentan, 253
Ambulation, 48
American College of Chest Physicians (ACCP) survey, 35
American Thoracic Society (ATS), 21
Aminoglycoside, 193
Amlodipine, 253
Amphotericin B
   for blastomycosis, 143
   for coccidioidomycosis, 145
   for histoplasmosis, 150
   for invasive pulmonary aspergillosis, 136
   for mucormycosis, 152
Anemic hypoxia, 40
Angiotensin-converting enzyme (ACE) inhibitors, associated with chronic cough, 64
Anidulafungin, in invasive pulmonary aspergillosis, 136
Annual flu vaccines, 164
ANPSG. *See* All-night polysomnogram (ANPSG)
Anterior mediastinum, 5
Antibiotic de-escalation, in HAP, 120–123
Antibiotics
   for asthma, 79
   for bronchiectasis, 69
   for COPD, 89, 92–93

Antibody–drug conjugates (ADCs), 308
Antibody-mediated rejection, lung transplantation, 333–335, 335t
Anticholinergic agents, 91
Anti-inflammatory reliever (AIR) therapy, 72
Antileukotriene agents, 75
Antineoplastic therapy–induced pulmonary disease
  classification, 308, 309t
  diagnosis, 310
    clinical presentation, 310
    Common Terminology Criteria for Adverse Events (CTCAE v5.0), 310, 311t
    criteria for, 310–311
    differential, 311
    history, 310
    imaging for, 311–312
    procedures for, 312
  epidemiology, 308
  medications for treatment, 312
  outcome/prognosis, 312
  overview, 308
  pathophysiology of, 310
  risk factors, 310
  treatment, 312
Antiphospholipid antibody syndrome (APLS), 208
Antisialogogues, during bronchoscopy, 35
Antithymocyte globulin (ATG), in lung transplantation, 331–332
Anxiolytics, 104
Aorta, CXR evaluation, 5
APAP. *See* Auto-titrating positive airway pressure (APAP)
APLS. *See* Antiphospholipid antibody syndrome (APLS)
Apnea, 270
Apnea–hypopnea index (AHI), 270
Apophysomyces, 133
ARD. *See* Acute respiratory disease (ARD)
Arm claudication, 216
Armodafinil, 274
Asbestos-associated lung disease
  diagnosis of, 296–297
    asbestosis, 296
    MPM, 297
    pleural disease, 297
  and lung cancer, 297
  overview, 294–296
  tobacco smoking and, 297
Asbestosis, 296
Aspergilloma
  diagnosis of, 138
  diagnostic testing for, 139
  overview, 138
  risk factors for, 138
  treatment of, 139
Aspergillosis, 133–134
Aspergillus, 133
Aspergillus flavus complex, 133
Aspergillus fumigatus complex, 133
Aspergillus niger complex, 133
Aspergillus spp., 133–134
Aspergillus terres complex, 133
Aspirin, 217, 218
Asthma, 31, 56
  acute asthma exacerbations, 77–80
    clinical presentation, 77
    diagnostic testing of, 77–78
    management of, 78–80
  allergic rhinitis and, 76
  cough, 63
  diagnosis of, 66, 70–72
    clinical presentation, 70–71
    fractional exhaled nitric oxide (F_ENO), measurement of, 72
    history, 70–71
    imaging with CXR, 72
    PFT, 72
    physical examination, 71
    testing, 71–72
  direct and indirect cost of asthma in US, 70
  exacerbations, 70
  morbidity/mortality, 70
  obesity as risk factor for, 77
  overview, 70
  PVFMD symptoms overlap with, 77
  symptoms of, 70
  treatment of, 68, 72–77
    AIR therapy for, 72
    biologic therapies for, 73, 74t–75t, 76
    GINA for, 72–73
    lifestyle modification for, 76–77
    medications for, 72–76, 74t–75t
    multimorbidity management for, 76–77
    nonpharmacologic therapies for, 76
    nonpreferred alternative therapies for, 72–73
    SMART for, 73
ASV. *See* Adaptive/auto-servo ventilation (ASV)
Atrial septostomy, 256
Atropine, during bronchoscopy, 35
ATS. *See* American Thoracic Society (ATS)
Atypical *pneumonia,* 338
Auto-titrating positive airway pressure (APAP), 274
Avacopan, 222

AVAPS. *See* Average volume-assured pressure support (AVAPS)
Average volume-assured pressure support (AVAPS), 51, 53–54
AVRS. *See* Acute viral rhinosinusitis (AVRS)
Azathioprine (AZA)
 for eosinophilic granulomatosis with polyangiitis, 227
 for granulomatosis with polyangiitis, 222
 in lung transplantation, 329
 in takayasu arteritis, 217
Azithromycin, 76, 193
 in lung transplantation, 332

B

Bacterial *pneumonia,* 62
 lung transplantation and, 337–338
Bacterial rhinosinusitis, 62
BAL. *See* Bronchoalveolar lavage (BAL)
Baloxavir, 176
Baricitinib, 172–173
Basiliximab, in lung transplantation, 331
Behçet disease, 218
Benralizumab, 74t
Benzodiazepines, 35, 104
Berylliosis. *See* Chronic beryllium disease (CBD)
Beta2 (β2)-agonist, 91
Bilateral lung transplantation (BLT), 328
Bilevel positive airway pressure (BiPAP), 52–53, 274
Biomass fuel combustion fumes, 302
BiPAP. *See* Bilevel positive airway pressure (BiPAP)
Bird fancier's disease, 304
Bisphosphonate therapy, 194
Blastomyces, 133
Blastomyces dermatitidis, 141
Blastomyces gilchristii, 141
Blastomyces helicus, 141
Blastomyces spp., 141–142
Blastomycosis
 diagnosis
  clinical presentations, 142
  testing for, 142–143
 overview, 141–142
 treatment, 143
Bleomycin, 308, 309t, 310–312
BLT. *See* Bilateral lung transplantation (BLT)
Bordetella pertussis, 64
Bortezomib, in lung transplantation, 332
BOS. *See* Bronchiolitis obliterans syndrome (BOS)
Bosentan, 253
Bronchial thermoplasty (BT), 76

Bronchiectasis, 19, 64, 69
Bronchiolitis, 162
Bronchiolitis obliterans syndrome (BOS), 332
Bronchitis, 161
 acute, 161
 chronic, 161
Bronchoalveolar lavage (BAL), 37, 119, 209, 305
 in cryptococcosis, 146
 in EPGA, 226
 in ILD, 284
Bronchoprovocation testing, 71
Bronchoscopy
 flexible, 202
 for hemoptysis, 201–202
 rigid, 202
BT. *See* Bronchial thermoplasty (BT)
Bullectomy, 95
Bupropion, 103–104
Buspirone, 104

C

Calcium channel blockers (CCBs), for pulmonary hypertension, 253
Calcium supplementation, 194
Candida albicans, 143
Candidal infections, 339–340
Candida spp., 133, 143
Candidiasis, 143
CAP. *See* Community-acquired pneumonia (CAP)
Carcinogens, 98
Cardiogenic pulmonary edema (CPE), 54
Cardiopulmonary exercise testing (CPET), 251
Carmustine, 311
Caspofungin, in invasive pulmonary aspergillosis, 136
CBD. *See* Chronic beryllium disease (CBD)
Central access devices, CXR evaluation, 6
Central apnea–hypopnea index (CAHI), 270
Central apneas, 270
Central hypopneas, 271
Central sleep apnea (CSA), 270
 associated conditions, 272
 classification, 270–271
 definitions, 270
 diagnosis
  clinical presentation, 272–273
  criteria for, 273
  differential, 273
  history, 272
  HSAT for, 274

Central sleep apnea (CSA) (*Continued*)
  laboratories testing for, 273
  physical examination for, 272–273
  procedures for, 273–274
  PSG for, 273–274
 epidemiology, 271
 etiology, 271
 overview, 270
 pathophysiology of, 271
 prevention from, 272
 risk factors for, 272
 treatment
  lifestyle/risk modification, 275
  medications, 274
  nonpharmacologic therapies, 274
Central venous catheters (including dialysis catheters), 6
Cephalosporin, 193
CF. *See* Cystic fibrosis (CF)
CFTR. *See* Cystic fibrosis transmembrane conductance regulator gene (CFTR)
Chapel Hill Consensus Conference, 213
Chest computed tomography
 in ABPA, 141
 approach for reading, 16–19
  basic lung parenchymal patterns, 17–19
  high-attenuation lung parenchymal pattern, 18–19
  low-attenuation lung parenchymal pattern, 19
  lung window, 17
  nodular lung parenchymal pattern, 18
  reticular lung parenchymal pattern, 18
  soft tissue window, 17
 in chronic necrotizing aspergillosis, 137
 common indications for, 10
 comparison to prior CT studies, 10
 in diffuse alveolar hemorrhage, 209
 in granulomatosis with polyangiitis, 221
 for hemoptysis, 200–201
 high-resolution, 12
 in hypoxemic respiratory failure, 45
 initial assessment, 10–13
  body region, 10–11
  contrast, 11–12
  CT scans and protocols, 12
  ordering CT, 10–12
  preparing patient, 12–13
 interpretation of, 10, 13–16
  basic anatomy, 13–16
  hila and lung anatomy, 15
  mediastinal anatomy, 14–15
  pleural, diaphragm, and chest wall anatomy, 15–16
  window levels, 13
  window width, 13
 in interstitial lung disease, 283–284
 low-dose, 12
 overview, 10
 in *pneumocystis* pneumonia, 153
 in pulmonary hypertension, 250
 in subacute aspergillosis, 137
Chest pain, 280–281
Chest radiography
 in interstitial lung disease, 283
 in pleural diseases, 263
Chest wall deformity, 55–56
Chest x-ray (CXR)
 for ABPA, 141
 for asthma, 72
 for chronic necrotizing aspergillosis, 137
 for coccidioidomycosis, 145
 in diffuse alveolar hemorrhage, 209
 general principles, 1
 in granulomatosis with polyangiitis, 221
 for hemoptysis, 200
 in hypoxemic respiratory failure, 45
 initial assessment, 1–3
  degree of inspiration, 1–2
  patient position, 2
  patient rotation, 1
  radiation dose, 2
  study quality, 2–3
 interpretation of, 3–7
  aorta, 5
  diaphragm, 4
  extrapulmonary masses, 6
  hila, 5
  lungs, 6
  mediastinum, 4–5
  medical devices, 6
  old films *vs.* current study, 7
  osseous structures, 3
  pleural space, 5
  upper abdomen, 3–4
 lung disease, evaluation of, 7–9
  diffuse lung disease, 9
  lobar collapse, 8
  pneumothorax, 8–9
  radiographic densities, 7
  radiographic signs, 7–8, 7t
 overview, 1
 for *pneumocystis* pneumonia, 153
 in pulmonary embolism, 234
 in pulmonary hypertension, 250
 radiation dose of, 2
 for subacute aspergillosis, 137
 views, 2–3
  anteroposterior (AP), 3
  lateral decubitus (LD), 3
  lateral (LAT), 2–3
  posteroanterior (PA), 2

Cheyne–Stokes breathing (CSB) pattern, 270
Chickenpox vaccine, 165
Chronic beryllium disease (CBD), 305
Chronic bronchitis, 68, 161
Chronic corticosteroids, 76
Chronic cough, 62, 63t
Chronic idiopathic pancreatitis, 189
Chronic necrotizing aspergillosis, 137–138
Chronic obstructive pulmonary disease (COPD), 21
  associated conditions, 85
  chronic, treatment of, 90–95
    anticholinergic agents, 91
    beta2 (β2)-agonist, 91
    bronchodilator therapy, 90–91
    chronic antibiotic treatment, 92–93
    combination therapy, 91
    inhaled corticosteroids, 91–92
    lifestyle/risk modification, 95
    long-acting inhaled medical therapy, 91
    lung transplantation, 95
    LVRS, 95
    medications, 90–93
    methylxanthines, 92
    nedocromil and leukotriene modifiers, 93
    other nonpharmacologic therapies, 93–94
    oxygen therapy, 93–94, 94t
    PDE4 selective inhibitors, 92
    pulmonary rehabilitation, 94
    surgical management, 94–95
    systemic corticosteroids, 92
    vaccines, 92
  with chronic bronchitis, 64
  classification, 83, 84t
  definition, 83
  diagnosis of, 85–87
    cardiac testing, 87
    clinical presentation, 85–86
    criteria, 86
    differential, 86
    history, 85
    imaging, 86
    laboratory testing, 86
    physical examination, 85–86
    procedures for, 86–87
    pulmonary function tests, 86–87
    pulse oximetry assessment, 87
  epidemiology of, 83
  exacerbation, 62
  genetic disorders and, 84–85
  Global Obstructive Lung Disease 2024 (GOLD) classification of, 83, 84t
  noninvasive ventilation in, 55
  overview, 83
  pathophysiology of, 84
  phenotype, 298
  prognosis for, 95
  risk factors, 84–85
  role of airway infections in, 84
  smoking cessation and, 95, 98
  symptoms of, 85–86
  treatment of, 87–90
    acute exacerbations, 87, 87t
    antibiotics for, 89
    bronchodilator therapy for, 88
    corticosteroids for, 88
    follow-up, 90
    inhaled SAACs for, 88
    inhaled SABA for, 88
    medications, 88–89
    methylxanthines for, 89
    NIPPV, 89–90, 90t
    other nonpharmacologic therapies, 89–90
    oxygen, 89
Chronic rhinosinusitis, 189
Chronic silicosis, 300–301
Chylothorax, 260, 268
Ciprofloxacin, 193
Circulatory hypoxia, 40
Clinical Pulmonary Infection Score, 119
Clonidine, 104
CMV. *See* Cytomegalovirus (CMV)
Coal dust-associated pulmonary disease, 298–299
  diagnosis of, 298–299
  overview, 298
  prevalence of, 298
Coal workers' pneumoconiosis, 298
Coccidioides, 133
Coccidioides immitis, 143
Coccidioidomycosis
  diagnosis of, 144
  diagnostic testing for, 144–145
  overview, 143–144
  primary manifestations, 144
  treatment of, 145
Combined pulmonary fibrosis and emphysema (CPFE), 287
Community-acquired pneumonia (CAP)
  classification, 107
  definition, 107
  diagnosis of, 108–110
    clinical presentation, 108
    differential, 109
    imaging study for, 110
    laboratories testing for, 110
    procedures for, 110
    testing, 109–110, 109t

Community-acquired pneumonia (CAP) (*Continued*)
  epidemiology, 107–108
  etiology for, 108
  monitoring/follow-up, 113
  outcome/prognosis, 113–114
  pathophysiology, 108
  prevention, 108
  risk factors, 108
  treatment, 110–113
    antimicrobial therapy for, 113
    empiric therapy for, 111f
    medications for, 111–112
    other nonpharmacologic therapies for, 112–113
    recognized guidelines for, 107
    steroids for, 112–113
    surgical management, 113
Community-acquired respiratory viruses, 339
Congestive heart failure, 69
Connective tissue disease-related interstitial lung disease and interstitial pneumonia with autoimmune features (CTD-ILD), 287–288
Continuous positive airway pressure (CPAP), 51–52
COP. *See* Cryptogenic organizing pneumonia (COP)
COPD. *See* Chronic obstructive pulmonary disease (COPD)
Corticosteroids, 173, 215, 217
  for COPD, 88
  for ILD, 289
  inhaled, 72, 91–92
  in lung transplantation, 328–329
Cough, 44, 280
  ACE inhibitors and, 64
  acute, 61
  asthma, 63
  bronchiectasis, 64
  chronic, 62, 63t
  classification of, 61–65
  COPD with chronic bronchitis, 64
  diagnosis of, 65–67
    additional testing, 67
    asthma, 66
    clinical presentation, 65–66
    criteria, 66
    CXR, 67
    differential, 66
    echocardiography, 67
    gastrointestinal evaluation, 67
    GERD, 66
    history, 65–66
    physical examination, 66
    pulmonary function tests, 67
    sinus CT scan, 67
    upper airway cough syndrome, 66
  etiologies of, 65
  exacerbation of underlying disease process, 62
    allergic rhinitis, 62
    COPD exacerbation, 62
  exposure, 62
  gastroesophageal reflux disease, 63
    diagnosis of, 66
    treatment of, 68
  hypersensitivity syndrome, 64
  infectious, 61–62
    bacterial pneumonia, 62
    viral, 61
    viral/bacterial rhinosinusitis, 62
  less common causes of, 64–65
  nonasthmatic eosinophilic bronchitis, 64
  overview, 61
  pathophysiology of, 65
  rare causes of, 65
  special considerations, 69
  treatment of, 67–69
    asthma, 68
    bronchiectasis, 69
    chronic bronchitis, 68
    congestive heart failure, 69
    GERD, 68
    interstitial lung disease, 69
    lung cancer, 69
    medication-induced cough, 68
    nonasthmatic eosinophilic bronchitis, 68–69
    sinusitis, 68
    somatic cough disorder (psychogenic cough), 69
    upper airway cough syndrome, 68
  upper airway cough syndrome (postnasal drip), 62–63
COVID-19 (Coronaviruses), 64, 171–174
  classification by severity, 172
  clinical presentation, 171–172
  diagnosis of, 172
  epidemiology, 171
  nucleic acid amplification testing (NAAT) for, 172
  treatment of, 172–174
  vaccines, 92, 163
  virology, 171
CPAP. *See* Continuous positive airway pressure (CPAP)
CPE. *See* Cardiogenic pulmonary edema (CPE)
CPET. *See* Cardiopulmonary exercise testing (CPET)

CPFE. *See* Combined pulmonary fibrosis and emphysema (CPFE)
Crazy paving, 284
Cryptococcosis
 cryptococcal antigen testing for, 146
 culture of BAL fluid in, 146
 diagnosis of, 145–146
 diagnostic testing for, 146
 overview, 145
 radiographic findings of, 146
 treatment of, 146, 147t–148t
Cryptococcus, 133
Cryptogenic OP, 311
Cryptogenic organizing pneumonia (COP), 286
CSA. *See* Central sleep apnea (CSA)
CTD-ILD. *See* Connective tissue disease-related interstitial lung disease and interstitial pneumonia with autoimmune features (CTD-ILD)
Cunninghamella, 133
Cyclophosphamide, 311–312
Cyclosporine (CsA), in lung transplantation, 330
Cystic fibrosis (CF)
 acute exacerbation of, 187
 adequate nutrition in, 194
 chronic sinusitis and, 194
 clinical presentation
  acute exacerbation of CF, 187
  chronic lower airway infections, 187
  chronic sinusitis, 187
  DIOS, 188
  endocrine and reproductive, 188
  exocrine pancreatic insufficiency, 188
  gastroesophageal reflux disease, 188
  pneumothorax, 187
  respiratory failure, 188
 complications
  hemoptysis, 196
  pneumothorax, 195–196
 definition, 185
 diabetes mellitus in, 188, 194
 diagnosis, 187–190
  clinical presentation, 187–188
  criteria for, 189
  differential, 189
  testing, 189–190
 DIOS and, 194
 epidemiology, 185
 inflammation in, 193
 osteoporosis in adult, 188, 194
 pathophysiology, 185–186
 replacement of pancreatic enzymes in, 194
 special considerations, 195
 treatment, 190–195
  antibiotics, 192–193
  for chronic respiratory failure, 193–194
  endocrine and reproductive, 194
  gastrointestinal, 194
  inhaled recombinant DNase, 192
  lung transplantation, 194–195
  pulmonary, 190–194
Cystic fibrosis transmembrane conductance regulator gene (CFTR), 185–186, 190
Cystic lung diseases, 19, 288–289
Cytomegalovirus (CMV), 174–175
 clinical presentation, 174
 diagnosis, 174–175
 epidemiology, 174
 in lung transplantation, 337–338
 treatment for, 175
 virology, 174
Cytoplasmic ANCA (c-ANCA), 220–221
Cytotoxic hypoxia, 40

D

DADA2 syndrome, 217
DAH. *See* Diffuse alveolar hemorrhage (DAH)
D-dimer, 233–234
Dead space ventilation, 43
Deep venous thrombosis (DVT), 230–241
 definition, 230
 definitions of risk levels in acute, 236t
 diagnosis
  clinical presentation, 231–232, 232t
  contrast-enhanced CT scan for, 234
  CXR for, 234
  D-dimer for, 233–234
  differential, 232
  electrocardiography for, 234
  imaging studies for, 234–235
  laboratory testing for, 234
  modified Wells criteria for, 232t
  testing for, 232–235, 234f
  TTE for, 235
  venous CUS for, 235
  V/Q scanning for, 235
 epidemiology of, 230
 etiology of, 230–231
 follow-up, 241
 incidence of, 230
 monitoring, 241
 overview, 230
 pathophysiology of, 231
 prognosis, 241
 risk factors for, 231, 231t
 risk stratification, 236

Deep venous thrombosis (DVT) (*Continued*)
  severity index score, 238
  treatment of, 236–241, 237f
    advanced therapies for, 240
    anticoagulation therapy for, 238–239
    complications of therapy, 240–241
    DOACs for, 238
    general principles for, 236–238, 237f
    inferior vena cava (IVC) filters for, 240
    low–molecular-weight heparin for, 238–239
    PE response teams for, 239
    respiratory and circulatory support for, 238
    systemic thrombolytic therapy for, 239–240
    unfractionated heparin for, 238–239
    warfarin for, 238–239
Dexamethasone, 172
Diaphragm, 4
Diffuse alveolar hemorrhage (DAH)
  diagnosis of, 205, 207–210
    clinical presentation, 205, 207
    differential, 206f, 207–208, 207t
    fiberoptic bronchoscopy for, 209
    imaging studies for, 209
    laboratory evaluation for, 208–209
    microscopic findings for, 210
    procedures for, 209–210
    pulmonary function testing for, 209
    surgical lung biopsy for, 209
  etiologies, 205, 206f, 206t
  overview, 205
  pathogenesis of, 205
  treatment of, 210
Diffuse lung disease, 9
Diffusing capacity of lung for carbon monoxide (DLCO), 30
DILD. *See* Drug-induced interstitial lung disease (DILD)
Diltiazem, 253
Dimorphic fungi, 133
DIOS. *See* Distal intestinal obstruction syndrome (DIOS)
Distal intestinal obstruction syndrome (DIOS), 188
DLCO. *See* Diffusing capacity of lung for carbon monoxide (DLCO)
DPI. *See* Dry powder inhaler (DPI)
Drug-induced interstitial lung disease (DILD), 308, 309t
Dry powder inhaler (DPI), 72
Dual-organ lung transplantation, 324
Dupilumab, 75t
DVT. *See* Deep venous thrombosis (DVT)

E

Efficiency of gas exchange, 30
EGPA. *See* Eosinophilic granulomatosis with polyangiitis (EGPA)
Electronic cigarettes, 98, 102
Elexacaftor-Tezacaftor-Ivacaftor (ETI), 190–191
Empyema, 260, 267
Endobronchial biopsy, 37
Endobronchial ultrasound, 38
Endothelin receptor antagonists (ERAs), 253
  for pulmonary hypertension, 253
Endotracheal tubes (ETs), CXR evaluation, 6
Enteroviruses (EV), 179–180
  clinical presentation, 180
  diagnosis, 180
  epidemiology, 179
  treatment, 180
  virology, 179
Environmental exposures, 62
Eosinophilic granulomatosis with polyangiitis (EGPA)
  diagnosis of
    BAL for, 226
    biopsy for, 226
    clinical presentation, 224–225
    criteria for, 225
    differential, 225
    imaging studies for, 225
    laboratories testing for, 224–225
    procedures, 225
    testing for, 224
    tissue biopsy for, 226
  overview, 224
  treatment of, 225–226
Eosinophilic pneumonias, 288, 312
Eosinophilic (T2-high) phenotype, 75
EPAP. *See* Expiratory positive airway pressure (EPAP)
Epinephrine, 79
Epoprostenol (IV), 254
Epstein–Barr virus (EBV), 339
ERAs. *See* Endothelin receptor antagonists (ERAs)
ETs. *See* Endotracheal tubes (ETs)
EV. *See* Enteroviruses (EV)
Everolimus, 311–312
Exertional dyspnea, 279
Expiratory positive airway pressure (EPAP), 51, 53
Exposures, cough, 62
Extended-spectrum penicillin, 193
Extrapleural spaces, CXR evaluation, 5–6
Extrapulmonary masses, CXR evaluation, 6
Extrinsic allergic alveolitis. *See* Hypersensitivity pneumonitis (HP)

F

Facemasks, 47
F508del, 186
Fentanyl, during bronchoscopy, 35
FEV1. *See* Forced expiratory volumes in 1 second (FEV1)
FFS. *See* Five factor score (FFS)
Fiberoptic bronchoscopy (FOB), 209
  cardiac evaluation in patients, 35
  complications of, 39
  diagnosis of, 37–38
  indications for, 34t
  monitoring, 36
  overview, 34
  postprocedure, 37
  pre-bronchoscopy evaluation, 35
  procedural medications in, 35–36
    antisialogogues, 35
    benzodiazepines, 35
    opiates, 35
    propofol, 36
    topical anesthesia, 35
  relative contraindications to, 35t
  technique, 36–37
  treatment of, 38
    anastomotic stricture/dehiscence, management of, 38
    argon plasma coagulation for, 38
    cryotherapy for, 38
    foreign body removals, 38
    one-way endobronchial valves, placement of, 38
    therapeutic aspiration of secretions, 38
    tracheobronchial narrowing, 38
Fibrosing mediastinitis, 151
"Five A's" program, 98–99
Five factor score (FFS), 226
Fixed upper airway obstruction, 27, 27f
Fleischner Society Guidelines, 319
Flexible bronchoscopy, 202
Flow–volume loops
  normal PFTs, 22–23, 22f
  in obstructive ventilatory defects, 26, 26f
  in restrictive ventilatory defects, 29, 30f
Fluconazole, for coccidioidomycosis, 145
FOB. *See* Fiberoptic bronchoscopy (FOB)
Forced expiratory volumes in 1 second (FEV1), 22–23
Forced vital capacity (FVC), 22–23
Formoterol, 72
"Four A's" program, 98–99
Fractional exhaled nitric oxide (F_ENO), measurement of, 72
Fungal *pneumonia*, lung transplantation and, 339–340
Fungal pulmonary infections
  aspergilloma, 138–139
  aspergillosis, 133–134
    allergic bronchopulmonary, 139–141
    chronic necrotizing, 137–138
    invasive pulmonary, 134–136
    subacute, 137–138
  blastomycosis, 141–143
  candidiasis, 143
  coccidioidomycosis, 143–145
  cryptococcosis, 145–146
  fusariosis, 146–149
  histoplasmosis, 149–151
  mucormycosis, 151–152
  overview, 133
  Pneumocystis pneumonia, 152–154
Fusariosis
  diagnosis of, 148–149
  overview, 146, 148
  treatment of, 149
Fusarium, 133
FVC. *See* Forced vital capacity (FVC)

G

Gabapentin, 69
Gastroesophageal reflux disease (GERD)
  asthma and, 76
  cough, 63
  diagnosis of, 66
  treatment of, 68
GCA. *See* Giant-cell arteritis (GCA)
Geneva score, 232t
GERD. *See* Gastroesophageal reflux disease (GERD)
GGO. *See* Ground glass opacity (GGO)
Giant-cell arteritis (GCA), 214
GINA. *See* Global Initiative for Asthma (GINA)
Global Initiative for Asthma (GINA), 72–73
Glucocorticoids, 226
  for ABPA, 141
  sparing agent, 216
GPA. *See* Granulomatosis with polyangiitis (GPA)
Gram-negative *pneumonia*, 337
Gram-positive *pneumonia*, 338
Granulomatosis with polyangiitis (GPA)
  classification, 219
  diagnosis
    clinical presentation, 219–220
    criteria for, 220
    fiberoptic bronchoscopy for, 221
    imaging studies for, 221
    laboratory testing for, 220–221
    procedures for, 221
    renal biopsy for, 221
    testing for, 220–221
  overview, 219
  treatment of, 221–222

Granulomatous mediastinitis, 151
Ground-glass nodule, 314, 315f
Ground glass opacity (GGO), 18, 283

H
Haemophilus influenza, 116, 157
HAP. *See* Hospital-acquired pneumonia (HAP)
Hazardous agents in workplace, 294t
HCAP. *See* Health care–associated pneumonia (HCAP)
Health care–associated pneumonia (HCAP), 115–116
Heamophilus influenza, 62
Heart–lung transplantation, 328
Heliox, 80–81
Hemoptysis, 138, 196, 280
  common causes of, 199, 201t
  definition, 199
  diagnosis of, 199–202
    bronchoscopy for, 201–202
    clinical presentation, 200
    differential, 200, 201t
    imaging studies for, 200–201
    laboratories testing for, 200
    procedures for, 201–202
  massive, 199, 202
  overview, 199
  risk factors for, 199
  treatment of, 202–204
    airway protection and stabilization for, 202–203
    bronchial artery embolization for, 203
    control of bleeding, 203
    localization of bleeding, 203
    massive hemoptysis, 202
    nonmassive hemoptysis, 202
    pulmonary angiography for, 203
    surgery for, 203–204
Hemothorax, 260, 268
Heparin-induced thrombocytopenia (HIT), 240–241
Herpesviruses (HSV-1, EBV, VZV), 175
High-flow nasal cannulas, 47
High-resolution CT (HRCT), 12
Hila, CXR evaluation, 5
Histoplasma, 133
Histoplasmosis, 149–151
  complications, 151
  diagnosis of, 149–150
  diagnostic testing for, 150
  overview, 149
  treatment of, 150
Histoplasmosis capsulatum, 149–150
HIT. *See* Heparin-induced thrombocytopenia (HIT)
Home sleep apnea testing (HSAT), 274
Honeycombing, 19, 283
Hospital-acquired pneumonia (HAP), 115–116
  definition, 115
  diagnosis, 118–120
    clinical presentation, 118–119
    testing for, 119–120
  early-onset, 116
  epidemiology, 116
  etiology, 116
  late-onset, 116
  pathogenesis of, 117
  treatment, 120–122
    duration of, 122
    medications for, 120–122, 121t
Hounsfield unit (HU), 13
HP. *See* Hypersensitivity pneumonitis (HP)
HRCT. *See* High-resolution CT (HRCT)
HSAT. *See* Home sleep apnea testing (HSAT)
HU. *See* Hounsfield unit (HU)
Hypercapnic respiratory failure, 40, 52
Hyperinflation, 26
Hypersensitivity pneumonitis (HP), 287, 302–305
  causative agents, 303t
  diagnosis of, 303–305
    bird fancier's disease, 304
    farmer's lung, 304
    testing for, 304–305
  overview, 302–303
  treatment, 305
Hypnotic agents, 35
Hypopneas, 270, 271
Hypoxemia, 40
Hypoxemic hypoxia, 40
Hypoxemic respiratory failure
  classification, 40
  CPAP in, 52
  CT chest in, 45
  CXR in, 45
  definition, 40
  diagnosis of, 44–45
    clinical presentation of, 44
    criteria, 44–45
    diagnostic testing, 44
    history, 44
    imaging, 45
    laboratory evaluation, 45
    physical examination, 44
    procedures, 45
  etiology of, 41–44, 42f
    alveolar hypoventilation, 41
    decreased barometric pressure/fraction of inspired oxygen, 41

diffusion limitation, 43
right-left shunts, 43–44
ventilation/perfusion mismatch, 43
follow-up, 49
low mixed venous oxygen content, 44
monitoring, 48
pathophysiology of, 40–41
patient education, 49
treatment of, 45–48
  ambulation for, 48
  facemasks for, 47
  high-flow nasal cannulas for, 47
  incentive spirometry for, 48
  low-flow oxygen delivery devices for, 46
  mobilization for, 48
  nasal cannulas for, 46
  nonrebreather facemasks for, 48
  oxygen delivery devices for, 46–48
  pulmonary flutter valves for, 48
  reservoir nasal cannulas for, 46–47
  venturi masks for, 47
Hypoxia, 40

I

ICIs. *See* Immune checkpoint inhibitors (ICIs)
ICS. *See* Inhaled corticosteroid (ICS)
Idiopathic bronchiectasis, 189
Idiopathic pulmonary fibrosis, 285–286
Iloprost, 254
Immune checkpoint inhibitors (ICIs), 308
Immunoglobulin deficiency, 189
Immunoglobulin (Ig)-E, 73
IMV. *See* Invasive mechanical ventilation (IMV)
Incentive spirometry, 48
Industrial bronchitis, 298–299
Infectious cough, 61–62
  bacterial pneumonia, 62
  viral, 61
  viral/bacterial rhinosinusitis, 62
Infliximab, 173
Influenza vaccination, 92
Influenza virus, 175–177
  clinical presentation, 176
  diagnosis of, 176
  epidemiology, 176
  treatment, 176–177
  virology, 175
Inhaled aztreonam, 193
Inhaled corticosteroid (ICS), 72, 91–92
Inhaled maintenance corticosteroid (ICS) therapy, 91–92
Interferon beta, 311
Interleukin (IL)-4, 73
Interleukin (IL)-5, 73
Interleukin (IL)-13, 73

Interleukin-2 receptor antagonists, in lung transplantation, 331
Interstitial lung disease (ILD), 65, 69
  classification, 277, 278t–279t, 279
  diagnosis
    BAL in, 284
    chest radiography for, 283
    clinical presentation, 279–282
    for combined pulmonary fibrosis and emphysema, 287
    for CTD-ILD, 287–288
    for cystic lung diseases, 288–289
    for eosinophilic pneumonias, 288
    high-resolution chest CT for, 283–284
    history, 279–281
    for hypersensitivity pneumonitis, 287
    for idiopathic pulmonary fibrosis, 285–286
    laboratory testing for, 282
    lung sampling for, 284–285
    for nonspecific interstitial pneumonia, 286
    for organizing pneumonia, 286
    overview of, 279, 280f
    physical examination for, 281–282
    physiologic testing for, 282
    for progressive pulmonary fibrosis, 287
    for sarcoid interstitial lung disease, 288
    surgical lung biopsy, 285
    transbronchial cryobiopsy, 285
    transbronchial forceps biopsy in, 284–285
  epidemiology, 277, 279
  etiology, 279
  HRCT in, 283–284
  pathogenesis, 279
  treatment
    advance care planning and palliative care, 290
    antifibrotic therapy, 289–290
    immunosuppressive therapy for, 289–290
    nonpharmacologic therapies for, 290
    other pharmacologic therapies for, 290
    overview of, 289
Invasive mechanical ventilation (IMV), 50–51, 80
Invasive pulmonary aspergillosis (IPA), 134–136
  characterization, 134
  diagnosis of, 134, 135t

Invasive pulmonary aspergillosis (IPA) (*Continued*)
   diagnostic testing for, 135–136
   risk factors for, 134
   treatment of, 136
IPA. *See* Invasive pulmonary aspergillosis (IPA)
Isavuconazole, 138
Itraconazole, 138, 141, 143, 150
Ivacaftor, 191
IV immunoglobulin (IVIG), 217, 222
IV vancomycin, 193

K

Kawasaki disease (KD), 217
KD. *See* Kawasaki disease (KD)
Keratoconjunctivitis, 170

L

LAMAs. *See* Long-acting muscarinic antagonists (LAMAs)
Latent (inactive) TB/TBI, 125
   criteria for positive TST, 126t
   diagnosis of, 125, 127
   risk of reactivation, 126t
   treatment of, 127
Leflunomide, in lung transplantation, 332
Left heart catheterization (LHC), 251
Leukotriene modifiers, 93
LHC. *See* Left heart catheterization (LHC)
Lidocaine, during bronchoscopy, 36
Linezolid, 193
Listeria and Nocardia infections, 338
LLN. *See* Lower Limit of Normal (LLN)
Lobar collapse, CXR evaluation, 8
Long-acting inhaled medical therapy, 91
Long-acting muscarinic antagonists (LAMAs), 76
Lorazepam, during bronchoscopy, 35
Low-dose CT, 12
Lower Limit of Normal (LLN), 21
Lower respiratory tract infections (LRTIs), 161–162
   bronchiolitis, 162
   bronchitis, 161
   pneumonia, 162
Low-flow oxygen delivery devices, 46
Low–molecular-weight heparin (LMWH), 238–239
LRTIs. *See* Lower respiratory tract infections (LRTIs)
Luftsichel sign, 8
Lumacaftor-Ivacaftor, 191
Lung cancer, 69
Lung disease, CXR evaluation, 7–9
   diffuse lung disease, 9
   lobar collapse, 8
   pneumothorax, 8–9
   radiographic densities, 7
   radiographic signs, 7–8, 7t
      air bronchogram sign, 8
      luftsichel sign, 8
      Silhouette sign, 7, 7t
Lung parenchymal patterns, computed tomography, 17–19
   high-attenuation pattern, 18–19
   low-attenuation pattern, 19
   nodular pattern, 18
   reticular pattern, 18
Lungs, CXR evaluation, 6
Lung transplantation, 95
   bilateral, 328
   complications
      acute rejection, 332–333
      allograft rejection, 334t
      antibody-mediated rejection, 333–335, 335t
      chronic rejection, 335–337, 336t
      GI, 341
      hyperacute rejection, 332
      hypercoagulability, risk for, 340
      infections, 333–340
      malignancy, risk for, 340
      primary graft dysfunction, 340
      PTLD, 340
      recurrent primary disease, 341
      venous thromboembolism, risk for, 340
   contraindications to, 325t
   donor and candidate selection for, 324–328
   donor selection for, 327–328, 327t
   indications and timing of referral by diagnosis, 324–326
      COPD/emphysema, 325–326
      cystic fibrosis, 326
      pulmonary arterial hypertension, 326
      pulmonary fibrosis/interstitial lung disease, 326
   infection in, 337
      bacterial *pneumonia*, 337–338
      fungal *pneumonia*, 339–340
      viral *pneumonia*, 338–339
   organ allocation for, 326–327
   outcomes, 341
   overview, 324
   recipients for, 324, 326–327
   single, 328
   surgical considerations, 328

treatment
  alemtuzumab for, 332
  antithymocyte globulin for, 331–332
  azathioprine for, 329
  azithromycin for, 332
  bortezomib for, 332
  corticosteroids for, 328–329
  cyclosporine for, 330
  immunosuppressive therapy, 328
  interleukin-2 receptor antagonists for, 331
  leflunomide for, 332
  mycophenolate mofetil for, 329–330
  rituximab for, 332
  sirolimus for, 331
  tacrolimus for, 330–331
Lung volume reduction surgery (LVRS), 95
LVRS. *See* Lung volume reduction surgery (LVRS)

M

Macitentan, 253
Magnesium sulfate, 79
Malignancy, 65
Malignant pleural mesothelioma (MPM), 297
Mallinckrodt Institute of Radiology (MIR), 1
Mammalian target of rapamycin (mTOR), 308
  inhibitors for ILD, 289
Mask leak, 51
Massive hemoptysis, 199, 202
Maximal voluntary ventilation (MVV), 31
Mediastinum, CXR evaluation, 4–5
  mediastinal borders, 4
  mediastinal lines, 4
  mediastinal masses, 5
Medical devices, CXR evaluation, 6
Medication-induced cough, 68
Meperidine, during bronchoscopy, 35
Mepolizumab, 74t, 226
Metapneumovirus, 177
Methacholine challenge testing, 31–33
Methacholine dilution schedule, 32t
Methicillin-resistant *S. aureus,* 193
Methicillin-sensitive *Staphylococcus aureus,* 116
Methotrexate, 217, 227, 311
  for ILD, 289
Methylprednisolone, 79
  for histoplasmosis, 150
Methylxanthines, 76
  for acute asthma exacerbations, 79
  for COPD, 89, 92
MIA. *See* Minimally invasive adenocarcinoma (MIA)
Micafungin, in invasive pulmonary aspergillosis, 136

Microscopic polyangiitis (MPA)
  definition, 223
  diagnosis of
    clinical presentation, 223
    criteria for, 223–224
    testing for, 224
  overview, 223
  treatment of, 224
Midazolam, during bronchoscopy, 35
Middle East respiratory syndrome virus (MERS-CoV), 171
Middle mediastinum, 5
Minimally invasive adenocarcinoma (MIA), 314
MIR. *See* Mallinckrodt Institute of Radiology (MIR)
MIS-C. *See* Multisystem inflammatory syndrome in children (MIS-C)
Mixed apneas, 270
Mobilization, 48
Modafinil, 274
Modified Fagerström Test for Nicotine Dependence, 98
Molnupiravir, 172
Montelukast, for asthma, 75
Moraxella catarrhalis, 62, 161
Mosaic attenuation, 19
MPM. *See* Malignant pleural mesothelioma (MPM)
MTOR. *See* Mammalian target of rapamycin (mTOR)
Mucor, 133
Mucormycosis
  diagnosis of, 151
  diagnostic testing of, 151–152
  overview, 151
  treatment of, 152
Multisystem inflammatory syndrome in children (MIS-C), 217
MVV. *See* Maximal voluntary ventilation (MVV)
Mycobacterial pulmonary disease, entities of, 125
Mycobacterium abscessus, 130–131
Mycobacterium avium complex lung disease, 130
Mycobacterium kansasii, 131
Mycophenolate mofetil (MMF), in lung transplantation, 329–330

N

NAAT. *See* Nucleic acid amplification testing (NAAT)
NAEPP. *See* National Asthma Education and Prevention Program (NAEPP)
Nakaseomyces glabrata, 143

Naloxone/naltrexone, 104
Nasal cannulas, 46
Nasogastric tubes, 6
National Asthma Education and Prevention Program (NAEPP), 73
Necrotizing sarcoid granulomatosis, 218
Nedocromil modifiers, 93
Neuromuscular disease, 55–56
Nicotine, 97
Nicotine fading, 105
Nicotine gum, 101
Nicotine inhalers, 102
Nicotine lozenges, 102
Nicotine nasal sprays, 102
Nicotine patches, 101
Nicotine replacement therapy, 100–102
  course of treatment, 100
  electronic cigarettes, 102
  nicotine gum, 101
  nicotine inhalers, 102
  nicotine lozenges, 101
  nicotine nasal sprays, 102
  nicotine patches, 101
  underuse (not overuse) of, 100
  uses, 100
Nifedipine, 253
Nintedanib, for ILD, 289
Nirmatrelvir-ritonavir, 172
Nirsevimab, 179
NISP. *See* Nonspecific interstitial pneumonia (NISP)
NIV. *See* Noninvasive ventilation (NIV)
Nodules, 284
Nonasthmatic eosinophilic bronchitis, 64, 68–69
Noninvasive positive pressure ventilation (NPPV), 50, 80
Noninvasive ventilation (NIV)
  classification, 51–54
    AVAPS, 53–54
    BiPAP, 52–53
    CPAP, 52
  clinical application of, 50–51
  common modes, initial settings for, 57t
  contraindications to, 51t
  definition, 50
  initiation of, 57–58
  special considerations and monitoring, 58
  specific disease indications for, 54–57
    acute hypoxemic respiratory failure trauma, 56
    asthma, 56
    chest wall deformity, 55–56
    COPD, 55
    CPE, 54

  neuromuscular disease, 55–56
  palliative noninvasive ventilation, 56–57
  postextubation respiratory failure, 55
Non-nicotine pharmacotherapies, 103–104
  anxiolytics, 104
  bupropion, 103–104
  tricyclic antidepressants, 104
  varenicline, 103
Nonrebreather facemasks, 48
Nonspecific interstitial pneumonia (NISP), 286
Nontuberculous mycobacterial (NTM) pulmonary disease, 125
Nontuberculous pulmonary disease, 128–129
  diagnosis, 129
  treatment of, 129–131
    Mycobacterium abscessus, 130–131
    Mycobacterium avium complex lung disease, 130
    Mycobacterium kansasii, 131
Normal pulmonary function tests, 22–23
  FEV_1, 23
  flow–volume loops, 22–23, 22f
  FVC, 23
  lung volumes, 23
Nosocomial pneumonia (NP)
  classification, 115
  definition, 115
  diagnosis, 118–120
    clinical presentation, 118–119
    testing for, 119–120
  epidemiology, 116
  etiology, 116–117
  pathophysiology, 117
  prevention, 118, 118t
  risk factors, 117, 118t
  treatment, 120–122
    duration of, 122
    medications for, 120–122, 121t
NP. *See* Nosocomial pneumonia (NP)
NPPV. *See* Noninvasive positive pressure ventilation (NPPV)
Nucleic acid amplification testing (NAAT), 172

O

Obesity, 76
Obesity hypoventilation (OHV), 270
  associated conditions, 272
  classification, 270–271
  definitions, 270
  diagnosis
    clinical presentation, 272–273
    criteria for, 273

differential, 273
history, 272
HSAT for, 274
laboratories testing for, 273
physical examination for, 272–273
procedures for, 273–274
PSG for, 273–274
epidemiology, 271
etiology, 271
overview, 270
pathophysiology of, 271
prevention from, 272
risk factors for, 272
treatment
  lifestyle/risk modification, 275
  medications, 274
  nonpharmacologic therapies, 275
Obstructive apneas, 270
Obstructive hypopneas, 271
Obstructive sleep apnea (OSA)
  associated conditions, 272
  classification, 270–271
  definitions, 270
  diagnosis
    clinical presentation, 272–273
    criteria for, 273
    differential, 273
    history, 272
    HSAT for, 274
    laboratories testing for, 273
    physical examination for, 272–273
    procedures for, 273–274
    PSG for, 273–274
  epidemiology, 271
  etiology, 271
  overview, 270
  pathophysiology of, 271
  prevention from, 272
  risk factors for, 272
  treatment
    lifestyle/risk modification, 275
    medications, 274
    nonpharmacologic therapies, 274
Obstructive ventilatory defects (OVDs), 23–26
  air trapping, determining, 26
  bronchodilator reversibility, assessing for, 25
  flow–volume loop in, 26, 26f
  hyperinflation, determining, 26
  quantifying, 25, 25t
Occupational lung disease
  asbestos-associated lung disease, 294–297
  chronic beryllium disease, 305
  coal dust-associated pulmonary disease, 298–299
  hypersensitivity pneumonitis, 302–305
  overview, 293
  potentially hazardous agents in workplace, 294t
  sample occupational history, 295t
  silica-associated lung disease, 299–300
  Silo Filler's disease, 305
  workplace- and environment-associated bronchial reactivity, 300–302
Occupation exposures, 62
OHV. *See* Obesity hypoventilation (OHV)
Omalizumab, 73, 74t
OP. *See* Organizing pneumonia (OP)
Opiates, during bronchoscopy, 35
OPOs. *See* Organ procurement organizations (OPOs)
OPTN. *See* Organ procurement and transplantation network (OPTN)
Organizing pneumonia (OP), 286
Organ procurement and transplantation network (OPTN), 324
Organ procurement organizations (OPOs), 324
OSA. *See* Obstructive sleep apnea (OSA)
Oseltamivir, 176
Osseous structures of thorax, 3
Osteopenia, 194
OVDs. *See* Obstructive ventilatory defects (OVDs)
Oxygen delivery devices, 46–48
  facemasks for, 47
  high-flow nasal cannulas, 47
  low-flow oxygen delivery devices, 46
  nasal cannulas, 46
  nonrebreather facemasks, 48
  pulmonary flutter valves, 48
  reservoir nasal cannulas, 46–47
  venturi masks, 47
Oxygen therapy, 43, 89, 93–94, 94t

P

PAH. *See* Pulmonary arterial hypertension (PAH)
Palivizumab, 179
Palliative noninvasive ventilation, 56–57
PAP titration, 274
Parainfluenza virus (PIV), 177–178
Parenteral bronchodilators, 79
Paroxysmal vocal fold motion disorder (PVFMD), 77
Part-solid nodule, 314, 315f
Pauci-immune crescentic glomerulonephritis, 221
PCC. *See* Post-COVID conditions (PCC)
PDE-5Is block phosphodiesterase, 254

PDE4 selective inhibitors, 92
PE. *See* Pulmonary embolism (PE)
PEEP. *See* Positive end-expiratory pressure (PEEP)
Peramivir, 176
PE response teams (PERT), 239
Perinuclear ANCA (p-ANCA), 221
PERT. *See* PE response teams (PERT)
PE severity index (PESI) score, 238
PEXIVAS trial, 222
PFTs. *See* Pulmonary function tests (PFTs)
PGD. *See* Primary graft dysfunction (PGD)
PH. *See* Pulmonary hypertension (PH)
Pharyngitis, 160–161
Pharyngoconjunctival fever, 170
Piperacillin, 193
Pirfenidone, for ILD, 289
Pitchia kudriavzevii, 143
PIV. *See* Parainfluenza virus (PIV)
Plasma exchange (PLEX), 222
Plethysmography, 71
Pleural diseases, 297
  complications, 268
  definition, 260
  diagnosis of, 262
    chest radiograph for, 263
    clinical presentation, 262–263
    criteria for, 263
    CT for, 263
    differential, 263
    history, 262–263
    imaging studies for, 263
    laboratories testing for, 264–265, 264t, 265t
    physical examination for, 263
    procedures for, 264
    testing for, 263–265
    ultrasound for, 263
  epidemiology, 260
  etiology of, 260, 261t, 262
  overview, 260
  pathophysiology, 262
  referral, 269
  risk factors for, 262
  special considerations, 268
  treatment, 265, 266f, 267–268
    for chylothorax, 268
    for empyema, 267
    for hemothorax, 268
    for malignant pleural effusion, 267
    medications for, 265–266
    other nonpharmacologic therapies for, 267
    for pleural effusions, 267
    for pneumothorax, 268

Pleural effusion, 260, 297. *See also* Pleural diseases
Pleural fluid drainage chamber, 266f
Pleural space, CXR evaluation, 5
Pleural thickening, 297
Pneumocystis jirovecii, 133, 152–153
Pneumocystis jirovecii pneumonia, 340
Pneumocystis jirovecii prophylaxis (PJP), 338
Pneumocystis pneumonia
  diagnosis of, 152–153
  diagnostic testing of, 153
  overview, 152
  treatment of, 153–154
Pneumonia, 44, 162
  HAP, 115–116
  HCAP, 115–116
  nosocomial
    classification, 115
    clinical presentation, 118–119
    definition, 115
    diagnosis, 118–120
    duration of treatment, 122
    epidemiology, 116
    etiology, 116–117
    medications for treatment, 120–122, 121t
    pathophysiology, 117
    prevention, 118, 118t
    risk factors, 117, 118t
    testing for, 119–120
    treatment, 120–122
  Pneumocystis, 152–154
  VAP, 115–116
  vHAP, 115–116
Pneumothorax, 195–196, 260, 268
  CXR evaluation of, 8–9
Polysomnography, 251
Popcorn lung, 302
Posaconazole
  for mucormycosis, 152
  for subacute aspergillosis, 138
Positive end-expiratory pressure (PEEP), 51–52
Post-COVID conditions (PCC), 180–181
Posterior mediastinum, 5
Postextubation respiratory failure, 55
Postinfectious chronic cough, 64
Posttransplant lymphoproliferative disorder (PTLD), 340
Potts shunts, 256
PPF. *See* Progressive pulmonary fibrosis (PPF)
Prednisone, 79
Prednisone with azathioprine, 218
Primary ciliary dyskinesia, 189

Primary graft dysfunction (PGD), 340
Primary large-vessel vasculitides, 215–217
Primary medium-vessel vasculitides, 217
Primary vasculitis, 213
Progressive massive fibrosis, 298
Progressive pulmonary fibrosis (PPF), 287
Propofol, during bronchoscopy, 36
Prostanoids, 254
Pruning, 250
Pseudomonas aeruginosa, 116
Psychogenic cough, 65
Psychological addiction, 97
PTLD. *See* Posttransplant lymphoproliferative disorder (PTLD)
Pulmonary arterial hypertension (PAH). *See also* Pulmonary hypertension (PH)
  definition, 244
  diagnostic approach to, 252f
  treatment, 253–255
    diuretic therapy, 255
    inotropic agents for, 255
    vasodilator therapy, 253–255
Pulmonary edema, 44
Pulmonary embolism (PE)
  definition, 230
  diagnosis
    clinical presentation, 231–232, 232t
    contrast-enhanced CT scan for, 234
    CXR for, 234
    D-dimer for, 233–234
    differential, 232
    electrocardiography for, 234
    imaging studies for, 234–235
    laboratory testing for, 234
    modified Wells criteria for, 232t
    testing for, 232–235, 234f
    TTE for, 235
    venous CUS for, 235
    V/Q scanning for, 235
  epidemiology of, 230
  etiology of, 230–231
  follow-up, 241
  incidence of, 230
  monitoring, 241
  overview, 230
  pathophysiology of, 231
  prognosis, 241
  risk factors for, 231, 231t
  risk levels in acute PE, definitions of, 236t
  risk stratification, 236
  severity index score, 238
  treatment of, 236–241, 237f
    advanced therapies for, 240
    anticoagulation therapy for, 238–239
    complications of therapy, 240–241
    DOACs for, 238
    general principles for, 236–238, 237f
    inferior vena cava (IVC) filters for, 240
    low–molecular-weight heparin for, 238–239
    PE response teams for, 239
    respiratory and circulatory support for, 238
    systemic thrombolytic therapy for, 239–240
    unfractionated heparin for, 238–239
    warfarin for, 238–239
Pulmonary fibrosis, 311
Pulmonary flutter valves, 48
Pulmonary function tests (PFTs)
  for diagnosis of asthma, 71
  diffusing capacity, 30–31
  maximal voluntary ventilation, 31
  methacholine challenge testing, 31–33
  normal, 22–23
    FEV_1, 23
    flow–volume loops, 22–23, 22f
    FVC, 23
    lung volumes, 23
  normal values and reference ranges, 20–21
    lower limit of normal method, 21
    percent predicted method, 20–21
  obstructive ventilatory defects, 23–26
    air trapping, determining, 26
    bronchodilator reversibility, assessing for, 25
    flow–volume loop in, 26, 26f
    hyperinflation, determining, 26
    quantifying, 25, 25t
  overview, 20
  patterns, 23, 24f
  restrictive ventilatory defects, 28–29
    flow–volume loop in, 29, 30f
    quantifying severity by percentile for, 30t
  standardization of, 21–22
    acceptability criteria, 22
    reproducibility criteria, 22
  upper airway obstruction, 27–28
    fixed, 27, 27f
    variable, 27–28, 28f
Pulmonary hypertension (PH)
  classification, 244, 245t–246t
  definition, 244
  diagnosis
    approach for, 248f
    cardiac MRI for, 250
    cardiopulmonary exercise testing for, 251
    chest CT for, 250

Pulmonary hypertension (PH) (*Continued*)
  clinical presentation, 247–248
  criteria for, 249
  CXR for, 250
  electrocardiography for, 249
  history for, 247
  left heart catheterization for, 251
  PFT for, 250–251
  physical examination for, 248
  polysomnography for, 251
  procedures for, 250–251
  RHC for, 251
  testing for, 249–250
  transthoracic echocardiography for, 249–250
  ventilation/perfusion scan for, 250
 epidemiology, 245–246
 hemodynamic definitions of, 244, 244t
 monitoring/follow-up, 256
 pathophysiology of, 246–247
 prognosis in, 257
 referral for, 256
 treatment of, 251–256, 252f
  algorithm, 252f
  atrial septostomy, 256
  of groups 2–4, 251–253
  lifestyle/risk modification for, 256
  liver transplantation, 256
  other nonpharmacologic therapies, 255
  pharmacologic therapy for group 1, 253–255
  Potts shunts, 256
  septal defect closure, 256
  surgical, 255–256
  transplant surgery, 255–256
Pulmonary rehabilitation, 94
Pulmonary shunt, 43
Pulmonary tuberculosis (TB), 125
 active TB, 125
 latent (inactive) TB, 125
Purulent sputum, 44
PVFMD. *See* Paroxysmal vocal fold motion disorder (PVFMD)

R

Radial endobronchial ultrasound, 38
Radiation dose of CXR, 2
Radiographic signs, 7–8, 7t
 air bronchogram sign, 8
 luftsichel sign, 8
 Silhouette sign, 7, 7t
Radiotherapy, 308
RBC. *See* Red blood cell (RBC)
RDI. *See* Respiratory disturbance index (RDI)
Red blood cell (RBC), 43

Remdesivir, 172
RERA. *See* Respiratory effort-related arousal (RERA)
Reservoir nasal cannulas, 46–47
Residual volume (RV), 23
Reslizumab, 74t
Respiratory disturbance index (RDI), 270
Respiratory effort-related arousal (RERA), 270
Respiratory failure
 classification of, 40
 definition, 40
 hypoxemic. *See* Hypoxemic respiratory failure
Respiratory syncytial virus (RSV), 164–165, 178–179
 clinical presentation, 178
 diagnosis, 178
 epidemiology, 178
 treatment, 178–179
 virology, 178
Restrictive ventilatory defects (RVDs), 28–29
 flow–volume loop in, 29, 30f
 quantifying severity by percentile for, 30t
Rhinosinusitis
 diagnosis, 157
 etiology, 157
 management, 160
Rhinoviruses (RV), 179–180
 clinical presentation, 180
 diagnosis, 180
 epidemiology, 179
 treatment, 180
 virology, 179
Rhizomucor, 133
Rhizopus, 133
Ribavirin, 163, 179
Right-left shunts, 43–44
Rigid bronchoscopy, 202
Riociguat, 254
Rituximab (RTX), 222
 for granulomatosis with polyangiitis, 218
 for lung transplantation, 332
Rounded atelectasis, 297
RSV. *See* Respiratory syncytial virus (RSV)
RV. *See* Residual volume (RV); Rhinoviruses (RV)
RVDs. *See* Restrictive ventilatory defects (RVDs)

S

SAAC. *See* Short-acting anticholinergic (SAAC)
Saksenaea, 133
Sarcoid interstitial lung disease, 288
Scedosporium/Lomentospora, 133
SDB. *See* Sleep-disordered breathing (SDB)

Secondary vasculitides, 218
Secondary vasculitis, 213
Second-hand smoke, 97
Selexipag, 254
Septal defect closure, 256
Serologic markers, 208–209
Severe acute respiratory syndrome virus-1 (SARS-CoV-1), 171
Severe acute respiratory syndrome virus-2 (SARS-CoV-2), 171
Short-acting anticholinergic (SAAC), 88
Short-acting beta-agonist (SABA) monotherapy, 72–73, 88
Shwachman–Diamond syndrome, 189
Sildenafil, 254
Silhouette sign, 7, 7t
Silica-associated lung disease, 299–300
  diagnosis of, 299–300
    accelerated silicosis, 300
    acute silicosis, 300
    chronic silicosis, 300–301
  overview, 299
Silo Filler's disease, 305
Single lung transplantation (SLT), 328
Single maintenance and reliever therapy (SMART), 73
Sinusitis, 68
Sirolimus, for lung transplantation, 331
Sleep-disordered breathing (SDB)
  associated conditions, 272
  classification, 270–271
  definitions, 270
  diagnosis
    clinical presentation, 272–273
    criteria for, 273
    differential, 273
    history, 272
    HSAT for, 274
    laboratories testing for, 273
    physical examination for, 272–273
    procedures for, 273–274
    PSG for, 273–274
  epidemiology, 271
  etiology, 271
  overview, 270
  pathophysiology of, 271
  prevention from, 272
  risk factors for, 272
  treatment
    lifestyle/risk modification, 275
    medications, 274
    nonpharmacologic therapies, 274–275
Sleep-related hypoventilation, 270–271
SLT. *See* Single lung transplantation (SLT)

SMART. *See* Single maintenance and reliever therapy (SMART)
Smoking cessation
  associated conditions, 98
  asthma and, 76
  bupropion in, 103–104
  carcinogens in, 98
  in COPD, 95
  diagnosis of, 98–99
    criteria, 98–99
    Modified Fagerström Test for Nicotine Dependence for, 98
  e-cigarette and, 98
  epidemiology of, 97
  monitoring/follow-up of, 105
  pathophysiology of, 97
  prevalence of, 97
  prognosis for, 105
  rates of, 97
  risk of, 98
  treatment of, 100–105
    alternative therapies, 105
    behavioral counseling, 104–105
    nicotine replacement therapy for, 100–102
    non-nicotine pharmacotherapies for, 103–104
    other nonpharmacologic therapies for, 104–105
  varenicline in, 103
Solid spiculated nodule, 314, 315f
Solitary pulmonary nodule (SPN)
  definition, 314
  diagnosis
    biomarker evaluation, 321
    biopsy, 321–322
    clinical manifestations, 316
    clinical presentation, 314–317
    differential, 317, 318t
    follow-up interval and next steps in management, 319–320
    history in patient, 314–316
    imaging studies for, 317, 319
    laboratory evaluation for, 317
    physical examination, 316–317
    risk stratification, 320–321
    symptoms, 316
  guidelines
    for incidental SPN, 320t
    for incidental subsolid SPN, 320t
    for nodule management in lung cancer screening, 321t
  overview, 314
  treatment, 322
  workup by risk assessment, 316f

Soluble guanylate cyclase (sGC) stimulators, 254
Somatic cough disorder (psychogenic cough), 69
Speech therapy, 69
Spirometry, 23, 71
Split-night PSG, 273–274
SPN. *See* Solitary pulmonary nodule (SPN)
Staphylococcus aureus, 338
Steroids, 178
    in community-acquired pneumonia, 112–113
Streptococcus pneumoniae, 62, 116, 157, 161
Subacute aspergillosis, 137–138
    diagnosis of, 137
    diagnostic testing for, 137
    overview, 137
    treatment of, 138
Sublingual immunotherapy, 76
Surgical resection
    for chronic necrotizing aspergillosis, 138
    for invasive pulmonary aspergillosis, 136
    for subacute aspergillosis, 137
Swan–Ganz catheters, 6
Systemic corticosteroids, 92

T

Tacrolimus, for lung transplantation, 330–331
Tadalafil, 254
Takayasu arteritis, 216
Tazobactam, 193
TB. *See* Pulmonary tuberculosis (TB)
TBC. *See* Transbronchial cryobiopsy (TBC)
TBNA. *See* Transbronchial needle aspirations (TBNA)
Telangiectasias, 248
Terbutaline, 79
Tetrahydrocannabinol (THC), 98
Tezacaftor-Ivacaftor, 191
Tezepelumab, 75, 75t
Third-hand smoke, 97
Thymic stromal lymphopoietin (TSLP), 73, 75t
TKIs. *See* Tyrosine kinase inhibitors (TKIs)
TLC. *See* Total lung capacity (TLC)
TNF inhibitors, 217–218
Tobacco and inhalational abuse
    associated conditions, 98
    bupropion in, 103–104
    diagnosis of, 98–99
        criteria, 98–99
        Modified Fagerström Test for Nicotine Dependence for, 98
    epidemiology of, 97
    monitoring/follow-up of, 105
    overview, 97
    pathophysiology of, 97
    prevalence of, 97
    prognosis for, 105
    treatment of, 100–105
        alternative therapies, 105
        behavioral counseling, 104–105
        nicotine replacement therapy for, 100–102
        non-nicotine pharmacotherapies for, 103–104
        other nonpharmacologic therapies for, 104–105
        varenicline in, 103
Tobacco smoking, 297
Tobramycin, 193
Tocilizumab, 173
Tonsillitis, 160–161
    in infants, 170
Topical anesthesia, during bronchoscopy, 35
Total lung capacity (TLC), 23
Tracheal aspirates, for HAP/VAP, 120
Tranexamic acid (TXA), 202
    for aspergilloma, 139
Transbronchial cryobiopsy (TBC), 285
Transbronchial lung biopsy, 37
Transbronchial needle aspirations (TBNA), 38
Transthoracic echocardiography (TTE), 235
    for PH, 249–250
Trastuzumab, 311
Treprostinil, 254
Tricyclic antidepressants, 104
Trimethoprim-sulfamethoxazole (TMP-SMX), 153, 223
TSLP. *See* Thymic stromal lymphopoietin (TSLP)
TTE. *See* Transthoracic echocardiography (TTE)
Tyrosine kinase inhibitors (TKIs), 308

U

UFH. *See* Unfractionated heparin (UFH)
Unfractionated heparin (UFH), 238–239
United network for organ sharing (UNOS), 324
UNOS. *See* United network for organ sharing (UNOS)
Upper abdomen, 3–4
Upper airway cough syndrome, 62–63, 68
Upper airway obstruction, 27–28
    fixed, 27, 27f

variable, 27–28, 28f
  extrathoracic obstruction, 28, 29f
  intrathoracic obstruction, 28, 28f
Upper respiratory tract infections (URTIs), 157, 160–161
  pharyngitis/tonsillitis, 160–161
  rhinosinusitis, 157, 160
URTIs. *See* Upper respiratory tract infections (URTIs)

V

Vaccination, 92, 164–165
  adenovirus, 165
  annual flu, 164
  chickenpox, 165
  influenza, 164
  RSV, 164–165
  SARS-CoV-2, 164
  varicella zoster virus, 165
Vacuoles, E1 enzyme, X-linked, autoinflammatory, somatic (VEXAS) syndrome, 217
VAP. *See* Ventilator-acquired pneumonia
Varenicline, 103
Variable upper airway obstruction, 27–28, 28f
  extrathoracic obstruction, 28, 29f
  intrathoracic obstruction, 28, 28f
Varicella zoster virus (VZV), 339
Vasculitis
  classification, 213, 214t
  definition, 213
  diagnosis, 214–215
  epidemiology, 213–214
  primary, 213
  secondary, 213, 218
  special considerations, 215–218
    Behçet disease, 218
    primary large-vessel vasculitides, 215–217
    primary medium-vessel vasculitides, 217
    secondary vasculitides, 218
  treatment of, 215
Vasodilator therapy, 253–255
Vemurafenib, 311
Venous compression ultrasonography, 235
Venous thromboembolism (VTE), 230–231
Ventilated hospital–acquired pneumonia (vHAP), 115–116
Ventilator-acquired pneumonia (VAP), 115–116
Venturi masks, 47
Verapamil, 253
VHAP. *See* Ventilated hospital–acquired pneumonia (vHAP)
Vinblastine, 311
Viral infections, 62

Viral infectious cough, 61
Viral *pneumonia,* lung transplantation and, 338–339
Viral respiratory infections
  classification in normal host, 157–162
    LRTIs, 161–162
    URTIs, 157, 160–161
  common respiratory viruses, 157, 158t–159t
  complications
    cough, postviral, 180
    post-COVID conditions, 180–181
    wheeze/asthma, postviral, 180
  diagnosis of, 165, 165t–166t, 167
  overview, 157
  prevention, 164–165
    adenovirus vaccine, 165
    influenza vaccine, 164
    RSV vaccine, 164–165
    SARS-CoV-2 vaccine, 164
    vaccination, 164–165
    varicella zoster virus vaccine, 165
  in special adult populations, 162–164
    chronic lung diseases, 163
    immunocompromised, 163–164
    pregnancy, 162–163
  specific viral pathogens in
    adenovirus, 167, 169–170
    coronaviruses, 171–174
    cytomegalovirus, 174–175
    enteroviruses, 179–180
    herpesviruses (HSV-1, EBV, VZV), 175
    influenza virus, 175–177
    metapneumovirus, 177
    parainfluenza virus, 177–178
    respiratory syncytial virus, 178–179
    rhinoviruses, 179–180
  treatment of
    specific antiviral therapies for, 167, 168t–169t
    supportive care for, 167
  types, 158t–159t
Viral rhinosinusitis, 62
Viruses, in respiratory infections
  adenovirus, 167, 169–170
  coronaviruses, 171–174
  cytomegalovirus, 174–175
  enteroviruses, 179–180
  herpesviruses (HSV-1, EBV, VZV), 175
  influenza virus, 175–177
  metapneumovirus, 177
  parainfluenza virus, 177–178
  respiratory syncytial virus, 178–179
Vitamin D supplementation, 194

Voriconazole
  for chronic necrotizing aspergillosis, 138
  for invasive pulmonary aspergillosis, 136
  for subacute aspergillosis, 137
V/Q mismatch, 43
V/Q ratios, 43
V/Q scan, 235
VTE. *See* Venous thromboembolism (VTE)

W

Warfarin, 238–239
Wells score, 232t
Wheezing, 280
Workplace- and environment-associated bronchial reactivity, 300–302
  diagnosis, 301
  overview, 300–301
  treatment, 301–302
    biomass fuel combustion fumes, 302
    environmental, 301
    family and social problems, 302
    pharmacologic, 301
    popcorn lung, 302
    reports to patients and third parties, 301–302
    World Trade Center disaster, 302
World Trade Center disaster, 302

Y

Young syndrome, 189

Z

Zafirlukast, for asthma, 75
Zanamivir, for influenza virus, 176